Clinical Orthodontics

Clinical Orthodontics

Edited by Samuel James

STATES
ACADEMIC PRESS
www.statesacademicpress.com

States Academic Press,
109 South 5th Street,
Brooklyn, NY 11249, USA

Visit us on the World Wide Web at:
www.statesacademicpress.com

ISBN: 978-1-63989-113-9

Cataloging-in-Publication Data

Clinical orthodontics / edited by Samuel James.
p. cm.
Includes bibliographical references and index.
ISBN 978-1-63989-113-9
1. Orthodontics. 2. Dentistry. 3. Orthopedics. 4. Orthodontia. I. James, Samuel.
RK521 .C55 2022
617.643--dc23

Table of Contents

Preface

This book has been an outcome of determined endeavour from a group of educationists in the field. The primary objective was to involve a broad spectrum of professionals from diverse cultural background involved in the field for developing new researches. The book not only targets students but also scholars pursuing higher research for further enhancement of the theoretical and practical applications of the subject.

The specialty of dentistry that deals with the prevention, diagnosis and correction of misaligned bite patterns, and malpositioned teeth and jaws is known as orthodontics. It also involves the study of modifying facial growth termed as dentofacial orthopedics. Misalignment of jaws and teeth is common and the treatments involve using dental braces and other appliances to steadily move the jaws and teeth around. In severe cases, jaw surgery may also be used. Usually, the treatment of misaligned teeth takes about 1 to 3 years to complete, and the braces are slightly altered every 4 to 10 weeks by specialists. This book discusses the fundamentals as well as modern approaches of orthodontics. It strives to provide a fair idea about this discipline and to help develop a better understanding of the clinical studies within this field. This book aims to equip students and experts with the advanced topics and upcoming concepts in this area.

It was an honour to edit such a profound book and also a challenging task to compile and examine all the relevant data for accuracy and originality. I wish to acknowledge the efforts of the contributors for submitting such brilliant and diverse chapters in the field and for endlessly working for the completion of the book. Last, but not the least; I thank my family for being a constant source of support in all my research endeavours.

Editor

1

Accelerated Orthodontics

Anand K. Patil and Amrit Singh Maan

Abstract

Clinical orthodontics is ever dynamic branch of Dentistry. Traditionally orthodontics was always considered as aesthetic treatment of face & also needed for proper oral oral function. This treatment may take up 2–3 years of total duration. The chapter describes changing trends in this aspect wherein we speed up the treatment by various methods thus reducing the overall time duration. These modalities include alteration in bio mechanics, pharmacological, chemical & by biological means. It is also cautioned here that the clinician has to take up these changing trends based on sound clinical knowledge & evidence based applicability.

Keywords: biology of tooth movement, acceleration of tooth movement, prostaglandins, regional acceleration phenomena, corticotomy

1. Accelerated orthodontics

Orthodontic treatment in the present day does not just require to meet the demands of creating the functional harmony in occlusion and improving the aesthetic outlook of but is should also be completed in the most efficient duration that is accepted by the patient and the orthodontist. We live in a fast-paced world where the treatment duration has clearly made the field of orthodontic treatment to revolve around it. Accelerated orthodontic tooth movement is not something that has recently emerged; it has been studied and tried out for many years. In an attempt of producing faster tooth movement during orthodontic treatment, there are numerous methods of accelerating tooth movements that have been introduced over the years which range from surgical means to the use of laser therapy. Now let us look at each method explained in this chapter.

2. Methods of accelerated tooth movements

We can categorise the methods of accelerated tooth movement into the following categories:

A. Pharmacological methods

B. Surgical methods

C. Physical methods

2.1. Pharmacological methods

Orthodontic forces cause a fluid movement in the periodontal ligament space and distortion of the matrix and cells. There is release of molecules which initiate bone remodelling for tooth movement [1]. There are a number of researches on pharmacological agents that act as biomodulators for increased orthodontic tooth movement. These are examples of such biomodulators:

- Prostaglandin E_2 and Prostaglandin E_1
- Misoprostol
- 1,25-Dihydroxycholecalciferol
- Parathyroid hormones
- Intravenous immunoglobulins

Prostaglandin E_2 (PGE_2) is an arachidonic acid metabolite is an often-tested substance to increase orthodontic tooth movement [2]. Animal studies have shown PGE_2 to increase tooth movement and facilitate bone resorption [3–6]. Camacho and Velásquez Cujar conducted a study that showed that it required repeated injections due to its short half-life [7]. Particular synthases that are required for the synthesis of PGE_2 could be targeted to control the production of the prostaglandins [8].

Another prostaglandin that has been reported to speed up orthodontic tooth movement is Prostaglandin E_1 (PGE_1). Prostaglandin E_1 (PGE_1) has also been seen to be induced by mechanical stress and cause bone remodelling, Patil and his co-workers had shown that even minimal amounts of PGE_1 injection had significant increase in tooth movement [9]. Due to the hyperalgesia that accompanies with the local injection of $PGE_{1,}$ an analogue of it which is misoprostol was tried out. It was seen that it was effective in increasing orthodontic tooth movement (**Figure 1**) [10].

The parathyroid hormone (PTH) acts directly on osteoblasts and on osteoclasts indirectly by binding to the PTH type 1 receptor on osteoblasts. This causes the expression of insulin like growth factor 1. There is promotion of osteoblast survival, osteoblastogenesis and receptor activator for nuclear factor κ B ligand (RANKL) which induces osteoclast activation [2]. PTH facilitates bone remodelling in intermittent treatment by enhancing activities of osteoblasts and osteoclasts [11].

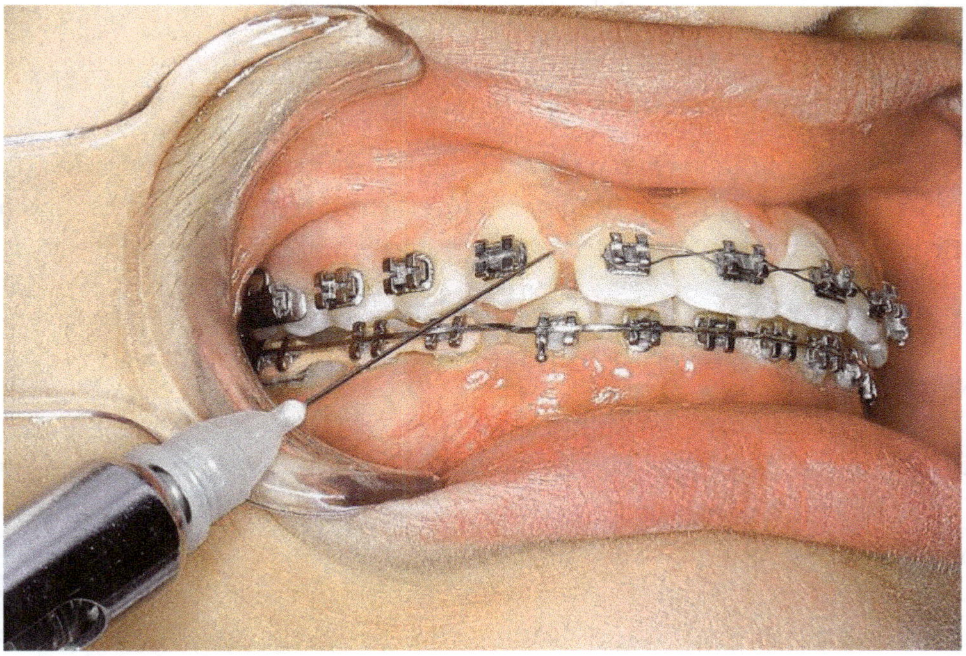

Figure 1. Injection of a biomodulator in the periodontium.

Calcitriol or 1,25-dihydroxycholecalciferol which is the most active metabolite of vitamin D acts in a similar fashion to PTH by facilitating osteoblastic proliferation and function [12]. Calcitriol facilitates alveolar bone remodelling which leads to increase in tooth movement while force application [6, 13].

Recently intravenous immunoglobulin (IVIg) preparations which are used in immunodeficient patients as replacement therapy. These preparations have been shown to induce COX-2 mediated PGE_2 and cytokine production [14, 15]. Future potential of these preparations could be used to modulate orthodontic movement via PGE_2 synthesis.

2.2. Surgical methods

Bichmalyr in 1931, put forward a surgical technique with orthodontic appliances for rapid correction of severe maxillary protrusion. First, wedges of bone were removed to reduce the volume for which the roots of the maxillary anterior teeth would require for retraction. Köle further looked into this technique in 1959 by including special movements like crossbite correction and space closure. He believed that he was able to move bony blocks using the crowns of teeth as handles as the blocks were connected by only less-dense medullary bone [16]. Currently there are few surgical methods being practiced, they are:

- Periodontally accelerated osteogenic orthodontics
- Piezocision
- Micro-osteoperforations

In 2001, Wilcko et al. had introduced a method which combines corticotomy surgery and alveolar bone grafting which is referred to as accelerated osteogenic orthodontics or recently termed as periodontally accelerated osteogenic orthodontics (PAOO) [16]. This procedure which enables rapid tooth movement is due to a healing event that was described by Frost [17] and termed as regional acceleratory phenomenon (RAP).

RAP is the acceleration of the normal regional healing process from the original injury. It usually occurs after osteotomy, bone-grafting procedure, arthrodesis and fractures and there might be involvement and activation of precursor cells required for healing at the injury site. RAP can increase both soft and hard tissue healing processes by two- to tenfold [17]. It usually starts in the first few days of injury, peaks at the first or second month and may last for 3–4 months [16].

Orthodontic treatment can be started 1 week before or within 2 weeks after the surgery. Surgery begins with flap reflection and decortication with low-speed round burs. Bone graft is then laid over these areas of corticotomies. The flaps are then closed and sutured [18]. Several studies have been done related to corticotomies, an example is one by Uzuner and her co-workers where they showed that canine retraction assisted by corticotomy had reduced duration of retraction by 20% ratio [19]. PAOO has shown to have reduced treatment time, produce lower cortical bone resistance leading to reduced root resorption, enhancement of post-orthodontic stability, increased bone support since there is supplementation of the bone graft. However, PAOO still has risks since it is an invasive procedure and is expensive [20–24].

Since the corticotomy procedure is still invasive, Dibart et al. introduced a new minimally invasive method called piezocision. Piezocision involves microincisions which are confined to the buccal side that allows the use of piezoelectric knife and selective tunnelling which enables hard and soft tissue grafting [25]. Piezocision is usually done a week after orthodontic appliance placement. The procedure involves vertical incisions made buccally and interproximally. The mid portion of the incision between the roots enables the piezoelectric knife to be inserted. A piezotome is then inserted in the gingival openings that were made and piezoelectrical corticotomy of 3 mm is made. Hard or soft tissue grafts can then be added via a tunnelling procedure (**Figure 2**) [26].

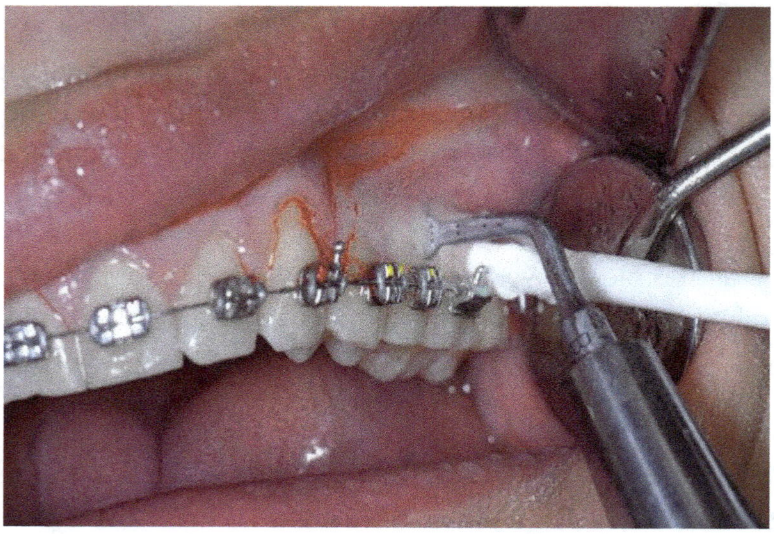

Figure 2. Piezocision.

Piezocision can be used as an adjunct to treat a number of malocclusions and aid in rapid orthodontic treatment in adults. Since it is much more minimally invasive than corticotomy, it is having high degree of patient acceptance, short surgical time and has less postoperative discomfort [25, 26]. Dibart and coworkers in 2013 showed that there was an increase in the rate of tooth movement in their animal study and preliminary human studies are being conducted to correlate with the animal studies [26, 27].

To further reduce the amount of invasive nature of surgical intervention, a method called micro-osteoperforation (MOP). It is procedure in which small pinhole-sized perforations are created within the alveolar bone surrounding the dentition. This initiates cytokine release to call in osteoclasts to increase bone resorption. Thus, acceleration of tooth movement occurs during orthodontic treatment. The site of perforation is within the attached gingiva and close to the target teeth on the mesial and distal aspect of the roots of the teeth which will be moved. The most favourable place for placement of the perforation is the buccal cortical plate but lingual plate can also be approached with a contra-angled appliance. Two to four perforations are ideal amounts with depths of 3–7 mm into the bone [28].

In 2013, Alikhani et al. showed that MOP increased expression of cytokines for osteoclast differentiation, increased canine retraction, reduced orthodontic treatment by 62% with mild discomfort in patients [29]. In an animal study, Alikhani and co-workers found that the expression of inflammatory markers and bone resorption was significant. Their human clinical trial found distalisation was twice as much with MOP than the forces alone [30].

2.3. Physical methods

Despite all the attempts in making surgical methods being minimally invasive, they still remain as an invasive procedure. This had led to discoveries in other tools that can accelerate tooth movement during orthodontic treatment. The two most common physical methods used in the present day are:

- Vibratory stimulus
- Low level laser therapy
- Low-intensity pulsed ultrasound

Bone has the ability to respond to the mechanical stimuli that is applied to it as a mechanism to withstand functional activity. Rubin et al. showed the rate of remodelling in mechanically loaded long bones have been increased following vibrations or low level mechanical oscillatory signals [31]. In 2008, Nishimura et al. did an animal study which gave an insight on how resonance vibration could be able to accelerate tooth movement through the expression of RANKL in the periodontal ligament [32].

A novel device that was introduced by OrthoAccel Technologies is the AcceleDent device. The device has an activator and a mouthpiece. The patient bites on the mouthpiece component when in use. The activator which is extraorally positioned generates and transmits vibrations to the teeth. It can provide 0.2 N of vibration at 30 Hz for 20 minutes. It was fabricated to work in tandem with existing bracket systems and not replace them. The device produces cyclic forces to move teeth within the alveolus via accelerated bone remodelling [33]. Pavlin and co-workers in 2015 showed low-level cyclic loading with AcceleDent increased the rate of orthodontic movement (**Figure 3**) [34].

Another treatment modality to speed up orthodontic tooth movement is by the use of low-level laser therapy (LLLT). Laser irradiation on tissues has a biostimulating effect with not more than 1°C rise in local temperature. Biostimulation potency of laser irradiation utilised by treatment are called low-level laser therapy [35]. Other than accelerating tooth movement, LLLT can enhance stability of orthodontic mini-implants [36], reduce post-adjustment pain [37], and induce bone growth in midpalatal suture area following rapid maxillary expansion [38].

Studies done by Fujita et al. and Yamaguchi et al. showed that LLLT enhances osteoclastogenesis on the compressed side of teeth being moved. There was stimulation of RANKL and macrophage colony-stimulating factor [39, 40]. Coordination of bone remodelling had been facilitated by RANKL and osteoprotegerin following orthodontic force with LLLT. LLLT stimulates bone formation on the tension side [41]. Kim et al. observed osteopontin localisation in the periodontal tissue in their study subjects, indicating LLLT may stimulate osteogenesis as well in orthodontic treatment [42]. Although much findings show LLLT stimulates osteoblast and osteoclast function, further studies are still required to optimise the effect of LLLT on tooth movement (**Figure 4**) [43].

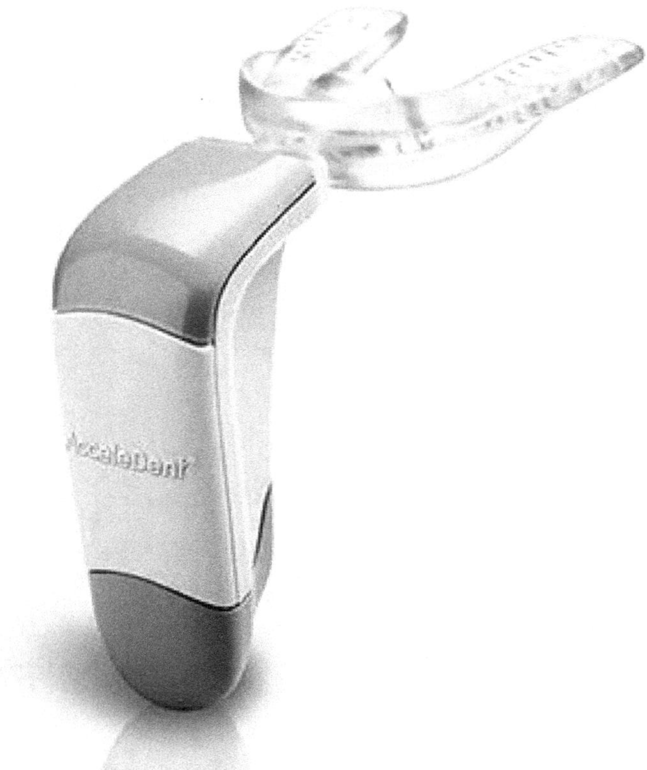

Figure 3. AcceleDent device.

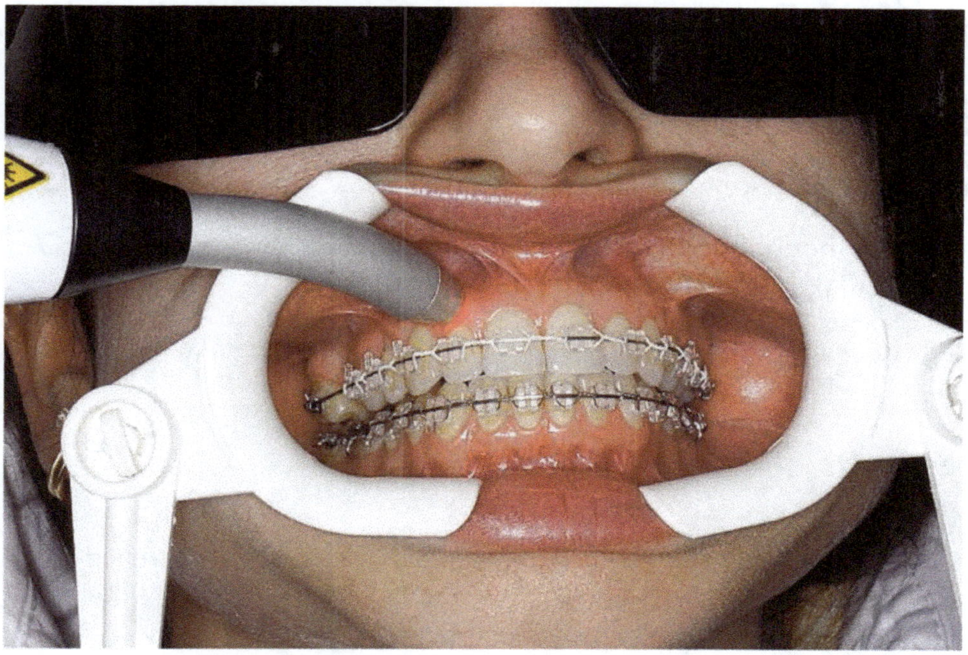

Figure 4. Low-level laser therapy.

Apart from physical agents, low-intensity pulsed ultrasound (LIPUS) has also been suggested. It uses mechanical energy which passes through the tissues as acoustic pressure waves [44]. This leads to biochemical changes at molecular and cellular levels. It can increase the healing of both soft tissue and hard tissue [45]. LIPUS is usually used at frequency pulses of 1.5 MHz with 200 μs pulse width, which is repeated at 1KHz a for 20 minutes a day with an intensity of 30 mW/cm^2 [46].

Recent studies on LIPUS using animal models by Xue et al. showed that there is induction of alveolar bone remodelling. The remodelling occurred due to an increase in the gene expression of HGF/Runx2/BMP-2 signalling pathway with LIPUS. This led to an increase in the velocity of tooth movement during orthodontic treatment [47]. El-Bialy et al. observed that LIPUS may reduce the root resorption that was orthodontically-induced by deposition of dentin and cementum to create a preventive layer from root resorption [48].

3. Conclusion

Over the years, the methods of reducing treatment time has risen along with its' demand. The options that are available on the orthodontist's plate are numerous ranging from surgical means to photostimulation. Much studies will still need to be done for newer methods to emerge and obtaining a clearer understanding on the methods that already exist. At present, the clinician should use all the knowledge obtained for deciding which treatment option is best for the patient to meet the healthcare needs of the patient and achieving an optimum treatment outcome.

Author details

Anand K. Patil[1]* and Amrit Singh Maan[2]

*Address all correspondence to: akptimes7@gmail.com

1 Department of Orthodontics and Dentofacial Orthodontics, SDM College of Dental Sciences and Hospital, Karnataka, India

2 SDM College of Dental Sciences and Hospital, Dharwad, Karnataka, India

References

[1] Krishnan V, Davidovitch ZE. Cellular, molecular, and tissue-level reactions to orthodontic force. American Journal of Orthodontics and Dentofacial Orthopedics. 2006;**129**(4):469, e1-e32

[2] Kouskoura T, Katsaros C, Gunten SV. The potential use of pharmacological agents to modulate orthodontic tooth movement (OTM). Frontiers in Physiology. 2017;**8**:67

[3] Yamasaki K, Shibata Y, Fukuhara T. The effect of prostaglandins on experimental tooth movement in monkeys (*Macaca fuscata*). Journal of Dental Research. 1982;**61**(12):1444-1446

[4] Yamasaki K, Shibata Y, Imai S, Tani Y, Shibasaki Y, Fukuhara T. Clinical application of prostaglandin E_1 (PGE_1) upon orthodontic tooth movement. American Journal of Orthodontics and Dentofacial Orthopedics. 1984;**85**(6):508-518

[5] Kale S, Kocadereli I, Atilla P, Aşan E. Comparison of the effects of 1,25 dihydroxycholecalciferol and prostaglandin E2 on orthodontic tooth movement. American Journal of Orthodontics and Dentofacial Orthopedics. 2004;**125**(5):607-614

[6] Leiker BJ, Nanda RS, Currier G, Howes RI, Sinha PK. The effects of exogenous prostaglandins on orthodontic tooth movement in rats. American Journal of Orthodontics and Dentofacial Orthopedics. 1995;**108**(4):380-388

[7] Camacho AD, Velásquez Cujar SA. Dental movement acceleration: Literature review by an alternative scientific evidence method. World Journal of Methodology. 2014;**4**(3): 151-162

[8] Forsberg L, Leeb L, Thorén S, Morgenstern R, Jakobsson P-J. Human glutathione dependent prostaglandin E synthase: Gene structure and regulation. FEBS Letters. 2000;**471**(1): 78-82

[9] Patil AK, Keluskar KM, Gaitonde SD. The clinical application of prostaglandin E1 on orthodontic tooth movement. Journal of Indian Orthodontic Society. 2005;**38**:91-98

[10] Sekhavat AR, Mousavizadeh K, Pakshir HR, Aslani FS. Effect of misoprostol, a prostaglandin E_1 analog, on orthodontic tooth movement in rats. American Journal of Orthodontics and Dentofacial Orthopedics. 2002;**122**(5):542-547

[11] Li F, Li G, Hu H, Liu R, Chen J, Zou S. Effect of parathyroid hormone on experimental tooth movement in rats. American Journal of Orthodontics and Dentofacial Orthopedics. 2013;**144**(4):523-532

[12] Reichel H, Koeffler HP, Norman AW. The role of the vitamin D endocrine system in health and disease. The New England Journal of Medicine. 1989;**320**(15):980-991

[13] Takano-Yamamoto T, Kawakami M, Kobayashi Y, Yamashiro T, Sakuda M. The effect of local application of 1,25-dihydroxycholecalciferol on osteoclast numbers in orthodontically treated rats. Journal of Dental Research. 1992;**71**(1):53-59

[14] Trinath J, Hegde P, Sharma M, Maddur MS, Rabin M, Vallat J-M, et al. Intravenous immunoglobulin expands regulatory T cells via induction of cyclooxygenase-2-dependent prostaglandin E_2 in human dendritic cells. Blood. 2013;**122**(8):1419-1427

[15] Djoumerska-Alexieva I, Roumenina L. Intravenous immunoglobulin with enhanced polyspecificity improves survival in experimental sepsis and aseptic systemic inflammatory response syndromes. Molecular Medicine. 2015;**21**(1):1

[16] Wilcko WM, Wilcko T, Bouquot JE, Ferguson DJ. Rapid orthodontics with alveolar reshaping: Two case reports of decrowding. The International Journal of Periodontics & Restorative Dentistry. 2001;**21**(1):9-19

[17] Frost HM. The regional acceleratory phenomenon: A review. Henry Ford Hospital Medical Journal. 1983;**31**(1):3-9

[18] Goyal A, Kalra JPS, Bhatiya P, Singla S, Bansal P. Periodontally accelerated osteogenic orthodontics (PAOO)—A review. Journal of Clinical and Experimental Dentistry. 2012; **4**(5):e292-e296

[19] Uzuner FD, Yücel E, Göfteci B, Gülsen A. The effect of corticotomy on tooth movements during canine retraction. Journal of Orthodontic Research. 2015;**3**:181-187

[20] Ferguson DJ, Makki L, Stapelberg R, Wilcko MT, Wilcko WM. Stability of the mandibular dental arch following periodontally accelerated osteogenic orthodontics therapy: Preliminary studies. Seminars in Orthodontics. 2014;**20**(3):239-246

[21] Wilcko MT, Wilcko WM, Pulver JJ, Bissada NF, Bouquot JE. Accelerated osteogenic orthodontics technique: A 1-stage surgically facilitated rapid orthodontic technique with alveolar augmentation. Journal of Oral and Maxillofacial Surgery. 2009;**67**(10):2149-2159

[22] Yalamanchi L, Yalamanchili P, Adusumilli S. Periodontally accelerated osteogenic orthodontics: An interdisciplinary approach for faster orthodontic therapy. Journal of Pharmacy & Bioallied Sciences. 2014;**6**(5):2

[23] Andrade IJ, Sousa AB, da Silva GG. New therapeutic modalities to modulate orthodontic tooth movement. Dental Press Journal of Orthodontics. 2014;**19**(6):123-133

[24] Uzuner FD, Darendeliler N. Dentoalveolar surgery techniques combined with orthodontic treatment: A literature review. European Journal of Dentistry. 2013;**7**:257-265

[25] Dibart S, Dibart J-P. Practical Osseous Surgery in Periodontics and Implant Dentistry. Chichester, West Sussex, UK: Wiley-Blackwell; 2011. pp. 195-197

[26] Dibart S, Keser E, Nelson D. Piezocision™-assisted orthodontics: Past, present, and future. Seminars in Orthodontics. 2015;**21**:170-175

[27] Dibart S, Yee C, Surmenian J, Sebaoun JD, Baloul S, Goguet-Surmenian E, et al. Tissue response during piezocision-assisted tooth movement: A histological study in rats. European Journal of Orthodontics. 2013;**36**(4):457-464

[28] Sangsuwon C, Alansari S, Nervina J, Teixeira CC, Alikhani M. Micro-osteoperforations in accelerated orthodontics. Clinical Dentistry Reviewed. 2018;**2**:4

[29] Alikhani M, Raptis M, Zoldan B, Sangsuwon C, Lee YB, Alyami B, et al. Effect of micro-osteoperforations on the rate of tooth movement. American Journal of Orthodontics and Dentofacial Orthopedics. 2013;**144**(5):639-648

[30] Alikhani M, Alansari S, Sangsuwon C, Alikhani M, Chou MY, Alyami B, et al. Micro-osteoperforations: Minimally invasive accelerated tooth movement. Seminars in Orthodontics. 2015;**21**(3):162-169

[31] Rubin C, Turner AS, Müller R, Mittra E, Mcleod K, Lin W, et al. Quantity and quality of trabecular bone in the femur are enhanced by a strongly anabolic, noninvasive mechanical intervention. Journal of Bone and Mineral Research. 2002;**17**(2):349-357

[32] Nishimura M, Chiba M, Ohashi T, Sato M, Shimizu Y, Igarashi K, et al. Periodontal tissue activation by vibration: Intermittent stimulation by resonance vibration accelerates experimental tooth movement in rats. American Journal of Orthodontics and Dentofacial Orthopedics. 2008;**133**(4):572-583

[33] Kau CH, Nguyen JT, English JD. The clinical evaluation of a novel cyclical force generating device in orthodontics. Orthodontic Practice US. 2010;**1**:10-15

[34] Pavlin D, Anthony R, Raj V, Gakunga PT. Cyclic loading (vibration) accelerates tooth movement in orthodontic patients: A double-blind, randomized controlled trial. Seminars in Orthodontics. 2015;**21**(3):187-194

[35] Walsh LJ. The current status of low level laser therapy in dentistry, part 1. Soft tissue applications. Australian Dental Journal. 1997;**42**(4):247-254

[36] Omasa S, Motoyoshi M, Arai Y, Ejima K-I, Shimizu N. Low-level laser therapy enhances the stability of orthodontic mini-implants via bone formation related to BMP-2 expression in a rat model. Photomedicine and Laser Surgery. 2012;**30**(5):255-261

[37] Bicakci AA, Kocoglu-Altan B, Toker H, Mutaf I, Sumer Z. Efficiency of low-level laser therapy in reducing pain induced by orthodontic forces. Photomedicine and Laser Surgery. 2012;**30**(8):460-465

[38] Cepera F, Torres FC, Scanavini MA, Paranhos LR, Filho LC, Cardoso MA, et al. Effect of a low-level laser on bone regeneration after rapid maxillary expansion. American Journal of Orthodontics and Dentofacial Orthopedics. 2012;**141**(4):444-450

[39] Fujita S, Yamaguchi M, Utsunomiya T, Yamamoto H, Kasai K. Low-energy laser stimulates tooth movement velocity via expression of RANK and RANKL. Orthodontics & Craniofacial Research. 2008;**11**(3):143-155

[40] Yamaguchi M, Fujita S, Yoshida T, Oikawa K, Utsunomiya T, Yamamoto H, et al. Low-energy laser irradiation stimulates the tooth movement velocity via expression of M-CSF and c-fms. Orthodontic Waves. 2007;**66**(4):139-148

[41] Yoshida T, Yamaguchi M, Utsunomiya T, Kato M, Arai Y, Kaneda T, et al. Low-energy laser irradiation accelerates the velocity of tooth movement via stimulation of the alveolar bone remodeling. Orthodontics & Craniofacial Research. 2009;**12**(4):289-298

[42] Kim J-Y, Kim B-I, Jue S-S, Park JH, Shin J-W. Localization of osteopontin and osterix in periodontal tissue during orthodontic tooth movement in rats. The Angle Orthodontist. 2012;**82**(1):107-114

[43] Kasai K, Chou MY, Yamaguchi M. Molecular effects of low-energy laser irradiation during orthodontic tooth movement. Seminars in Orthodontics. 2015;**21**(3):203-209

[44] Buckley MJ, Banes AJ, Levin LG, Sumpio BE, Sato M, Jordan R, et al. Osteoblasts increase their rate of division and align in response to cyclic, mechanical tension in vitro. Bone and Mineral. 1988;**4**(3):225-236

[45] Claes L, Willie B. The enhancement of bone regeneration by ultrasound. Progress in Biophysics and Molecular Biology. 2007;**93**(1-3):384-398

[46] Xue H, Zheng J, Chou MY, Zhou H, Duan Y. The effects of low-intensity pulsed ultrasound on the rate of orthodontic tooth movement. Seminars in Orthodontics. 2015;**21**(3):219-223

[47] Xue H, Zheng J, Cui Z, Bai X, Li G, Zhang C, et al. Low-intensity pulsed ultrasound accelerates tooth movement via activation of the BMP-2 signaling pathway. PLoS One. 2013;**8**(7)

[48] El-Bialy T, Lam B, Aldaghreer S, Sloan A. The effect of low intensity pulsed ultrasound in a 3D ex vivo orthodontic model. Journal of Dentistry. 2011;**39**(10):693-699

2

Surgery First Approach

Ayşe Gülşen

Abstract

The surgery first approach (SFA) was presented by some researchers in earlier years, but SFA in a combined treatment, with the surgery first and the orthodontic treatment second, as introduced by Brachvogel et al. and by Nagasaka et al., has gained attention in the past 10 years. The advantages of SFA were reported in the literature, and the research into this method continues. One of the advantages of the SFA is the shorter total treatment time, and another is that patients begin treatment with a much improved face esthetically. The protocol of presurgical orthodontics is well known in dentofacial anomalies, but in SFA, especially in complex cases, the meticulous treatment is very important. In this chapter, SFA will be discussed.

Keywords: surgery first, orthognathic surgery, orthodontics

1. Introduction

The treatment of skeletal discrepancies requires orthognathic surgery in combination with orthodontic treatment to improve malocclusion, function, facial, and smile esthetics.

In the 1960s, the surgeons performed orthognathic surgery without orthodontic treatment [1–3]. But it was clearly understood that mandibular or maxillary movement was limited without tooth movement. For example, amount of mandibular setback was limited by the overjet in Class III cases. To achieve a proper setback and to have a good the occlusal and facial esthetics results, orthodontic alignment of malaligned teeth and solving the compensation of teeth to the malposed jaws are required before surgery [4–6]. After the 1970s, orthognathic surgery in combination with orthodontic treatment began to have good standards and showed popularity [7–11].

In conventional orthognathic surgery approach, the surgery follows the orthodontic treatment (orthodontic-first approach). Teeth are tended to compensate for skeletal discrepancies to have functional occlusion. The presurgical orthodontic treatment is needed to solve the dental decompensation that reveals the true extent of the skeletal deformity to align the teeth and to fit the maxilla and mandible into a good occlusion after surgery [11, 12]. Following the orthodontic treatment, orthognathic surgery corrects the skeletal discrepancy to obtain a good jaw alignment with good facial proportions. As the direction of presurgical orthodontic treatment is opposite to that of natural dental compensation forces, the orthodontic treatment time is said to require time to overcome the natural compensation forces [13]. The presurgical orthodontic treatment period which includes aligning dental occlusion, reversing incisor decompensation, correcting tooth rotation, and arch coordination lasts for 12–36 months depending on the complexity of case and also for a period after the surgery [13].

In last 10 years, surgery first approach (SFA) has begun to be implemented in some centers [14] and created broader interest [15–20].

The surgery first approach (SFA) is the orthognathic surgery approach that the orthognathic surgery precedes the orthodontic treatment. In the beginning of the treatment, surgery is performed without orthodontic preparation, and the orthodontic treatment is done after the surgery.

Historically, the SFA was presented by some researchers in earlier years [2, 21–24], but SFA in a combined treatment, which was introduced officially by Brachvogel et al. [25] and by Nagasaka et al., has gained attention in the past 10 years [26].

Among the published studies about SFA regarding the type of malocclusion, Class III is the most prevalent. Class III with openbite and asymmetry cases with SFA are the other published studies. SFA in Class II cases and in some deformities like TMJ disorders or condylar hyperplasia is rare [27–29].

2. The advantages of SFA

The advantages of SFA reported in literature continue. One of the advantages of the SFA is the shorter total treatment time [13, 15, 30]. Other advantages are that patients begin treatment with a much improved face esthetically in the beginning of the treatment and that the patient's chief complaint, dental function, and facial esthetics are achieved and improved in the beginning of the treatment [31, 32] and a psychosocial benefit of improved body image in the beginning of the treatment instead of worsening the facial appearance because of the presurgical decompensation of incisors [31, 34]. Improved corporation of the patient during the treatment may be the other advantage of SFA due to rapid profile improvement [33, 35]. SFA is also preferred in early correction of obstructive sleep apnea patients. On the other side, due to the early correction of skeletal and soft tissue problems, orthodontic treatment may be easier due to normalized surrounding soft tissue [23]. It was reported that the patients with preexisting TMJ dysfunction might experience a significant improvement of TMD signs and symptoms after SFA [29].

One of the reasons for the shorter duration of treatment in SFA is the regional accelerated phenomenon (RAP) which is the increase of the osteoclastic and metabolic activities due to the surgery. Selective bone injury activates stimulus for anabolic and catabolic responses in the periodontium adjacent to the osteotomies performed during orthognathic surgery and increases bone reorganization [32, 36–45]. It was reported that RAP in humans began in a few days after surgery and peaked at 1–2 months and took 6 months to more than 24 months to subside [39]. Liou et al. also studied the causes of rapid postoperative orthodontic treatment time in SFA cases, and they found that the levels of serum alkaline phosphatase and C-terminal telopeptide of type I collagen (ICTP) increased, which supported the postoperative accelerated orthodontic tooth movement caused the orthognathic surgery [15]. Zingler et al. found that crevicular fluids in SFA cases were higher levels of bone remodeling factors for fracture healing [32].

The other reason for the shorter duration of treatment in SFA than in the conventional approach may be improvement of function. Choi and Bradley reported that teeth tended

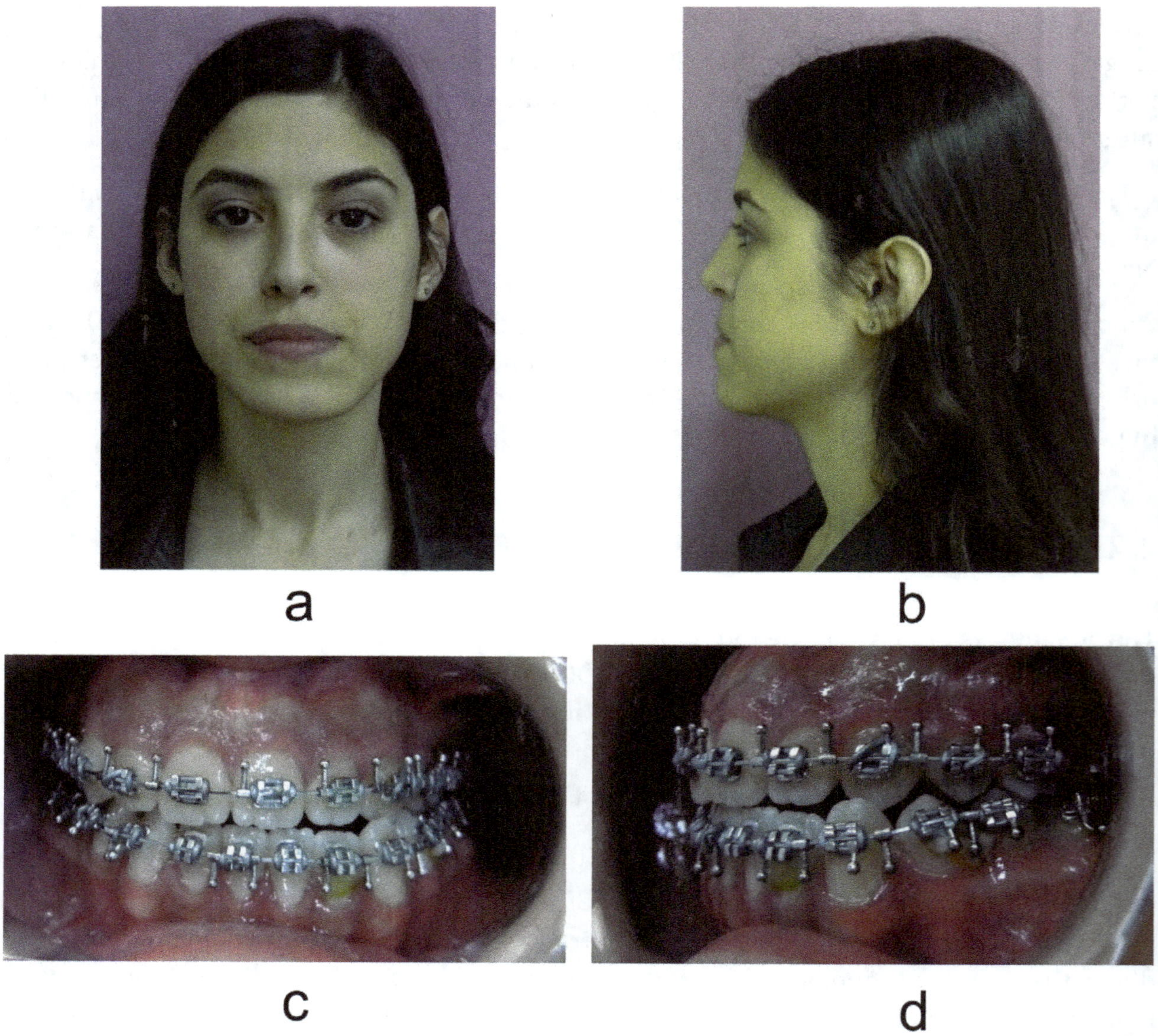

a b c d

Figure 1. a-d: Facial asymmetry case. Passive arch wires were inserted the day before surgery.

to move in the direction of decompensation to perform the function following the surgery [46]. Postoperative orthodontic direction and function improve the efficiency of decompensation. Additionally, orthodontic movement via a more rapid natural dental adaptation by facilitating natural compensation may be performed easier with less occluded occlusion.

Orthodontic treatment time depends on the complexity of case. The shortest reported treatment time is 4 months (**Figure 1a-d, 2a-d**) but generally it takes 6–12 months [17, 26, 28, 33, 35, 47–50]. Tooth extraction is the factor that influences the total treatment time [13], and in some cases, the time range was reported between 10 and 19 months [51–53].

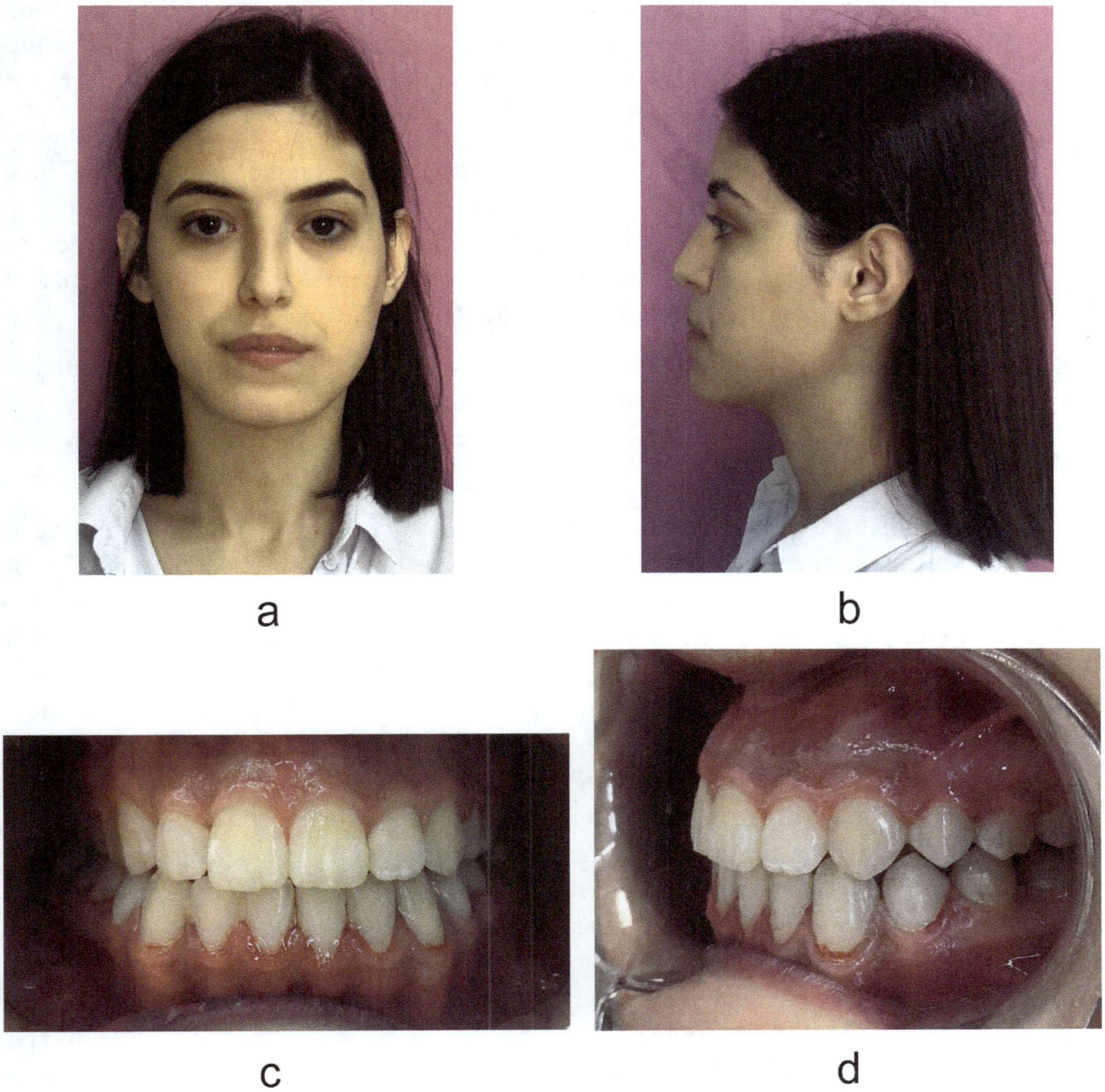

Figure 2. a-d: Three months later after surgery. Total treatment time 3 and half months.

3. Treatment plan in SFA

SFA is indicated more common in some cases like well-aligned to mildly crowded anterior teeth, flat to mildly curve of Spee, and normal to mildly proclined/retroclined incisor inclination. The protocol of presurgical orthodontics is well known in conventional approach [4, 8]; however, treatment plan including orthodontic treatment is questioned in SFA especially in complex cases. The orthodontic management and treatment plan are different in SFA compared with the conventional approaches.

In treatment plan, accurate and detailed prediction of the postoperative orthodontic treatment is required at the beginning of all treatment [50]. Following the analysis of occlusion with model mounting, of detailed clinical and cephalometrics, presurgical orthodontic setup that is useful for accurate prediction and simulation of postsurgical orthodontics and cephalometric setup may be required before the surgery [13, 51].

The model surgery is a setup according to the cephalometric and molar relationship. Three stable occlusion points between the upper and lower dentitions are required [38]. Liou et al. reported that the molar relationship could be set up in Class I in cases of nonextraction or bimaxillary first premolar extraction, Class III in cases of lower first premolar extraction, and Class II in cases of maxillary first premolar extraction [16].

Following cephalometric, model, and clinical diagnosis, the aim is to optimize the position of facial components to attain the most desirable results in esthetics, function, and stability. The skeletal movements in all anteroposterior, vertical, and transverse directions are determined to obtain good facial proportions, smile esthetics, and occlusion.

Liou et al. have made some suggestions in treatment plan of SFA [16]. In Class III cases, to correct the decompensation of maxillary incisor, first premolar extraction and retraction of anterior teeth can be done by orthodontics or by anterior segmental osteotomy. If the case has moderately retroclined and crowded lower incisors, the molars in a Class I relationship with an excessive incisor overjet can be planned. In cases with severe crowding and retroclination in mandible, first premolar extraction and lower anterior setback osteotomy can be planned. In Class III cases with deep curve of Spee, leveling of Spee can be corrected before the surgery or can be corrected with lower anterior segmental osteotomy surgically to avoid upward-forward rotation of mandible postoperatively, which is not preferred in Class III cases. The chin cap therapy may be used to prevent the skeletal postsurgical relapse after surgery for 3 months [16]. In Class II cases, in mandibular retrognathia with deep curve of Spee, mandibular advancement with surgical intrusion of anterior segment to advance mandible properly or mandibular advancement followed by orthodontically intrusion of lower incisor postsurgically is proposed to obtain a better chin profile. Otherwise, the mandible cannot be advanced properly and lower face can be longer with correction of posterior openbite after surgery, and this cannot be preferred in some long face case. But in some cases where advancements are not required much, correction of posterior openbite only with posterior extrusion can be preferred [54].

4. Time for orthodontic bonding and force application

On the basis of simulated model surgery setup, surgical guidance splint is prepared. Before the surgery, orthodontic bracket bonding/banding is placed but no arch wire is used. Bonding orthodontic bracket was reported as immediately before surgery [26, 47, 48], 1 week before surgery [16, 26, 38], and 1–2 months before surgery [50]. Some studies reported the usage of passive archwire before the surgery [49, 50, 52, 53, 55]. Passive arch can be used 1–3 days before the surgery [17, 35]. In some cases, the orthodontist can prefer minimal orthodontic preparation during 6 months [49] before the surgery, and then, they are continuing the orthodontic treatment after the surgery. Intermaxillary fixation of jaws during the surgery can be done by bony screws following the surgical guidance splints placements in cases without arch wires [47, 50, 51]. Kim et al. maintained intermaxillary fixation without surgical splint for 2 weeks but used intermaxillary elastic [50]. The osteotomized bones are fixed by rigid fixation.

Postoperatively, surgical splint is left for 2–4 weeks [34, 50, 53], and intermaxillary elastics usage may begin after orthodontic wire was placed.

There is no definitive consensus about postsurgical orthodontic force application time. But generally, the orthodontic treatment in SFA begins in 1 or 2 weeks after surgery. The surgical splint and inter-maxillary fixation were removed for the tooth movement. Liao et al. reported that postsurgical orthodontics begun immediately after surgery [17]. This is beneficial to shorten the orthodontic treatment time due to the regional accelerated phenomena. The studies showed that the orthognathic surgery triggers a 3- to 4-month period of higher osteoclastic activity, serum findings, and metabolic changes and that in the dentoalveolar bone postoperatively [15, 56]. Archwire changes took place every 2–3 weeks. Arch coordination may be managed with transpalatal elastics or active transpalatal arch. In segmental surgery patients, passive continuous arches which were placed before surgery are changed with sectional arches at first orthodontic appointment after surgery.

5. Relapse in SFA

The short- and long-term relapse rates in SFA have been investigated, and the results are good by comparison with the conventional surgical approach with a maximum follow-up of 3 years [19, 57–59]. Without presurgical orthodontics, the patients may have likely to develop unstable occlusion after surgery leading to relapse. However, some of the comparative studies between conventional and surgery first approach showed no statistical differences in relapse and almost equal for those achieved using the more traditional orthodontics-first approach [17, 19, 51, 53, 59–63]. Advancement of fixation system enabled more stabilized results due to more stable fixation of bony segments. On the other side, based on one research and on the meta-analysis, SFA showed more relapses than in the conventional approach [57, 64]. Larger overbite, a deeper curve of Spee, a greater negative overjet, and a greater mandibular setback were reported to affect stability in SFA cases [59].

Although there are benefits of the SFA, there are some difficulties like the prediction of final occlusion, instability of postsurgical transient occlusion [10, 65], the requirement of presurgical orthodontic setup before surgery in some complex cases, and requirement of frequent orthodontic appointment due to RAP. The treatment plan requires detailed and meticulous planning.

6. Conclusion

The surgery first approach is an alternative method that may be more satisfying for orthodontists and patients by minimizing the treatment time required for orthodontic treatment compared to conventional approach.

Author details

Ayşe Gülşen

Address all correspondence to: aysegulsen1968@gmail.com

Department of Plastic Reconstructive and Esthetic Surgery, University of Gazi, Ankara, Turkey

References

[1] Obwegeser HL. Surgical correction of small or retrodisplaced maxillae. The "dish-face" deformity. Plastic and Reconstructive Surgery. 1969;**43**:351-365

[2] Poulton DR, Taylor RC, Ware WH. Cephalometric x-ray evaluation of the vertical osteotomy correction of mandibular prognathism. Oral Surgery, Oral Medicine, and Oral Pathology. 1963;**16**:807-820

[3] Poulton DR, Ware WH. Surgical-orthodontic treatment of severe mandibular retrusion. II. American Journal of Orthodontics. 1973;**3**:237-255

[4] Bell WH, Creekmore TD. Surgical-orthodontic correction of mandibular prognathism. American Journal of Orthodontics. 1973;**63**:256-270

[5] Bell WH, Proffit WR, White RP. Surgical Correction of Dentofacial Deformities. Philadelphia: Saunders; 1980. pp. 1-3

[6] Worms FW, Isaacson RJ, Speidel TM. Surgical orthodontic treatment planning: Profile analysis and mandibular surgery. The Angle Orthodontist. 1976;**46**:1-25

[7] Profit WR, White RP Jr. Who needs surgical-orthodontic treatment? The International Journal of Adult Orthodontics and Orthognathic Surgery. 1990;**5**:81-89

[8] Proffit WR, Miguel JA. The duration and sequencing of surgical-orthodontic treatment. The International Journal of Adult Orthodontics and Orthognathic Surgery. 1995;**10**:35-42

[9] Proffit WR, White RP, Sarver DM. Combining surgery and orthognathics: Who does what, when? In: Proffit WR, White RP, Sarver DM, editors. Contemporary Treatment of Dentofacial Deformity. St Louis, MO. Mosby; 2003. pp. 245-267

[10] Sabri R. Orthodontic objectives in orthognathic surgery: State of the art today. World Journal of Orthodontics. 2006;**7**:177-191

[11] Grubb J, Evans C. Orthodontic management of dentofacial skeletal deformities. Clinics in Plastic Surgery. 2007;**34**:403-415

[12] Liou EJW, Chen PH, Wang YC, Yu CC, Huang CS, , and Chen YR: Can a surgery-first orthognathic approach reduce the total treatment time time? Journal of Oral and Maxillofacial Surgery. 2011;**69**:771-780

[13] Jeong WS, Choi JW, Kim DY, Lee JY, Kwon SM. Can a surgery-first orthognathic approach reduce the total treatment time? International Journal of Oral and Maxillofacial Surgery. 2017;**46**:473-482

[14] Assael LA. The biggest movement: Orthognathic surgery undergoes another paradigm shift. Journal of Oral and Maxillofacial Surgery. 2008;**66**:419-420

[15] Liou EJ, Chen PH, Wang YC, Yu CC, Huang CS, Chen YR. Surgery-first accelerated orthognathic surgery: Postoperative rapid orthodontic tooth movement. Journal of Oral and Maxillofacial Surgery. 2011;**69**:781-785

[16] Liou EJ, Chen PH, Wang YC, Yu CC, Huang CS, Chen YR. Surgery- first accelerated orthognathic surgery: Orthodontic guidelines and setup for model surgery. Journal of Oral and Maxillofacial Surgery. 2011;**69**:771-780

[17] Liao YF, Chiu YT, Huang CS, Ko EW, Chen YR. Presurgical orthodontics versus no pre-surgical orthodontics: Treatment outcome of surgical-orthodontic correction for skeletal class III open bite. Plastic and Reconstructive Surgery. 2010;**126**:2074-2083

[18] Park SH, Hyon WS, Lee JK, Lee YK. Paradigm shift in orthognathic surgery: Surgery first orthognathic approach and aesthetic two-jaw surgery. Journal of the Korean Society for Aesthetic Plastic Surgery. 2010;**16**(1):9-14

[19] Park KH, Sandor GK, Kim YD. Skeletal stability of surgery-first bimaxillary orthognathic surgery for skeletal class III malocclusion, using standardized criteria. International Journal of Oral and Maxillofacial Surgery. 2016;**45**:35-40

[20] Park HM, Lee YK, Choi JY, Baek SH. Maxillaryincisorinclinationof skeletal Class III patients treated with extraction of the upper first premolars and two-jaw surgery: conventional orthognathic surgery vs surgery-first approach. The Angle Orthodontist. 2014;**84**:720-729

[21] Dingman RO. Surgical correction of developmental deformities of the mandible. Plastic and Reconstructive Surgery. 1946;**3**(2):124-146

[22] Epker BN, Fish L. Surgical-orthodontic correction of open-bite deformity. American Journal of Orthodontics. 1977;**71**:278-299

[23] Behrman SJ, Behrman DA. Oral surgeons' considerations in surgical orthodontic treatment. Dental Clinics of North America. 1988;**32**:481-507

[24] Lee RT. The benefits of post-surgical orthodontic treatment. British Journal of Orthodontics. 1994;**21**:265-274

[25] Brachvogel P, Berten JL, Hausamen JE. Surgery before orthodontic treatment: A concept for timing the combined therapy of skeletal dysgnathias. Deutsche Zahn-, Mund-, und Kieferheilkunde mit Zentralblatt. 1991;**79**(7):557-563

[26] Nagasaka H, Sugawara J, Kawamura H, Nanda R. "Surgery first" skeletal Class III correction using the Skeletal Anchorage System. Journal of Clinical Orthodontics. 2009;**43**:97-105

[27] Park KR, Kim SY, Park HS, Jung YS. Surgery-first approach on patients with temporomandibular joint disease by intraoral vertical ramus osteotomy. Oral Surgery, Oral Medicine, Oral Pathology, Oral Radiology. 2013 Dec;**116**(6):e429-e436

[28] López DF, Aristizábal JF, Martínez-Smit R. Condylectomy and "surgery first" approach: An expedited treatment for condylar hyperplasia in a patient with facial asymmetry. Dental Press Journal of Orthodontics. 2017;**22**(4):86-96

[29] Pelo S, Saponaro G, De Angelis P, Gasparini G, Garagiola U, Moro A. Effect of surgery first orthognathic approach on the temporomandibular joint. The Journal of Craniofacial Surgery. 2018;**29**(3):671-675

[30] Uribe F, Adabi S, Janakiraman N, Allareddy V, Steinbacher D, Shafer D, et al. Treatment duration and factors associated with the surgery-first approach: A two-center study. Progress in Orthodontics. 2015;**16**:29-35

[31] Pelo S, Gasparini G, Garagiola U, Cordaro M, Di Nardo F, Staderini E, et al. Surgery-first orthognathic approach vs traditional orthognathic approach: Oral health-related quality of life assessed with 2 questionnaires. American Journal of Orthodontics and Dentofacial Orthopedics. 2017;**152**(2):250-254

[32] Zingler S, Hakim E, Finke D, Brunner M, Saure D, Hoffmann J, et al. Surgery-first approach in orthognathic surgery: Psychological and biological aspects. Journal of Cranio-Maxillo-Facial Surgery. 2017;**45**:1293-1301

[33] Hernández-Alfaro F, Guijarro-Martínez R, Molina-Coral A, Badía-Escriche C. "Surgery first" in bimaxillary orthognathic surgery. Journal of Oral and Maxillofacial Surgery. 2011;**69**:e201-e207

[34] Feu D, de Oliveira BH, Palomares NB, Celeste RG, Migue JAM. Oral health-related quality of life changes in patients with severe Class III malocclusion treated with the 2-jaw surgery-first approach. American Journal of Orthodontics and Dentofacial Orthopedics. 2017;**151**:1048-1057

[35] Hernandez-Alfaro F, Guijarro-Martinez R, MA P-G. Surgery first in orthognathic surgery: what have we learned? A comprehensive workflow based on 45 consecutive cases. Journal of Oral and Maxillofacial Surgery. 2014;**72**:376-390

[36] Hajji SS. The Influence of Accelerated Osteogenic Response on Mandibular Crowding. St. Louis, Missouri: St. Louis University, Center for Advanced Dental Education. 2000:1-49

[37] Wilcko WM, Wilcko T, Bouquot JE, Ferguson DJ. Rapid orthodontics with alveolar reshaping: two case reports of decrowding. The International Journal of Periodontics & Restorative Dentistry. 2001;**21**:9-19

[38] Villegas C, Uribe F, Sugawara J, Nanda R. Expedited correction of signi cant dentofacial asymmetry using a "surgery first" approach. Journal of Clinical Orthodontics. 2010;**44**:97-103

[39] Bogoch E, Gschwend N, Rahn B, Moran E, Perren S. Healing of cancellous bone osteotomy in rabbits—Part I: Regulation of bone volume and the regional acceleratory phenomenon in normal bone. Journal of Clinical Orthodontics. 1993;**11**:285-289

[40] Yaffe A, Fine N, Binderman I. Regional accelerated phenomenon in the mandible following mucoperiosteal flap surgery. Journal of Periodontology. 1994;**65**:79-83

[41] Bogoch E, Gschwend N, Rahn B, Moran E, Perren S. Healing of cancellous bone osteotomy in rabbits—Part II: Local reversal of arthritis-induced osteopenia after osteotomy. Journal of Orthopaedic Research. 1993;**11**:292-298

[42] Frost MH. The biology of fracture healing: An overview for clinicians part I. Clinical Orthopaedics. 1989;**248**:283-293

[43] Frost MH. The biology of fracture healing: An overview for clinicians part II. Clinical Orthopaedics. 1989;**248**:294-309

[44] Staffilino H, Levy S, Gargiulo A.: Histologie study of cellular mobilization and repair following a periosteal retention operation via split thickness mucogingival flap surgery. Journal of Periodontology. 1966;**37**:117-131

[45] Pfeifer JS. The reaction of alveolar bone to flap procedure in man. Periodontics. 1965;**3**:135-140

[46] Choi JW, Bradley JP. Surgery first orthognathic approach without presurgical orthodontic treatment: Questions and answers. The Journal of Craniofacial Surgery. 2017 Jul;**28**(5):1330-1333

[47] Sugawara J, Aymach Z, Nagasaka DH, Kawamura H, Nanda R. "Surgery first" orthognathics to correct a skeletal class II malocclusion with an impinging bite. Journal of Clinical Orthodontics. 2010;**44**:429-438

[48] Sugawara J, Aymach Z, Nagasaka DH, Yu CC, Chen PH, Liou EJ, et al. A surgery-first approach in surgical-orthodontic treatment of mandibular prognathism–a case report. Chang Gung Medical Journal. 2009;**33**:699-705

[49] Wang YC, Ko EW, Huang CS, Chen YR, Takano-Yamamoto T. Comparison of transverse dimensional changes in surgical skeletal Class III patients with and without presurgical orthodontics. Journal of Oral and Maxillofacial Surgery. 2010;**68**:1807-1812

[50] Baek SH, Ahn HW, Kwon YH, Choi JY. Surgery- first approach in skeletal class III malocclusion treated with 2-jaw surgery: Evaluation of surgical movement and postoperative orthodontic treatment. The Journal of Craniofacial Surgery. 2010;**21**:332-338

[51] Choi JW, Lee JY, Yang SJ, Koh KS. The reliability of a surgery-first orthognathic approach without presurgical orthodontic treatment for skeletal class III dentofacial deformity. Annals of Plastic Surgery. 2015;**74**:333-341

[52] Ko EW, Hsu SS, Hsieh HY, Wang YC, Huang CS, Chen YR. Comparison of progressive cephalometric changes and postsurgical stability of skeletal Class III correction with and without presurgical orthodontic treatment. Journal of Oral and Maxillofacial Surgery. 2011;**69**:1469-1477

[53] Kim CS, Lee SC, Kyung HM, Park HS, Kwon TG. Stability of mandibular setback surgery with and without presurgical orthodontics. Journal of Oral and Maxillofacial Surgery. 2014;**72**:779-787

[54] Kochar GD, Chakranarayan A, Londhe SM, Varghese B, Jayan B, Chopra SS, et al. Management of skeletal class II malocclusion by surgery-first approach. The Journal of Craniofacial Surgery. 2017;**29**(3):671-675

[55] Kim JY, Jung HD, Kim SY, Park HS, Jung YS. Postoperativestability for surgery-first approach using intraoral vertical ramus osteotomy: 12 month follow-up. The British Journal of Oral & Maxillofacial Surgery. 2014;**52**:539-544

[56] Sebaoun JD, Ferguson DJ, Wilcko MT, Wilcko WM. Alveolar osteotomy and rapid orthodontic treatments. L'Orthodontie Française. 2007;**78**:217-225

[57] Mah DH, Kim SG, Oh JS, You JS, Jung SY, Kim WG, et al. Comparative study of postoperative stability between conventional orthognathic surgery and a surgery-first orthognathic approach after bilateral sagittal split ramus osteotomy for skeletal Class III correction. Journal of the Korean Association of Oral and Maxillofacial Surgeons. 2017;**43**:23-28

[58] Park HM, Yang II-H, Choi JY, Lee JH, Kim MJ, Baek SH. Postsurgical relapse in Class III patients treated with two-jaw surgery: Conventional three-stage method versus surgery-first approach. The Journal of Craniofacial Surgery. 2015;**26**:2357-2563

[59] Ko EW, Lin SC, Chen YR, Huang CS. Skeletal and dental variables related to the stability of orthognathic surgery in skeletal class III malocclusion with a surgery-first approach. Journal of Oral and Maxillofacial Surgery. 2013;**71**:e215-e223

[60] Huang CS, Hsu SSP, Chen YR. Systematic review of the surgery-first approach in orthognathic surgery. Biomedical Journal. 2014;**37**(4):184-190

[61] Guo J, Wang T, Han JJ, Jung S, Kook MS, Park HJ, et al. Corrective outcome and transverse stability after orthognathic surgery using a surgery-first approach in mandibular prognathism with and without facial asymmetry. Oral Surgery, Oral Medicine, Oral Pathology, Oral Radiology. 2018;**5**:22-30

[62] Jeong WS, Lee JY, Choi JW. Large-scale study of long-term vertical skeletal stability in a surgery-first orthognathic approach without presurgical orthodontic treatment: Part II. The Journal of Craniofacial Surgery. 2018;**29**(4):953-958

[63] Lian YK, Hsieh AMC, Tsai MS, Jiang HR, Yen CY, Hsia YJ, et al. Treatment efficiency and stability of skeletal class III malocclusion with a surgery-first approach. Orthodontics & Craniofacial Research. 2018;**21**(2):90-95

[64] Wei H, Liu Z, Zang J, Wang X. Surgery-first/early-orthognathic approach may yield poorer postoperative stability than conventional orthodontics-first approach: A systematic review and meta-analysis. Oral Surgery, Oral Medicine, Oral Pathology, Oral Radiology. 2018;**126**(2):107-116

[65] Diaz PM, Garcia RG, Gias LN, Aquirre- Jaime A, Pe´rez JS, de la Plata MM, et al. Time used for orthodontic surgical treatment of dentofacial deformities in white patients. Journal of Oral and Maxillofacial Surgery. 2010;**68**:88-92

3

Temporomandibular Joint Pathology and its Indication in Clinical Orthodontics

Bakr M. Rabie, Jeremy Ho and Qianfeng Li

Abstract

Temporomandibular joint (TMJ) pathology has been an area of study in dentistry specifically a research interest in clinical orthodontics in which treatment option has been a dilemma for practitioners. Discussion between 'dos' and 'don'ts' in growth modification has drawn spread however opposite opinions from different schools of thoughts in whether growth modification itself is working. To provide a better illustration of biological process within TMJ, this chapter discussed aspects including overall condylar growth; the histological structure of endochondral bone of condyle; extracellular factors that regulate proliferation, differentiation, hypertrophy, terminal maturation and apoptosis of chondrocytes; and molecular regulation of the entire process. An understanding of the pathology, histology, cellular and molecular events related to the morphology and growth of TMJ forms through reading over this chapter; the emphasis of the mechanotransduction mediators and the influence of mechanical strain on the level of expression of genes were presented in details. Novel studies using virus vector stimulating condylar growth through enhancing angiogenesis within a time limit were discussed; also clinical implications in treatment options in relation to mandibular advancement were briefly compared.

Keywords: temporomandibular joint pathology, condylar growth, orthodontics, gene therapy, growth modification

1. Introduction

More than 700 of 6000 known hereditary syndromes involve dental or craniofacial disorders; temporomandibular disorders (TMDs) are one subgroup [1]. TMDs are a class of musculoskeletal disorders related to mouth opening and closing, chewing and other mandibular processes necessitating the involvement of the temporomandibular joint (TMJ) and any of its associated structures [2]. Currently, one of the most widely used diagnostic criteria remains to be the RDC/TMJ criteria, axis 1 diagnoses by Manfredini et al. which classifies TMJ cases into one of three categories: musculoskeletal issues [3], TMJ disc displacements and joint pain (arthralgia). There are also other classifications of TMDs which focus on inflammation, injury and systemic conditions (**Table 1**) [3–5].

As TMDs have implications on the quality of life and well-being of affected individuals and their families, it is of major interest to clarify the etiology of TMDs. Several issues have arisen with the understanding of the etiology, treatment options and preventative measures of TMDs. There is a great variability in symptoms of TMDs (ranging from pain and inflammation to limitations of jaw movements) which can even vary in prevalence between genders—as

---

I. Musculoskeletal issues

A. Myofascial pain: pain or ache in the jaw, temples, face, preauricular area or inside the ear at rest or during function and pain in response to palpation of three muscle sites of the mandible with at least one of the painful sites on the same side as the complaint of pain [3, 4]

B. Myofascial pain with limited opening: myofascial pain with pain-free unassisted mandibular opening 40 mm and maximum assisted opening (passive stretch) 5 mm greater than pain-free unassisted opening [3, 4]

C. Ankylosis: joint stiffness potentially from disease and injury or a consequence of surgery [4, 5] and can be divided into fibrous, fibro-osseous and osseous conditions [4, 5]

II. TMJ disc displacements

A. Disc displacement with reduction: reciprocal clicking in TMJ or clicking in TMJ on both vertical ranges of motion in two of three consecutive trials [3, 4]

B. Disc displacement without reduction with limited opening: history of significant limitation in opening, maximum unassisted opening 35 mm, passive stretch increases opening by 4 mm over maximum unassisted opening, contralateral excursion 7 mm or uncorrected deviation to ipsilateral side on opening and the absence of joint sound or joint sounds not meeting criteria for disc displacement with reduction [3, 4]

C. Disc displacement without reduction, without limited opening: history of limitation of mandibular opening, maximum unassisted opening 35 mm, passive stretch increases opening by 5 mm over maximum unassisted opening, contralateral excursion 7 mm, the presence of joint sounds not meeting criteria for disc displacement with reduction, imaging conducted by either arthrography or magnetic resonance reveals disc displacement without reduction [3, 4]

III. Arthralgia, osteoarthritis and osteoarthrosis

A. Arthralgia: pain in one or both joint sites during palpation; one or more self-reports of pain; for simple cases, coarse crepitus must be absent [3, 4]

B. Osteoarthritis of the TMJ: arthralgia, coarse crepitus in the joint or radiologic signs of arthrosis, classified as a degenerative joint disorder [3–5]

C. Osteoarthrosis of the TMJ: the absence of all signs of arthralgia; coarse crepitus in the joint or radiologic signs of arthrosis; classified as a degenerative joint disorder [3–5]

III. External causes

A. Inflammation: can be acute, chronic or, a third option, infectious, which can be nonspecific or specific to a type of disease [3, 4]

B. Tumors: can be benign or malignant [4, 5]

C. Systemic conditions: include rheumatoid, juvenile and psoriatic arthritis, scleroderma and mixed connective tissue disease [4, 5]

Table 1. General classification of temporomandibular disorders (TMDs).

Etiological factors of TMDs
A. Predisposing factors: factors of structure (decrease in calibration, disc erosion or improper alignment, patterns of occlusion and bruxism); tissue quality; systemic diseases such as rheumatoid arthritis (RA), gout and fibromyalgia; facial typology; as well as age [5, 7]
B. Triggering factors: trauma at the macro and micro levels (e.g. injury to the jaw joint, osteoarthritis), bruxism as well as excess ability of articular tolerance [5, 7]
C. Perpetuating factors: underlying behavioral, social and emotional stresses [7]

Table 2. Classification of etiological factors of TMJ [5, 7].

females have been found to be more susceptible to TMDs compared to males [6]. This has resulted in treatment options being too broad or general, such as cognitive behavior therapy, nonsteroidal anti-inflammatory drugs (NSAIDs) and physiotherapy [6]. While there have been efforts for classification of the etiological factors including a widely known classification by de Boever et al. (**Table 2**) [7], current literature has shifted its focus to anatomical and histological examination of the structures within the TMJ, to identify contributing factors for TMDs, which will be the focus of this chapter.

2. Anatomy of the TMJ

The temporomandibular joint (TMJ) is an articular disc between the cranium and mandible and, more specifically, centered within the orofacial system, a functional group of structures which includes the masticatory and stomatognathic systems as well as the maxilla-mandibular apparatus (**Figure 1**) [5, 8]. The TMJ contains the glenoid fossa, TMJ disc (center, anterior and

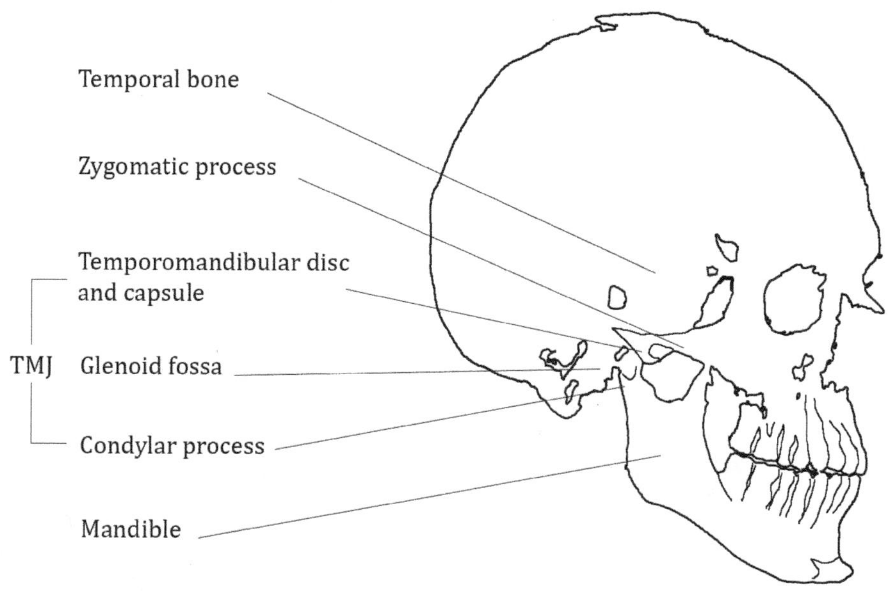

Figure 1. Schematic representation of the TMJ and associated structures in the human skull. The temporomandibular disc and capsule, glenoid fossa, neck of the condylar process and articular eminence (not labeled) are adjacent to each other and comprise the TMJ.

posterior), porous bone and mandibular condyle. It is a synovial joint and is unique in that it is one bone that is composed of two bilateral joints which cannot move independently of each other [6, 9]. Between the two joints is synovial fluid which promotes the hinge and sliding movements of the mandibular condyles required for mouth opening and closing and occlusion of the teeth [6].

The major function of the TMJ includes the coordination of individual tooth positions and other features of the orofacial system [8]. This is accomplished by lateral ligaments which are attached inside of joint capsules, being the structures which stabilize the intra-articular discs [10, 11]. The capsule is surrounded by fibrocartilage (rather than hyaline cartilage) and contrasts in thickness—the anteromedial and medial aspects are thin (0.7 mm), while the lateral and posterior aspects are thick (1.8 mm) [5, 9]. The capsule extends from the glenoid fossa to the neck of the mandible, preventing excessive displacement of the TMJ [5]. The majority of blood supply originates from the trail of superficial temporal, superior articular, anterior tympanic, and pterygoid arteries [5].

2.1. Glenoid fossa

The glenoid fossa is a concave portion of the temporal bone [8]. It borders the articular eminence anteriorly and the tympanic plate posteriorly [5, 9]. The glenoid fossa, similar to the disc and condyle, is a site of angiogenesis when subjected to mechanical stimuli [5, 9]. However, its histological composition has striking differences. Histological examination of the glenoid fossa has recorded fewer posterior layers of chondrocytes than the condyle. As chondrocytes are involved in chondrogenesis in the formation of cartilage to support the growth of the bone by means of endochondral ossification, the glenoid fossa may undergo a reduced level of endochondral ossification and a greater level of intramembranous ossification [5].

2.2. TMJ disc

The disc is fibrocartilaginous and biconcave and takes on a bow-tie morphology [5]. The two ridges of the disc are referred to as bands which attach to different structures. The smaller and shorter anterior band connects with the joint capsule, condylar head and articular eminence [5]. On the other hand, the larger and longer posterior band attaches to the condyle and the temporal bone [9]. The disc attaches to the capsule and neck of the condyle medially. The disc facilitates jaw opening in which the disc moves between the head of the mandible and the articular eminence [5].

2.3. Mandibular condyles

The articular surface of the mandible borders the anterior surface of the mandibular condyles [12]. The mandibular condyles are structures of the human mandible, covered with fibrous tissue composed of predominantly type I collagen, which present a surface for interaction with the articular disc of the temporomandibular joint, composed of avascular fibrous tissue including collagen and fibroblasts [12]. Below this resting, the fibrous layer of the condyles is four layers of cartilage: the proliferative, chondroblast, hypertrophic and erosive layers [12].

Extending further posteriorly than anteriorly, the condyles are convex laterally with a long axis situated medially and partially backwards [13]. The convex lateral extremities of the condyles are connected to small tubercles for attachment to the ligament of the TMJ [13].

Human condyles grow to 15–20 mm laterally and 8–10 mm anteroposteriorly in adulthood [5]. The growth of condyles is attributed to the condylar cartilage which acts as a template for bone growth [12]. The mandibular condyles are unique in that the cartilage (predominantly type II collagen) is known as secondary, compared to main and primary cartilage [12]. Another categorization of the condylar cartilage is articular [14]. However, unlike other types of the articular cartilage such as the synovial or epiphyseal cartilage, it has a striking difference of undergoing adaptive changes in response to external stimuli including mechanical or positional changes (e.g. repositioning of the condyles and/or the mandible, the functioning of the articular discs and the mechanical loading of the condyles) [15–17]. Some of the adaptive changes are related to growth and remodeling such as endochondral ossification and altering or regenerating chondrogenesis [14]. While these changes can occur during or after the natural growth period, there has been study that in adult rats, the remnant condylar cartilage serves more 'articular' function than 'growth' function as the adult rat condyle stops growth or becomes inactive of endochondral ossification [14]. Additionally, Luder studied adult human condyle structures and found that the cellular layers of organization did not resemble that of growing condyles and attributed the discrepancy to articular remodeling from mechanical loading [18]. As it was determined that articular tissue differed considerably between areas of loading and non-loading, Luder proposed that adult condyles should be divided differently and into three zones of organization—superficial, intermediate and deep [18]. Luder completed a follow-up study and found that features of the articular tissue in the condyles were subject to changes based on age [19]. Most tissue features were altered between 15 and 30 years of age and generally remained stable beyond this age range [19]. During this time, there was a progressive cartilaginification of the newly formed superficial zone, disappearance of the hypertrophic growth plate, appearance of the grid-fibrous fibrocartilage accompanied by a decline in endochondral ossification as well as formation of the subchondral bone plate [19]. From middle age to older age, there was a decrease in cellularity and some senescence and a progressive fibrosis of the intermediate zone. It was determined that the extent of maturation and remodeling and changes experienced in later age were related to articular load bearing [19].

Recently, there has been a spotlight on the mandibular condyles as major contributing factors to TMDs. As active growth sites of the mandible, impaired growth of the condyles has been associated with the development of TMDs [14]. Impairment of condylar development can result in mandibular asymmetry (e.g. hemifacial macrosomia and retrognathia) and problems in mastication, breathing and facial harmony which can lead to the onset of TMDs [14]. As it is evident that the etiological causes of TMDs are multifactorial, an evaluation of the influences and treatment options in the context of condylar growth is of great importance for affected individuals and their respective practitioners. Of major interest in condylar growth is the condylar cartilage for its influence in the growth of the mandible and its adaptive remodeling of the condyles in orthodontic intervention [14]. An understanding of the process of condylar growth and the involvement of cartilage in growth is therefore essential.

3. Steps in mandibular condylar growth

Given the fact that the anatomy of the condyles is clinically relevant in addressing TMDs, it is of importance to distil the major steps and cell types involved in the condylar growth process. There are two major processes involved in the growth of the mandibular condyles: chondrogenesis (cartilage formation) and osteogenesis (bone formation).

Mesenchymal cells eventually undergo one of two processes of osteogenesis by means of endochondral or intramembranous ossification, the latter of which is completed in the absence of the cartilage (**Figure 2**). In the former process, the mesenchymal cells will first differentiate into prechondrocytes which will mature into terminally hypertrophic chondroblasts [20–22]. This sequence of steps is collectively known as chondrogenesis. The chondroblasts eventually calcify and die, resulting in the bone replacing the cartilage by the bone through the invasion of osteoprogenitors which differentiate into osteoblasts [20]. This final step is known as endochondral ossification [23, 24]. Conversely, in intramembranous ossification, mesenchymal cells recruited from neovascularization migrate to the subperiosteal connective tissue and directly differentiate into osteoblasts to give rise to new bone (**Table 3**) [25].

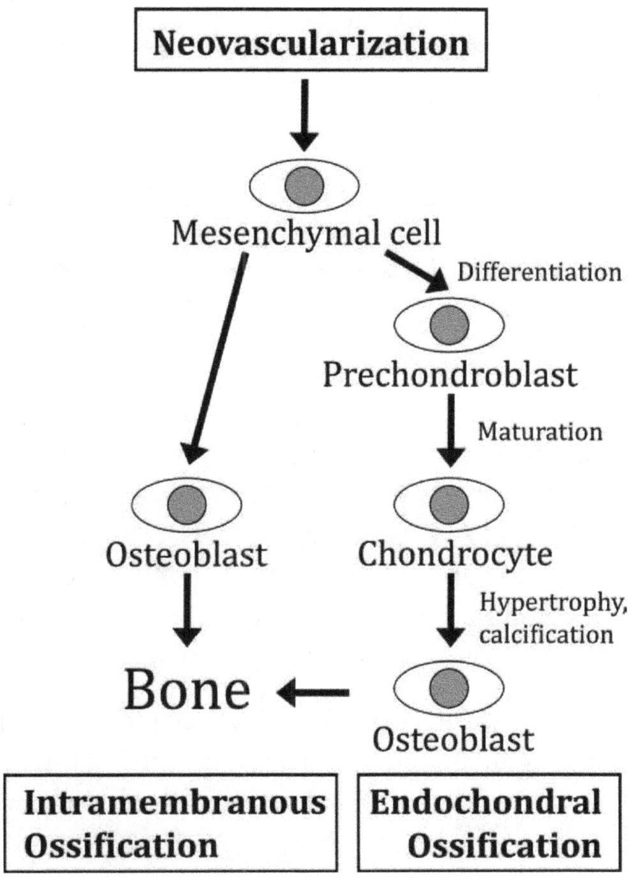

Figure 2. Schematic of the effects of VEGF during chondrogenesis, neovascularization and osteogenesis.

I. Chondrogenesis: mesenchymal cells

A. Fibrous layer [20]: differentiation into prechondroblasts [20]; can replicate up to 38 ± 4 times, and its quantity (dictated by various cellular and molecular factors) influences the growth potential [21, 26]; affected by mechanical forces [27]

B: Proliferative layer [21]: differentiates into chondroblasts and chondrocytes to maintain cartilage [21, 22]; affected by mechanical forces [27]

C: Erosive layer [21]: recruited with neovascularization and migrates to the subperiosteal connective tissue to directly give rise to osteoblasts through intramembranous ossification for the remodeling and repair of the bone [12, 21, 25, 28]

II. Chondrogenesis: prechondroblasts

Proliferative layer [12]: expresses type II collagen [12]; multipotential—can switch to differentiation of osteoblasts if articulate functioning is limited which can increase growth as articulate functioning retards growth versus condylar unloading which stimulates growth [23]

III. Chondrogenesis: hypertrophic chondrocytes

Hypertrophic layer, erosive layer [29–32]: maturation facilitates the transition from chondrogenesis to osteogenesis to serve as a regulatory point for growth [33], impacts cartilage formation and influences the growth of the condyle [34]; intercellular matrix calcification inhibits diffusion of nutrients, ultimately causing the death of the hypertrophic chondrocytes [20]

IV. Neovascularization

Refer to 3.1.

Va. Osteogenesis: endochondral ossification

Beneath erosive layer [20]: facilitates postnatal condylar growth and replaces degrading cartilage with the bone [20]

Vb. Osteogenesis: intramembranous ossification

Subperiosteal connective tissue [25]: unlike endochondral ossification, the cartilage is not present with this process of ossification which also serves the purpose for forming new bone [25]

Table 3. Analysis of the major processes involved in condylar growth and the corresponding stages within each process.

3.1. Neovascularization

Neovascularization is an essential step in endochondral or intramembranous ossification which occurs in the hypertrophic and erosive layers of the condylar cartilage as well as the glenoid fossa and the TMJ disc [28]. It is quantitatively correlated with endochondral ossification and is an indicator of osteogenesis in the replacement of dying cartilage with new bone [20]. Neovascularization functions by replenishing the population of mesenchymal cells for osteogenesis as blood vessels are the regions where progenitor cells are able to diffuse out and into the surrounding tissues [28].

While neovascularization has been determined to play a major role in condylar bone formation, it is of future interest to investigate the glenoid fossa and the TMJ disc, regions also characterized by mesenchymal cells and chondrocytes [5], as additional potential regions of neovascularization and subsequent bone growth. However, irrespective of anatomical location, an understanding of the factors influencing each of the steps in bone growth in the condyles and its associated regions is of major relevance for improving the management of TMDs.

4. Factors influencing condylar growth

Factors influencing the growth of condylar cartilage can be categorized into cellular (**Table 4**) and molecular factors (**Table 5**).

4.1. Factors at the cellular level

Cellular factors can be defined as factors that exert their activity at the extracellular level, including growth factors, cytokines, extracellular matrix (ECM) and other types of proteins. Growth factors and cytokines serve as local mediators in response to mechanical and inflammatory stimuli, while ECM serve as intercellular structural support [14].

I. Growth factors

A. Insulin-like growth factor (IGF): found in chondrocytes [35, 36], mediates growth and development of the cartilage and bone [14, 37]

B. Fibroblast growth factor (FGF): found in proliferating and chondroblast layers [14, 36]; regulates skeletal development and postnatal osteogenesis (e.g. FGF-2 promotes angiogenesis, inhibits the terminal differentiation of chondrocytes and reduces the formation of the bone) [14]

C. Vascular endothelial growth factor (VEGF): refers to 4.1.1

D. Connective tissue growth factor (CTGF): found in hypertrophic layer [38], regulates cartilage ECM and VEGF-A expression [38]; CTGF null or deficiency impairs endochondral ossification [39]

II. Cytokines

A. TGF-β: found in site of endochondral ossification, articular cartilage and growth plate [40, 41]; stimulatory and inhibitory roles dependent on concentration, culture period and state of cellular differentiation [42–44]; generally inhibits chondrocyte maturation and hypertrophy and alkaline phosphatase activity [45–47]

B. Bone morphogenetic protein (BMP): BMP-2 and BMP-4 are involved with cellular proliferation by regulating endochondral ossification [48]; activity of BMP-2 can be inhibited by Wnt signaling [14]

III. Extracellular matrix

A. Type II collagen: supports cartilage formation [12]

B. Type III collagen: regulates bone repair and development [49]; cross links are weaker than type I collagen and therefore can support replacement by type I collagen in remodeling [28]

C. Type X collagen: short-chain collagen [20]; correlated to the hypertrophic phenotype and marks the transition to osteogenesis [20]

IV. Other proteins

A. Parathyroid hormone-related protein (PTHrP): refers to 4.1.2

B. Indian hedgehog (Ihh): refers to 4.1.3

C. Matrix metalloproteinases (MMP-1, MMP-9): found in hypertrophic layer [50]; mediates the transition to osteogenesis, angiogenesis and further proliferation of the hypertrophic chondrocytes [20, 50]; facilitates remodeling of the bone by degrading matrix [51]

Table 4. Analysis of the cellular factors involved in condylar growth and, if applicable, the localizations of its respective activities.

I. Transcription factors
A. Core binding factor A1 (CBFA1): found in erosive layer [21]; essential for chondrocyte differentiation as the earliest regulator of transcription [21, 68, 69] can induce premature hypertrophy of chondrocytes [68]; mediates VEGF-A in endochondral ossification as its overexpression increases VEGF expression [38, 70]
B: SOX-9: refers to 4.2.1
II. Novel genes specific for condylar growth
A. Mustang, alpha B-crystallin (CryAB): associated with increased mesenchymal cell and osteoblast differentiation in response to mechanical strain [64]
B: Noggin: prevents apoptosis of chondrocytes [71]
C: Chondroadherin (CHAD): increases type II collagen expression in response to mechanical strain [64]
D: Nephroblastoma overexpressed (NOV): improves cartilage formation and integrity by positive modulation of type X collagen [64]
III. Other proteins
A: Wnt family: found in proliferative and hypertrophic layers [72]; controls mesenchymal cell differentiation into chondrocytes (e.g. Wnt1 and Wnt7a block chondrocyte differentiation, while Wnt4 blocks chondrogenesis but accelerates chondrocyte differentiation) [72–74]
B: Proliferating cell nuclear antigen (PCNA): found in hypertrophic layer [14]; increases the DNA replication of mesenchymal cells and is the marker for cell proliferation [14]
C: D-type cyclins: 'gatekeeper' of the G1 phase of the cell cycle which regulates the DNA replication of mesenchymal cells [72]

Table 5. Analysis of the molecular factors involved in condylar growth and, if applicable, the locations of its respective activities.

4.1.1. *Vascular endothelial growth factor (VEGF)*

VEGF is one of the most prominent regulators of mandibular condylar growth. It is found mainly in the hypertrophic layer of the condylar cartilage [24, 28, 52, 53], but traces have been discovered in the proliferative layer [54]. VEGF serves multiple functions in supporting the growth of the condyles including the coordination of the death of chondrocytes, function of chondroblasts, remodeling of ECM, secretion of growth factors and cytokines, angiogenesis as well as formation of the bone [12, 25, 26, 55].

Observing each of the functions of VEGF in greater detail, the coordination of chondrocyte death is accomplished by guiding of mesenchymal cell differentiation towards osteogenesis by bringing the cells to the mineralization front for calcification [24, 56, 57]. Additionally, VEGF-A has been the main isoform which facilitates the progression of angiogenesis [12]. VEGF in general supports rapid vascularization essential to healing and induction of bone associated with bone matrix that has been demineralized [58]. With respect to supporting bone formation, VEGF has been noted to increase mandibular length, and its expression has been correlated with the quantity of newly formed bone in the posterior of the condyle [12]. It is therefore evident that VEGF is a major therapeutic target of interest in research towards regulation of condylar growth.

4.1.2. Parathyroid hormone-related protein (PTHrP)

Another major regulator of condylar growth, PTHrP, is found in the transition zone between the proliferative and hypertrophic layers [59, 60]. It controls the condylar bone formation by facilitating and mediating the biomolecular pathway through which chondrogenic phenotype is shifted to osteogenesis [20]. This is accomplished by slowing down the hypertrophy of mature chondrocytes to promote further maturation and to provide more time to develop the cartilage in preparation for osteogenesis [33, 61]. By promoting further maturation and delaying the transition from chondrogenesis to osteogenesis, the population of chondrocytes continues to rise, leading to an increase in cartilage volume and subsequently bone formation.

Additionally, PTHrP induces the differentiation of mesenchymal cells through SOX-9, a transcription factor which serves to positively regulate the growth of the condyles [33].

4.1.3. Indian hedgehog (Ihh)

Compared to other factors at the cellular level, Ihh functions as a highly dynamic mechanotransduction factor which increases in expression in response to mechanical stimuli [12]. It is expressed by prechondroblasts and early hypertrophic chondrocytes in the proliferative layer [12, 62]. Ihh has a variety of effects on the TMJ and condyles including supporting early development [63] by regulating mesenchymal cell and chondrocyte proliferation and cartilage development (most notably type II collagen) in chondrogenesis as well as the transition to osteogenesis under mechanical strain [34, 64–66]. Interestingly, Ihh can also function as a molecular factor by shortening the turnover and enhancing the renewal of condylar cells [34] by upregulating cyclin D1, the 'gatekeeper' of the transition from the G1 to the S phases of the cell cycle [65, 67].

4.1.4. PTHr/Ihh negative feedback loop

Rabie et al. postulated that PTHrP and Ihh activities are linked through a negative feedback loop which regulates the development of the growth plate [5]. In the feedback loop, when PTHrP production is fleeting and not sufficiently stimulating chondrocytes, chondrocytes stop proliferating and maturing [66]. The chondrocytes begin to synthesize Ihh in the hypertrophic layer which acts on the chondrocytes by means of receptor-mediated signaling [66]. Ihh increases the proliferative rate of the chondrocytes and stimulates the production of PTHrP at the terminus of the bone. PTHrP then maintains the chondrocytes in a proliferative state and delays further maturation and differentiation which delays Ihh production [34]. As a result, the PTHrP/Ihh negative feedback loop modulates the pace of proliferation and differentiation of the chondrocytes to regulate cartilage and eventual bone formation [12].

4.2. Factors at the molecular level

Molecular factors can be defined as factors that operate within the cell by means of genetic and other intracellular factors. Such factors can be categorized into transcription factors, novel genes specific for condylar growth and other intracellular proteins. Transcription factors control genetic expression, while intracellular proteins control signal transduction and cell cycling pathways.

4.2.1. SOX-9

Targeted in PTHrP signaling, SOX-9 is a transcription factor that regulates the differentiation process from mesenchymal cells to hypertrophic chondrocytes [12]. Additionally, SOX-9 prevents premature differentiation and regulates type II collagen synthesis and cartilage formation through activation of the enhancer region of Col1a2 and Col2a1 [20, 75–77]. It is able to accomplish its activities by recognizing the DNA sequence of CCTTGAG and other members of the high mobility group (HMG) box class of DNA-binding proteins [71].

To understand how SOX-9 facilitates differentiation, it is vital to recognize that SOX-9 is expressed in mesenchymal cells, prechondroblasts and early differentiated chondrocytes but not in hypertrophic chondrocytes [78]. In mesenchymal cells, SOX-9 is required for differentiation into prechondroblasts. Later in the prechondroblast stage, SOX-9 supports the proliferation and further differentiation into early and proliferating chondrocytes. At the same time, SOX-9 regulates the expression of Noggin, an anti-apoptotic gene to support the proliferation of the chondrocytes [71]. After this stage, SOX-9 inhibits the transition from proliferative to hypertrophic chondrocytes to control subsequent endochondral ossification. Overall, SOX-9 is involved in cell proliferation of successive cell types in the earlier stages of chondrogenesis, but it also serves to prevent the hypertrophy of chondrocytes (**Figure 3**).

5. Interventions to address condylar growth

Given the working understanding of the stages and factors involved in condylar growth, researchers have found the condyles to be clinically relevant to the development and morphology of the orofacial complex [14, 20]. The condyles have been studied as a therapeutic target in addressing TMD and craniofacial issues in general. Two leading interventions to reactivate and control condylar growth have been the use of the recombinant adeno-associated virus (rAAV) vector and the application of mandibular advancement orthodontic appliances.

5.1. Intervention by the rAAV vector

The rAAV vector has become of interest in in vivo TMD therapy as it has been shown to overcome many limitations involved in the gene therapy of the cartilage and bone [79, 80]. Some advantages of the vector include reduced pathogenicity and immunogenicity, which supports long-term expression of transgenes which can be restricted to defined anatomical locations including specific oral tissues and success in transfecting many types of dividing and nondividing cells due to its size of 22–25 nm [55, 79, 81]. At this small size, rAAV-VEGF has been demonstrated as a suitable in vivo vector to significantly induce condylar growth by diffusing through the layers of the cell surface and infect with regular and hypertrophic chondrocytes to promote VEGF-mediated growth [79]. The systemic safety of the rAAV-VEGF vector has also been studied as exogenous VEGF was not identified in reverse-transcribed RNA samples of remote organs (e.g. heart, spleen and kidney) of transfected subjects [79].

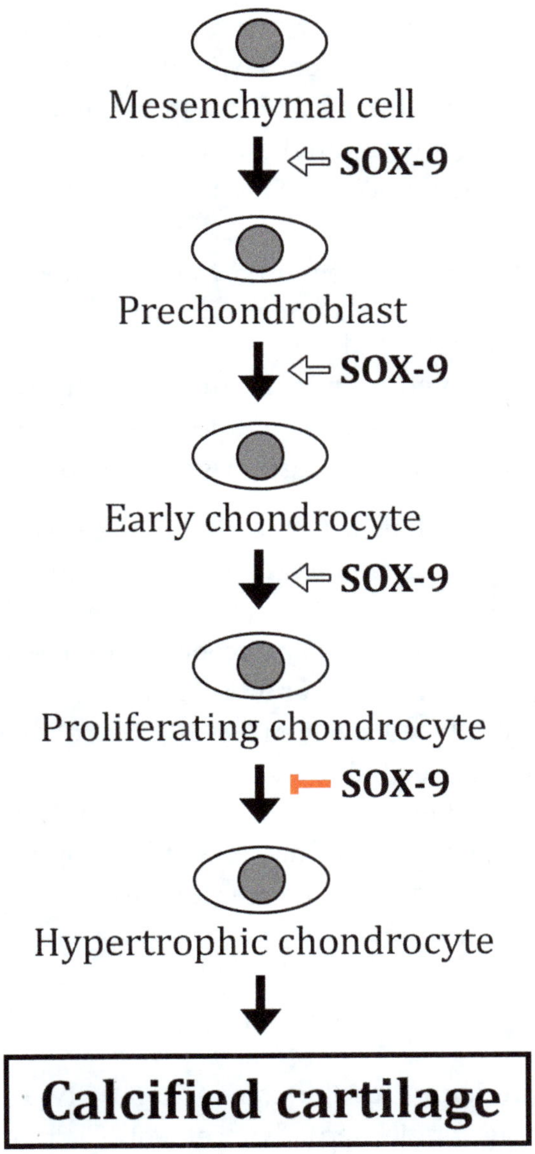

Figure 3. The roles of SOX-9 in each successive step of chondrogenesis towards endochondral ossification in the condyles. SOX-9 functions to commit mesenchymal cells to differentiate into prechondroblasts and supports the transition of prechondroblasts to early and proliferating chondrocytes but inhibits hypertrophy of the chondrocytes prior to the calcification of the cartilage.

Rabie et al. investigated the effect of in vivo rAAV-mediated VEGF administration on female Sprague–Dawley rats and found increases of the length of the condylar process axis (B-F) and the mandibular length from day 30 post-surgery and beyond [55]. The condylar width and length also increased during the same time period [55]. The growth of the condyle was upwards and backwards such that the greatest cellular response was found in the posterior condyle compared to the anterior surface [55]. This supported the adaptability of the condyle in directional changes in the growth of the mandible [24]. In addition, other studies have found a gain of function of VEGF, or VEGF gene has been associated with increases in neovascularization and regeneration of the bone in defective condyles [82, 83]. This has also reinforced the significance of rAAV-mediated VEGF as an appropriate option in contributing to neovascularization and endochondral ossification [28].

Most notably, it was determined that there was a delay in morphological effects of rAAV vector such that VEGF levels were increased on day 14 while chondrogenesis and osteogenesis occurred on days 21 and 30, respectively [55]. This finding had clinical implications in terms of understanding that gene therapy required a careful balance of inhibition or reinjection of the viral vector to address the potential consequences of overgrowth or relapse [55].

5.2. Intervention by mandibular advancement orthodontic devices

Recently, it has been proposed that condylar growth can be induced by forward mandibular advancement which has been noted to mirror natural growth [21]. Animal studies of mandibular advancement treatment on rats have reported the enhancement of chondrocyte maturation and endochondral ossification which give rise to new bone and condylar growth [84].

Three major factors of consideration include the age of the patient, the length of the treatment and stepwise versus single-step mandibular advancement. First, there have been recommendations of using functional appliances during or after the peak pubertal period to observe the greatest stability of treatment results [85–87]. Second, recommendations have been made to extend the commonly studied period of mandibular advancement of 6 months to 1 year in order to support the maturity of type I collagen [88–90]. Two other separate studies also noted that the treatment length was correlated to the maintenance of the effects of the orthodontic intervention [91, 92]. However, there have been mixed conclusions on the effect of lengthening the treatment period. Hagg et al. and Phan et al. found opposing trends of the length of treatment on the maxilla and the mandible, increasing the effect for the former and decreasing the effect for the latter [93, 94].

5.2.1. Stepwise versus single-step mandibular advancement

There has been extensive literature for the comparison of two approaches of mandibular advancement: stepwise versus single-step advancement. Currently, stepwise advancement has been determined as being the preferable therapy.

One of the reasons supporting stepwise advancement is the improvement in skeletal effect, most notably the sagittal jaw relationship with the maxilla, assuming a more forward positioned mandible due to more growth than single-step advancement [21, 95]. This improvement may be attributed to work completed by Petrovic et al. who found that the forward repositioning of the mandible periodically increases the rate and amount of growth in the condylar cartilage [96]. Van Lam and Rabie also found that stepwise treatment was correlated with significantly greater new bone formation [21].

From a cellular and molecular perspective, stepwise advancement that exceeded a minimum threshold of mechanical strain resulted in increases in Ihh, type II collagen, PTHrP and VEGF [34, 57, 97–100]. Thus, stepwise treatment involves repeated cycles of mechanical strain and increases neovascularization which results in increases in eventual new condylar bone formation [57]. Studies have shown that manipulating the amplitude of mechanical strain by stepwise advancement can significantly impact VEGF production by chondrocytes [55]. Moreover, the later stages of stepwise treatment are responsible for more VEGF production and subsequent condylar bone formation [57]. The extent of condylar growth modification from mandibular advancement has been determined through changes in measurements of the condyle and documented effects at the cellular and molecular levels (**Table 6**).

One modality of stepwise advancement in orthodontic treatment is the Herbst appliance; due to the advantages of stepwise treatment, it has been recommended to be included in an

---

I. Chondrogenesis

A. Mesenchymal cells: increase in quantity and rate of replication which is correlated to increased bone formation [12, 101]; cells deformed and oriented in the direction of the strain in the proliferative layers [84]

B: Prechondroblasts: reactivation of cells and chondrogenesis to promote growth of the condyle [12], which leads to an increase of osteogenesis [102, 103]

C: Hypertrophic chondrocytes: enhances but does not accelerate (a point that has not been clarified) [104] the hypertrophy of the cells towards osteogenesis [23]

D: Neovascularization: increased by means of VEGF expression which preceded the peaks of chondrogenesis and osteogenesis [55]; angiogenesis in the erosive layer during the enhanced, not accelerated (a point that has not been clarified) [104], transition towards osteogenesis [23]

II. Osteogenesis

Endochondral ossification: reactivation in the posterior aspect of the condyle leading to formation of new bone [12]

III. Cellular factors

A. IGF: increases expression of IGF-I and IGF-II [105]

B. VEGF: refers to 'neovascularization' in I (chondrogenesis)

C. Type II collagen: increases in expression [104]

D. Type X collagen: 540% increase in the posterior condyle which is correlated with 319% increase in bone formation [102, 106] by means of a similar temporal pattern when compared to natural growth [23]; maximal expression coinciding with that of Cbfa [88]

E. PTHrP: increases in expression which is associated with an increase in new chondrocyte population level [33]

F. Indian hedgehog (Ihh): immediate increase in expression due to deformation of the ECM and subsequent cellular cytoskeleton [62, 84, 107]; mechanical strain can reactivate dormant condylar growth [12], but the extent of reactivation of the condyle and glenoid fossa reduced with increasing age [108–110]; promotes chondrocyte proliferation, increased expression of cyclin D [72]

IV. Molecular factors

A. Cbfa1: upregulation of expression despite similar pattern of expression, coinciding with the maximal expression of type X collagen [21]

B. SOX-9: increases in expression which increased mesenchymal cell commitment to endochondral ossification [12, 33]

C. Novel condylar genes: increase in expression of Mustang, CryAB, NOV, Noggin and CHAD [64]

V. Morphology

Mandibular condyles: bending of the bone elongates [111, 112] the length and width of the condylar process and length of the mandible [55] with most change in direction posteriorly [24, 55]; there is potential to target the superior condylar layer to regulate upward condylar growth [55]

Table 6. Analysis of the factors affected by means of orthodontic mandibular advancement.

orthodontist's armamentarium [72]. The Herbst appliance has been evaluated with young adult patients and has yielded promising results in the treatment of Class II malocclusion [12]. It has been identified to operate by reactivating prechondroblast activity [12]. However, Pancherz has found several limitations of the Herbst appliance. The appliance has been met with concerns of relapse in cephalometric angle measurements after treatment [88, 90]. Additionally, it is most effective with Class II cases and thus cannot be used by individuals who have fully completed growth [90]. Thus, Pancherz has recommended the use of removable functional appliances post-treatment to maintain the effects from the Herbst appliance [90].

6. Conclusion

There have been considerable efforts to elucidate the etiological factors of TMDs and understand the factors regulating the growth of the TMJ and mandibular condyles at both the cellular and molecular levels. Current approaches to stimulating and controlling the growth of the condyles to address craniofacial abnormalities and/or TMDs have proven to be promising. Further research will be required to develop orthodontic treatment modalities that can be applied in a clinical setting on a case-to-case basis.

Author details

Bakr M. Rabie[1], Jeremy Ho[2] and Qianfeng Li[2*]

*Address all correspondence to: qianfengjennifer@gmail.com

1 Faculty of Dentistry, The University of Hong Kong, Hong Kong

2 The University of Hong Kong, Hong Kong

References

[1] Thyagarajan T, Totey S, Danton MJ, Kulkarni AB. Genetically altered mouse models: The good, the bad, and the ugly. Critical Reviews in Oral Biology and Medicine. 2003;**14**:154-174. DOI: 10.1177/154411130301400302

[2] Tanaka E, Detamore MS, Mercuri LG. Degenerative disorders of the temporomandibular joint: Etiology, diagnosis, and treatment. Journal of Dental Research. 2008;**87**:296-307. DOI: 10.1177/154405910808700406

[3] Manfredini D, Guarda-Nardini L, Winocur E, Piccotti F, Ahlberg J, Lobbezoo F. Research diagnostic criteria for temporomandibular disorders: A systematic review of axis I epidemiologic findings. Oral Surgery, Oral Medicine, Oral Pathology, Oral Radiology, and Endodontics. 2011;**112**:453-462. DOI: 10.1016/j.tripleo.2011.04.021

[4] Edvitar L, Oksana J, Ülle V-O. Temporomandibular joint arthroscopy versus arthrotomy. In: Bagaria V, editor. Regional Arthroscopy. Estonia: Tartu University, Tartu University Hospital; 2013. pp. 61-95. DOI: 10.5772/55011

[5] Schiffman E, Ohrbach R, Truelove E, et al. Diagnostic criteria for temporomandibular disorders (DC/TMD) for clinical and research applications: Recommendations of the International RDC/TMD Consortium Network and Orofacial Pain Special Interest Group. Journal of Oral & Facial Pain and Headache. 2014;**28**:6-27. DOI: 10.11607/jop.1151

[6] Sangani D, Suzuki A, VonVille H, Hixson JE, Iwata J. Gene mutations associated with temporomandibular joint disorders: A systematic review. OAlib. 2015;**2**:e1583. DOI: 10.4236/oalib.1101583

[7] de Boever JA, Carlsson GE, Klineberg IJ. Need for occlusal therapy and prosthodontic treatment in the management of temporomandibular disorders. Part I. Occlusal interferences and occlusal adjustment. Journal of Oral Rehabilitation. 2000;**27**:367-379. DOI: 10.1046/j.1365-2842.2000.00574.x

[8] Patil AS, Bindra GK. Morphology of the temporomandibular joint (TMJ) of sheep (*Ovis aries*). Open Journal of Veterinary Medicine. 2012;**2**:242-244. DOI: 10.4236/ojvm.2012.24039

[9] Alomar X, Medrano J, Cabratosa J, Clavero JA, Lorente M, Serra I, Monill JM, Salvador A. Anatomy of the temporomandibular joint. Seminars in Ultrasound, CT, and MR. 2007;**28**:170-183. DOI: 10.1053/j.sult.2007.02.002

[10] Maynard SJ, Savage RJG. The mechanics of mammalian jaws. The School Science Review. 1959;**40**:289-301

[11] Fanghänel J, Gedrange T. On the development, morphology and function of the temporomandibular joint in the light of the orofacial system. Annals of Anatomy—Anatomischer Anzeiger. 2007;**189**:314-319

[12] Xiong H, Rabie ABM, Hagg U. Mechanical strain leads to condylar growth in adult rats. Frontiers in Bioscience. 2005;**10**:65-73

[13] Gray H. Anatomy of the Human Body. 20th ed. Philadelphia: Lea & Febiger; 1918. 1396 p

[14] Leander D. Role of growth factors in the development of mandible. The Journal of Indian Orthodontic Society. 2011;**45**:51-60. DOI: 10.5005/jp-journals-10021-1010

[15] Kantomaa T, Ronning O. Growth mechanisms of the mandible. Dixon AD, Hoyte DA, Ronning O, editors. In: Fundamentals of Craniofacial Growth. New York: CRC Press; 1997. pp. 189-204

[16] Nakano H, Watahiki J, Kubota M, Maki K, Shibasaki Y, Hatcher D, Miller AJ. Micro X-ray computed tomography analysis for the evaluation of asymmetrical condylar growth in the rat. Orthodontics & Craniofacial Research. 2003;**6**:Suppl 1:168-172; discussion: 179-182

[17] Shen G, Rabie B, Hägg U. Neovascularization in the TMJ in response to mandibular protrusion. Chinese Journal of Dental Research. 2003;**6**:28-38

[18] Luder H. Frequency and distribution of articular tissue features in adult human mandibular condyles: A semiquantitative light microscopic study. The Anatomical Record. 1997;**248**:18-28. DOI: 10.1002/(SICI)1097-0185(199705)248:1<18::AID-AR3>3.0.CO;2-B

[19] Luder H. Age changes in the articular tissue of human mandibular condyles from adolescence to old age: A semiquantitative light microscopic study. The Anatomical Record. 1998;**251**:439-447. DOI: 10.1002/(SICI)1097-0185(199808)251:4<439::AID-AR3>3.0.CO;2-N

[20] Shen G, Hägg U, Rabie AB, Kaluarachchi K. Identification of temporal pattern of mandibular condylar growth: A molecular and biochemical experiment. Orthodontics & Craniofacial Research. 2005;**8**:114-122. DOI: 10.1111/j.1601-6343.2005.00316.x

[21] Van Lam S, Rabie AB. Mechanical strain induces Cbfa1 and type X collagen expression in mandibular condyle. Frontiers in Bioscience. 2005;**10**:2966-2971

[22] She TT, Rabie ABM. Expression of SOX9 in the mandibular condyle. Lecture presented at: 77th European orthodontic society congress; Ghent, Belgium: June 19-23. 2001

[23] Shen G, Zhao Z, Kaluarachchi K, Rabie AB. Expression of type X collagen and capillary endothelium in condylar cartilage during osteogenic transition — A comparison between adaptive remodelling and natural growth. European Journal of Orthodontics. 2006;**28**:210-216. DOI: 10.1093/ejo/cji123

[24] Rabie AB, Hägg U. Factors regulating mandibular condylar growth. American Journal of Orthodontics and Dentofacial Orthopedics. 2002;**122**:401-409. DOI: 10.1067/mod.2002.125713

[25] Yang YQ, Tan YY, Wong R, Wenden A, Zhang LK, Rabie AB. The role of vascular endothelial growth factor in ossification. International Journal of Oral Science. 2012;**4**:64-68. DOI: 10.1038/ijos.2012.33

[26] Bruder SP, Jaiswal N, Haynesworth SE. Growth kinetics, self-renewal, and the osteogenic potential of purified human mesenchymal stem cells during extensive subcultivation and following cryopreservation. Journal of Cellular Biochemistry. 1997;**64**:278-294. DOI: 10.1002/(SICI)1097-4644(199702)64:2<278::AID-JCB11>3.0.CO;2-F

[27] Rabie AB, Wong L, Tsai M. Replicating mesenchymal cells in the condyle and the glenoid fossa during mandibular forward positioning. American Journal of Orthodontics and Dentofacial Orthopedics. 2003;**123**:49-57. DOI: 10.1067/mod.2003.46

[28] Rabie AB, Leung FY, Chayanupatkul A, Hägg U. The correlation between neovascularization and bone formation in the condyle during forward mandibular positioning. The Angle Orthodontist. 2002;**72**:431-438. DOI: 10.1043/0003-3219(2002)072<0431:TCBNAB>2.0.CO;2

[29] Gerstenfeld LC, Shapiro FD. Expression of bone-specific genes by hypertrophic chondrocytes: Implication of the complex functions of the hypertrophic chondrocyte during endochondral bone development. Journal of Cellular Biochemistry 1996;**62**:1-9. DOI: 10.1002/(SICI)1097-4644(199607)62:1<1::AID-JCB1>3.0.CO;2-X

[30] Hashimoto S, Setareh M, Ochs RL, Lotz M. Fas/Fas ligand expression and induction of apoptosis in chondrocytes. Arthritis and rheumatism. 1997;**40**:1749-1755. DOI: 10.1002/1529-0131(199710)40:10<1749::AID-ART4>3.0.CO;2-D

[31] Garant PR. Oral Cells and Tissues. Quintessence: Illinois; 2003. 400 p. DOI: 10.1016/j.oraloncology.2004.06.001

[32] Chung U-I, Schipani E, McMahon AP, Kronenberg HM. Indian hedgehog couples chondrogenesis to osteogenesis in endochondral bone development. Journal of Clinical Investigation. 2001;**107**:295-304. DOI: 10.1172/JCI11706

[33] Rabie AB, Tang GH, Xiong H, Hägg U. PTHrP regulates chondrocyte maturation in condylar cartilage. Journal of Dental Research. 2003;**82**:627-631. DOI: 10.1177/154405910308200811

[34] Ng TC, Chiu KW, Rabie AB, Hägg U. Repeated mechanical loading enhances the expression of Indian hedgehog in condylar cartilage. Frontiers in Bioscience. 2006;**11**:943-948. DOI: 10.2741/1851

[35] Maor G, Hochberg Z, Silbermann M. Insulin-like growth factor I accelerates proliferation and differentiation of cartilage progenitor cells in cultures of neonatal mandibular condyles. Acta Endocrinologica. 1993;**128**:56-64. DOI: 10.1530/acta.0.1280056

[36] Fuentes MA, Opperman LA, Bellinger LL, Carlson DS, Hinton RJ. Regulation of cell proliferation in rat mandibular condylar cartilage in explant culture by insulin-like growth factor-I and fibroblast growth factor-2. Archives of Oral Biology. 2002;**47**:643-654. DOI: 10.1016/S0003-9969(02)00052-3

[37] Itoh K, Suzuki S, Kuroda T. Effects of local administration of insulin-like growth factor-I on mandibular condylar growth in rats. Journal of Medical and Dental Sciences. 2003;**50**:79-85. DOI: 10.11480/jmds.500111

[38] Dai J, Rabie AB. VEGF: An essential mediator of both angiogenesis and endochondral ossification. Journal of Dental Research. 2007;**86**:937-950. DOI: 10.1177/154405910708601006

[39] Ivkovic S, Yoon BS, Popoff SN, Safadi FF, Libuda DE, Stephenson RC, Daluiski A, Lyons KM. Connective tissue growth factor coordinates chondrogenesis and angiogenesis during skeletal development. Development. 2003;**130**:2779-2791. DOI: 10.1242/dev.00505

[40] Horner A, Kemp P, Summers C, Bord S, Bishop NJ, Kelsall AW, Coleman N, Compston JE. Expression and distribution of transforming growth factor-β isoforms and their signaling receptors in growing human bone. Bone. 1998;**23**:95-102. DOI: 10.1016/S8756-3282(98)00080-5

[41] Fukumura K, Matsunaga S, Yamamoto T, Nagamine T, Ishidou Y, Sakou T. Immunolocalization of transforming growth factor-betas and type I and type II receptors in rat articular cartilage. Anticancer Research. 1998;**18**:4189-4193

[42] Crabb ID, O'Keefe RJ, Puzas JE, Rosier RN. Synergistic effect of transforming growth factor β and fibroblast growth factor on DNA synthesis in chick growth plate chondrocytes. Journal of Bone and Mineral Research. 1990;**11**:1105-1112. DOI: 10.1002/jbmr.5650051103

[43] O'Keefe RJ, Crabb ID, Puzas JE, Rosier RN. Effects of transforming growth factor-β1 and fibroblast growth factor on DNA synthesis in growth plate chondrocytes are enhanced

by insulin-like growth factor-1. Journal of Orthopaedic Research. 1994;**12**:299-310. DOI: 10.1002/jor.1100120302

[44] Grimaud E, Heymann D, Redini F. Recent advances in TGF-β effects on chondrocyte metabolism. Potential therapeutic roles of TGF-β in cartilage disorders. Cytokine & Growth Factor Reviews. 2002;**13**:241-257. DOI: 10.1016/S1359-6101(02)00004-7

[45] Ballock RT, Heydemann A, Wakefield LM, Flanders KC, Roberts AB, Sporn MB. TGF-beta-1 prevents hypertrophy of epiphyseal chondrocytes: Regulation of gene expression for cartilage matrix proteins and metalloproteases. Developmental Biology. 1993;**158**:414-429. DOI: 10.1006/dbio.1993.1200

[46] Bohme K, Winterhalter KH, Bruckner P. Terminal differentiation of chondrocytes in culture is a spontaneous process and is arrested by transforming growth factor-β2 and basic fibroblast growth factor in synergy. Experimental Cell Research. 1995;**216**:191-198

[47] Ferguson CM, Schwarz EM, Reynolds PR, Puzas JE, Rosier RN, O'Keefe RJ. Smad2 and 3 mediate transforming growth factor-βl-induced inhibition of chondrocyte maturation. Endocrinology. 2000;**141**:4728-4735. DOI: 10.1210/endo.141.12.7848

[48] Ueno T. Kagawa T. Kanou M, Fujii T, Kukunaga J, Mizukawa N, Sugahara T, Yamamoto T. Immunohistochemical observations of cellular differentiation and proliferation in endochondral bone formation from grafted periosteum: Expression and localization of BMP-2 and -4 in the grafted periosteum. Journal of Craniomaxillofacial Surgery. 2003;**31**:356-361. DOI: 10.1016/j.jcms.2003.07.006

[49] Salo LA. Raustia AM. Type II and type III collagen in mandibular condylar cartilage of patients with temporomandibular joint pathology. Journal of Oral and Maxillofacial Surgery. 1995;**53**:39-45. DOI: 10.1016/0278-2391(95)90498-0

[50] Vu TH, Shipley JM, Bergers G, Berger JE, Helms JA, Hanahan D, Shapiro SD, Senior RM, Werb Z. MMP-9/gelatinase B is a key regulator of growth plate angiogenesis and apoptosis of hypertrophic chondrocytes. Cell. 1998;**93**:411-422. DOI: 10.1016/S0092-8674(00)81169-1

[51] Zheng LW, Ma L, Rabie AB, Cheung LK. Effect of recombinant human tissue inhibitor of matrix metalloproteinase-1 in rabbit mandibular distraction osteogenesis: A histological and immunohistochemical study. Journal of Cranio-Maxillo-Facial Surgery. 2006;**34**:277-282. DOI: 10.1016/j.jcms.2006.02.005

[52] Rabie AB, Shum L, Chayanupatkul A. VEGF and bone formation in the glenoid fossa during forward mandibular positioning. American Journal of Orthodontics and Dentofacial Orthopedics. 2002;**122**:202-209. DOI: 10.1067/mod.2002.125991

[53] Xiong H, Rabie AB, Hagg U. Neovascularization and mandibular condylar bone remodeling in adult rats under mechanical strain. Frontiers in Bioscience. 2005;**10**:74-82

[54] Gracia-Ramirez M, Toran N, Andaluz P, Carrascosa A, Audi L. Vascular endothelial growth factor is expressed in human fetal growth cartilage. Journal of Bone and Mineral Research. 2000;**15**:534-540. DOI: 10.1359/jbmr.2000.15.3.534

[55] Dai J, Bakr A, Rabie M. Gene therapy to enhance condylar growth using rAAV-VEGF. The Angle Orthodontist. 2008;**78**:89-94. DOI: 10.2319/102606-441.1

[56] Triffitt JT, Joyner CJ, Oreffo RO, Virdi AS. Osteogenesis: Bone development from primitive progenitors. Biochemical Society Transactions. 1998;**26**:21-27. DOI: 10.1042/bst0260021

[57] Leung FY, Rabie AB, Hagg U. Neovascularization and bone formation in the condyle during stepwise mandibular advancement. European Journal of Orthodontics. 2004;**26**:137-141. DOI: 10.1093/ejo/26.2.137

[58] Rabie AB. Vascular endothelial growth pattern during demineralized bone matrix induced osteogenesis. Connective Tissue Research. 1997;**36**:337-345. DOI: 10.3109/03008209709160232

[59] Lee K, Lanske B, Karaplis AC, Deeds JD, Kohno H, Nissenson RA, Kronenberg HM, Segre GV. Parathyroid hormone-related peptide delays terminal differentiation of chondrocytes during endochondral bone development. Endocrinology. 1996;**137**:5109-5118. DOI: 10.1210/endo.137.11.8895385

[60] Stevens DA, Williams GR. Hormone regulation of chondrocyte differentiation and endochondral bone formation. Molecular and Cellular Endocrinology. 1999;**151**:195-204. DOI: 10.1016/S0303-7207(99)00037-4

[61] de Crombrugghe B, Lefebvre V, Nakashima K. Regulatory mechanisms in the pathways of cartilage and bone formation. Current Opinion in Cell Biology. 2001;**13**:721-727. DOI: 10.1016/S0955-0674(00)00276-3

[62] Wu Q, Zhang Y, Chen Q. Indian hedgehog is an essential component of mechanotransduction complex to stimulate chondrocyte proliferation. The Journal of Biological Chemistry. 2001;**276**:35290-35296. DOI: 10.1074/jbc.M101055200

[63] Shibukawa Y, Young B, Wu C, Yamada S, Long F, Pacifi M, Koyama E. Temporomandibular joint formation and condyle growth require Indian hedgehog signaling. Developmental Dynamics. 2007;**236**:426-434. DOI: 10.1002/dvdy.21036

[64] Song Y, Wu C, Wing R, Wong K, Rabie ABM. Identification of the chondrogenic pathway in the mandibular condylar cartilage. Frontiers in Bioscience. 2009;**14**:1932-1938

[65] Long F, Zhang XM, Karp S, Yang Y, McMahon AP. Genetic manipulation of hedgehog signaling in the endochondral skeleton reveals a direct role in the regulation of chondrocyte proliferation. Development. 2001;**128**:5099-5108

[66] Kronenberg HM. Developmental regulation of the growth plate. Nature. 2003;**423**:332-336. DOI: 10.1038/nature01657

[67] Twyman R. Advanced Molecular Biology. Singapore: Springer; 1998. 510 p

[68] Rabie AB, Tang GH, Hagg U. Cbfa1 couples chondrocytes maturation and endochondral ossification in rat mandibular condylar cartilage. Archives of Oral Biology. 2004;**49**: 109-118. DOI: 10.1016/j.archoralbio.2003.09.006

[69] Tang GH, Rabie AB. Runx2 regulates endochondral ossification in condyle during mandibular advancement. Journal of Dental Research. 2005;**84**:166-171. DOI: 10.1177/154405910508400211

[70] Zelzer E, Glotzer DJ, Hartmann C, Thomas D, Fukai N, Soker S, Olsen BR. Tissue specific regulation of VEGF expression during bone development requires Cbfa1/Runx2. Mechanisms of Development. 2001;**106**:97-106. DOI: 10.1016/S0925-4773(01)00428-2

[71] Akiyama H, Chaboissier M-C, Martin JF, Schedl A, de Crombrugghe B. The transcription factor Sox9 has essential roles in successive steps of the chondrocyte differentiation pathway and is required for expression of Sox5 and Sox6. Genes & Development. 2002;**16**:2813-2828. DOI: 10.1101/gad.1017802

[72] Al-kalaly A, Wu C, Wong R, Rabie AB. The assessment of cell cycle genes in the rat mandibular condyle. Archives of Oral Biology. 2009;**54**:470-478. DOI: 10.1016/j.archoralbio.2009.01.020

[73] Rudnicki JA, Brown AM. Inhibition of chondrogenesis by Wnt gene expression in vivo and in vitro. Developmental Biology. 1997;**185**:104-118. DOI: 10.1006/dbio.1997.8536

[74] Church V, Nohno T, Linker C, Marcelle C, Francis-West P. Wnt regulation of chondrocyte differentiation. Journal of Cell Science. 2002;**115**:4809-4818. DOI: 10.1242/jcs.00152

[75] Nowak-Soliska E, Bakr A, Rabie M, Wong RWK, Lei SWY. The effect of naringin on early growth and development of the spheno-occipital synchondrosis as measured by the expression of PTHrP and Sox9—An in vitro model. European Journal of Orthodontics. 2013;**35**:826-831. DOI: 10.1093/ejo/cjs089

[76] Rabie AB, She TT, Harley VR. Forward mandibular positioning up-regulates SOX9 and type II collagen expression in the glenoid fossa. Journal of Dental Research. 2003;**82**:725-730. DOI: 10.1177/154405910308200913

[77] Cendekiawan T, Wong RW, Rabie AB. Temporal expression of SOX9 and type II collagen in spheno-occipital synchondrosis of mice after mechanical tension stimuli. The Angle Orthodontist. 2008;**78**:83-88. DOI: 10.2319/012507-36.1

[78] Zhao Q, Eberspaecher H, Lefebvre V, de Crombrugghe B. Parallel expression of Sox9 and Col2a1 in cells undergoing chondrogenesis. Developmental Dynamics. 1997;**209**:377-386. DOI: 10.1002/(SICI)1097-0177(199708)209:4<377::AID-AJA5>3.0.CO;2-F

[79] Rabie A, Dai J, Xu R. Recombinant AAV-mediated VEGF gene therapy induces mandibular condylar growth. Gene Therapy. 2007;**14**:972-980. DOI: 10.1038/sj.gt.3302943

[80] Dai J, Rabie AB. The use of recombinant adeno-associated virus for skeletal gene therapy. Orthodontics Craniofacial Research. 2007;**10**:1-14. DOI: 10.1111/j.1601-6343.2007.00381.x

[81] Dai J, Rabie AB. Recombinant adeno-associated virus vector hybrids efficiently target different skeletal cells. Frontiers in Bioscience. 2007;**12**:4280-4287. DOI: 10.2741/2387

[82] Street J, Bao M, deGuzman L, Bunting S, Peale Jr FV, Ferrara N, Steinmetz H, Hoeffel J, Cleland JL, Daugherty A, van Bruggen N, Redmond HP, Carano RA, Filvaroff EH. Vascular endothelial growth factor stimulates bone repair by promoting angiogenesis and bone turnover. Proceedings of the National Academy of Sciences of the United States of America. 2002;**99**:9656-9661. DOI: 10.1073/pnas.152324099

[83] Tarkka T, Sipola A, Jamsa T, Soini Y, Yla-Herttuala S, Tuukkanen J, Hautala T. Adenoviral VEGF-A gene transfer induces angiogenesis and promotes bone formation in healing osseous tissues. The Journal of Gene Medicine. 2003;**5**:560-566. DOI: 10.1002/jgm.392

[84] Rabie AB, Zhao Z, Shen G, Hägg EU, Robinson W. Osteogenesis in the glenoid fossa in response to mandibular advancement. American Journal of Orthodontics and Dentofacial Orthopedics. 2001;**119**:390-400. DOI: 10.1067/mod.2001.112875

[85] Ruf S, Pancherz H. Temporomandibular joint remodeling in adolescent and young adult during Herbst treatment: A prospective longitudinal magnetic resonance imaging and cephalometric radiographic investigation. American Journal of Orthodontics and Dentofacial Orthopedics. 1999;**115**:607-618. DOI: 10.1016/S0889-5406(99)70285-4

[86] Hansen K, Pancherz H, Hagg U. Long-term effects of the Herbst appliance in relation to the treatment growth period: A cephalometric study. European Journal of Orthodontics. 1991;**13**:471-481. DOI: 10.1093/ejo/14.4.285

[87] Von Bremen J, Pancherz H. Efficiency of class II, division 1 therapy in relation to treatment timing and modality. American Journal of Orthodontics and Dentofacial Orthopedics. 2002;**121**:31-37

[88] Pancherz H. Treatment of class II malocclusions by jumping the bite with the Herbst appliance: A cephalometric investigation. American Journal of Orthodontics and Dentofacial Orthopedics. 1979;**76**:423-442. DOI: 10.1016/0002-9416(79)90227-6

[89] Weislander L. Intensive treatment of severe class II malocclusion with a headgear-Herbst appliance in the early mixed dentition. American Journal of Orthodontics and Dentofacial Orthopedics. 1984;**86**:1-13. DOI: 10.1016/0002-9416(84)90271-9

[90] Pancherz H. The Herbst appliance—its biological effects and clinical use. American Journal of Orthodontics and Dentofacial Orthopedics. 1985;**87**:1-20. DOI: 10.1016/0002-9416(85)90169-1

[91] Hagg U, Du X, Rabie ABM. Growth modification of severe skeletal class II malocclusions by dentofacial orthopedics. Lecture presented at: 77th European Orthodontic Society Congress; Ghent, Belgium: June 19-23. 2001

[92] Wey MC, Bendeus M, Peng L, Hägg U, Rabie AB, Robinson W. Stepwise advancement versus maximum jumping with headgear activator. European Journal of Orthodontics. 2007;**29**:283-293. DOI: 10.1093/ejo/cjm018

[93] Hägg U, Du X, Rabie AB. Initial and late treatment effects of headgear-Herbst appliance with mandibular step- by-step advancement. American Journal of Orthodontics and Dentofacial Orthopedics. 2002;**122**:477-485. DOI: 10.1067/mod.2002.128218

[94] Phan KL, Bendeus M, Hägg U, Hansen K, Rabie AB. Comparison of the headgear activator and Herbst appliance--effects and post-treatment changes. European Journal of Orthodontics. 2006;**28**:594-604. DOI: 10.1093/ejo/cjl052

[95] Du X, Hägg U, Rabie AB. Effects of headgear Herbst and mandibular step-by-step advancement versus conventional Herbst appliance and maximal jumping of the mandible. European Journal of Orthodontics. 2002;**24**:167-174. DOI: 10.1067/mod.2002.127476

[96] Petrovic A, Stutzmann J, Gasson N. The final length of the mandible: Is it genetically predetermined? In: Craniofacial Biology. Craniofacial Growth Series. 2nd ed. The University of Michigan, Ann Arbor: 1981. p.105-126

[97] Rabie ABM, Al-Kalaly A. Does the degree of advancement during functional appliance therapy matter? European Journal of Orthodontics. 2008;**30**:274-282. DOI: 10.1093/ejo/cjm129

[98] Rabie AB, Wong L. Hägg U 2003c correlation of replicating cells and osteogenesis in the glenoid fossa during stepwise advancement. American Journal of Orthodontics and Dentofacial Orthopedics. 2003;**123**:521-526. DOI: 10.1016/S0889-5406(02)57033-5

[99] Ng AF, Yang YO, Wong RW, Hägg EU, Rabie AB. Factors regulating condylar cartilage growth under repeated load application. Frontiers in Bioscience. 2006;**11**:949-954

[100] Shum L, Rabie AB, Hägg U. Vascular endothelial growth factor expression and bone formation in posterior glenoid fossa during stepwise mandibular advancement. American Journal of Orthodontics and Dentofacial Orthopedics. 2004;**125**:185-190. DOI: 10.1016/S0889540603007194

[101] Rabie AB, Tsai MJ, Hägg U, Du X, Chou BW. The correlation of replicating cells and osteogenesis in the condyle during stepwise advancement. The Angle Orthodontist. 2003;**73**:457-465. DOI: 10.1043/0003-3219(2003)073<0457:TCORCA>2.0.CO;2

[102] Rabie AB, Xiong H, Hägg U. Forward mandibular positioning enhances condylar adaptation in adult rats. European Journal of Orthodontics. 2004;**26**:353-358. DOI: 10.1093/ejo/26.4.353

[103] Chayanupatkul A, Rabie AB, Hägg U. Temporomandibular response to early and late removal of bite-jumping devices. European Journal of Orthodontics. 2003;**25**:465-470. DOI: 10.1093/ejo/25.5.465

[104] Rabie AB, She TT, Hägg U. Functional appliance therapy accelerates and enhances condylar growth. American Journal of Orthodontics and Dentofacial Orthopedics. 2003;**123**:40-48. DOI: 10.1067/mod.2003.45

[105] Haijar D, Santos MF, Kimura ET. Propulsive appliance stimulates the synthesis of insulin-like growth factors I and II in the mandibular condylar cartilage of young rats. Archives of Oral Biology. 2003;**48**:635-642. DOI: 10.1016/S0003-9969(03)00128-6

[106] Rabie ABM, Shen G, Hägg U, Kalurachchi T. Type X collagen—A marker for endochondral ossification of the mandibular condyles. Quintessence orthodontics year book. Tokyo. 2000;**2000**:50-58

[107] Tang GH, Rabie ABM, Hagg U. Indian hedgehog: A mechanotransduction mediator in condylar cartilage. Journal of Dental Research. 2004;**83**:434-438. DOI: 10.1177/154405910408300516

[108] McNamara JA Jr, Hinton RJ, Hoffman DL. Histologic analysis of temporomandibular joint adaptation to protrusive function in young adult rhesus monkeys (*Macaca mulatta*). American Journal of Orthodontics and Dentofacial Orthopedics. 1982;**82**:288-298. DOI: 10.1016/0002-9416(82)90463-8

[109] Hinton RJ, McNamara JA Jr. Temporal bone adaptations in response to protrusive function in juvenile and young adult rhesus monkeys (*Macaca mulatta*). European Journal of Orthodontics. 1984;**6**:155-174. DOI: 10.1016/0002-9416(85)90183-6

[110] Woodside DG, Metaxas A, Altuna G. The influence of functional appliance therapy on glenoid fossa remodeling. American Journal of Orthodontics and Dentofacial Orthopedics. 1987;**92**:181-198. DOI: 10.1016/0889-5406(87)90411-2

[111] Raab-Cullen DM, Akhter MP, Kimmel DB, Recker RR. Periosteal bone formation stimulated by externally induced bending strains. Journal of Bone and Mineral Research. 1994;**9**:1143-1152. DOI: 10.1002/jbmr.5650090803

[112] Xiong H, Hägg U, Tang GH, Rabie ABM. The effect of continuous bite-jumping in adult rats: A morphological study. The Angle Orthodontist. 2004;**74**:86-92. DOI: 10.1043/0003-3219(2004)074<0086:TEOCBI>2.0.CO;2

4

Stability of Diastemas Closure after Orthodontic Treatment

Marcos Jimmy Carruitero Honores

Abstract

The prevalence of diastemas varies greatly according to age and ethnic group. In permanent dentition, it varies from 1.7 to 38%. Its etiology is multifactorial. In the deciduous and mixed dentition phases, interincisal diastemas are considered normal. There are several approaches used in the treatment of anterosuperior diastemas, which vary according to the present etiologic factor. Orthodontic treatment also has the function of treating any other associated occlusal problem and helping in the elimination of parafunctional habits. Some authors agree that orthodontic closure of diastemas without subsequent surgery for removing the abnormal labial brake greatly increases the frequency of relapse in the postretention period, while others concluded that the fibrotomy of periodontal fibers together with the retainer had a positive effect on the stability of space closure. Buccal and lingual teeth inclinations have greater tendency to relapse, while mesial and distal movements, with a period of containment, are stable movements. Removable retainers are not considered a good choice. Depending on the type of initial malocclusion, the use of retainers throughout life is recommended. Fixed retention is often cited as the only satisfactory method to promote stability at the closure of previous diastemas.

Keywords: diastemas closure, stability, diastema, relapse, corrective orthodontics

1. Introduction

The presence of diastemas in the anterosuperior region used to be considered unpleasant, being one of the main reasons why patients seek orthodontic treatment. However, some studies report that the stability of the orthodontic closure of the diastemas, particularly of the median diastema in the permanent denture phase, is low. Long-term stability is one of the main objectives in orthodontic treatment; however, it is one of the most difficult to reach.

In the anterosuperior region, this stability is especially desired and verified by patients. Most of the publications on anterosuperior diastemas consist of clinical cases and reviews of the literature on the etiology of the problem and its possible treatments. But, there is a shortage in the literature of studies on the stability of the treatment of the upper interincisal subjects. The present chapter seeks to evaluate the recurrence of the upper interincisal diastemas, the factors associated to the relapse and stability, some treatment proposals, and considerations for retention.

2. Definition and epidemiology of diastemas

At the beginning of the last century, Angle [1] described median diastema as a common form of malocclusion where there is a space between the upper central incisors and, very rarely, between the lower central incisors. According to the author, the width of this space usually varies from 1 to 4 mm and always presents an unpleasant appearance, and may interfere with speech, depending on the width. Later, according to Bishara [2], diastemas were described as just clinically visible spaces between two or more adjacent teeth.

In publishing the Six Keys for normal occlusion, Andrews [3] stated in Key V that there must be fair points of contact throughout the dental arch, in the absence of dental size discrepancy. According to this information, diastemas are also considered a malocclusion by Andrews.

2.1. General prevalence

The prevalence of diastemas varies greatly according to age and ethnic group [4, 5]. In permanent dentures, the prevalence of diastemas varies from 1.7 to 38% [4].

2.2. Prevalence according to age

The literature demonstrates that the prevalence of diastemas decreases with age, mainly due to the development of occlusion. Richardson et al. [6] observed 5307 children between 6 and 14 years of age and, as a result, obtained a prevalence of 38% of children with median diastemas above 6 years of age, 56% at 8 years, and 18% at 14 years.

In a longitudinal study, Bergström et al. [7] aimed to observe the behavior of median diastemas in relation to the presence of the labial frenulum, in children of age 9 years on average, followed up after 2, 5, and 10 years. In the first two follow-ups, the group submitted to the removal of the labial frenulum presented a larger number of cases with closed diastemas than the control group. However, 10 years after the first consultation, there was no difference between groups. The authors found that the number of children with diastema declined with age and that there were a considerable number of individuals where diastemas closed from 14 to 19 years.

Steigman and Weissberg [8] found a prevalence of 50% in 1279 adolescents with spaced permanent dentures, ranging in age from 12 to 18 years. On the other hand, Steigman et al. [9]

found that the number of diastemas per individual decreased with age, but 79% of the pre-existing spaces remained, resulting in a percentage of 38% of young adults with spacing between the teeth.

2.3. Prevalence according to gender

Richardson et al. [6] observed a higher percentage of 6-year-old girls with median diastemas; however, at age 14, the opposite occurred. The authors believe that this is due to an earlier maturation of the girls in relation to the boys.

The findings of Steigman and Weissberg [8] corroborate those of the other authors, since they found dimorphism only in the subgroup between 14 and 16 years. There was no difference between genders in the 12- to 14-year-old and 16- to 18-year-old groups. Another study published by Steigman et al. [9] supported this finding, demonstrating that there was no difference between genders regarding the number of spaces in the arches in a sample of patients aged 16–22 years. It was also found that the number of diastemas decreased with age in both genders, but this occurred earlier in females than in males.

2.4. Prevalence according to race

In an epidemiological study on the prevalence of diastemas in white and black ethnic groups, Richardson et al. [6] observed, in a sample of children between 6 and 14 years of age, a higher frequency of diastemas in blacks at almost all ages. A prevalence of 23% of blacks at 14 years of age with diastema was found, differing from 14% of whites of this age with central interincisive spaces.

Similarly, Lavelle [4] found a higher incidence of central interincisive diastemas in melanodermas (5.5%) than in leucodermas (3.4%) and a lower incidence in xanthomas (1.7%). Likewise, McVay and Latta [5] found a very significant difference between the prevalence of blacks (29%) compared to the percentage of 20% of adults presenting this space in both the white and yellow race.

3. Diastemas and occlusion development

It is a consensus in the literature that, during the development of occlusion, in the deciduous and mixed dentition stages, the presence of diastemas is a characteristic of normality [2, 10–14]. Nevertheless, Richardson et al. [6] suggested that median diastemas are more than a phase of development eliminated over time, due to the high prevalence found in 18% of adolescents with medium diastemas. Edwards [15] stated that if the median space is greater than 2 mm, it is unlikely to close spontaneously. It was observed in a longitudinal study in adolescents that there was stability in most of the existing diastema, although some were eliminated even after the eruption of permanent canines [9].

3.1. Primary dentition

Authors have suggested that these spaces in the primary dentition are normal and would have the function of assisting in the eruption of permanent teeth [10, 16]. In describing the biogenetic course of the deciduous dentition, Baume [11] classified the dental arches according to the spaces designated by him as type I, with anterior spaces, and type II, without such spaces. In this work, the author cites that one type cannot progress to the other.

Moyers [14] reported that there is a generalized spacing in the anterior region of the upper and lower arches in the deciduous dentition, which increases significantly after this dentition has been completed.

3.2. Mixed dentition

In the mixed dentition phase, the diastemas continue to appear as a physiological characteristic, mainly the diastema between the permanent maxillary incisors. The germs of these teeth remain separated within the maxilla, respecting the intermaxillary suture interposed between them [16].

Broadbent [12] published a study of 5000 individuals observed over 12 years. The author called the "ugly duckling stage" the period that ranges from the eruption of the upper incisors, around the age of 7 years, until approximately 10 years of age, when the upper canines erupt. At this stage, the lateral incisors remain with the converging roots until the maxilla size is sufficient to assume a more vertical position. With sufficient increase in the size of the subnasal area, and in the presence of normal growth, the canines move down, forward, and laterally to the lateral incisor roots. Correction of the ugly duckling stage will occur in the period between 8 and 12 years of age.

Burstone [13], observing the normal changes during development, identified that during the "ugly duckling phase" of Broadbent [12], protrusion of the crowns, overjet, and anterosuperior spaces occurs. He also reported that the upper central interincisive diastema would be closed with the eruption of the other permanent teeth, especially the canines, and that the overjet of the incisors would be corrected by the pressure of the labial musculature and the irruption of the other permanent teeth.

3.3. Permanent dentition

In the permanent dentition, the etiology of the diastemas is multifactorial [2, 16–19] and can be associated to the following factors: abnormal labial frenulum [1, 2, 16, 17, 20–22], microdontia, agenesis of maxillary incisors [2, 10, 16, 17, 20], dental discrepancy [2, 17, 23], shape of the anterior teeth (barrel) [10], brachyfacial pattern [17], a positive tooth-bone discrepancy [2, 16, 17], overbite, congenital anomalies such as soft tissue fissure, hybrid brake, or supernumerary teeth [2, 10, 16, 24], cysts and tumors [2, 24], periodontal disease [2, 25], macroglossia or neuromuscular imbalance of the tongue [10], acromegaly [26, 27], and orthodontic treatment [2, 20, 24].

The etiology of diastemas is also very well explored in a review article published by Bishara [2]. In this study, the authors divided diastemas into two categories, according to the etiology: (1) those not caused by orthodontic treatment, present before its accomplishment; and (2) those that appeared during or after orthodontic treatment. In the first category, the etiological factors mentioned are: physiological spaces in the deciduous dentition; developmental spaces in the mixed dentition phase, which are closed, according to the authors, after the canine eruption; genetic factors such as large jaws and small teeth; tooth size, interarch discrepancy, agenesis, and micro-diseases; characteristics relating to ethnic groups; low insertion of the upper labial frenulum, preventing the mesial migration of the maxillary central incisors during canine eruption; dental rotations; supernumerary teeth, among which a classic example is the mesiodens; pathological conditions, such as proximal caries, periodontitis, cysts, and tumors; and, finally, the deleterious habits, exemplified by the lingual interposition and sucking lip. In the second category, the author refers to dental extractions and occasional dental size discrepancies, caused by extractions as diastematic agents during orthodontic treatment.

Steigman et al. [9] evaluated the stability of permanent denture spaces during adolescence in untreated patients, and also investigated the association of tooth spacing with tooth size and dental arch dimensions. They observed that women with spaced dentition had smaller dental widths and similar arch dimensions than those without dental spacing. In them, the spaces were equally distributed in both arches. On the other hand, in men, there was an equivalence of the dental dimensions, but the intercanine distances and superior interpremolars were greater in those with a spaced dentition. This is the reason why, in males, a greater number of spaces were found in the maxilla than in the mandible.

Oesterle and Shellhart [27] mentioned that the presence of generalized spaces in the dental arches may be the result of discrepancies between the size of the teeth and their respective apical bases, muscular imbalances, deleterious habits, and loss or absence of teeth. The large jaw and/or jaw combination with normal or slightly reduced teeth size is related to inherited characteristics, but may also be a sign of endocrine imbalances, which result in excess growth hormone, such as acromegaly.

Gass et al. [18], when evaluating the correlation between the heredity and the presence of the medium diastemas in leucodermas and melanodermas, found that the genetic expression was more significant for the whites than for the black ones, where the existence of an interincisive diastema is more related to environmental factors, such as excessive protrusion of the incisors, a predisposing periodontal tissue, habits, and absence of teeth. However, in relation to the stability of the treatment, an association between heredity and median diastema recurrence has been reported [28].

In the same year, Mondelli et al. [24], in a comprehensive review work describing the etiology and the various diastema treatments, add that there are diastemas of iatrogenic etiology. As examples, the authors cited the rapid expansion of the maxilla and a type of mechanics inadequate for diastema closure, where an elastic band is positioned on the central incisors, but slides in the cervical direction, causing periodontal damage and root approximation, with consequent divergence of the crowns, making the diastema even wider.

4. Treatment of anterosuperior diastemas

In the deciduous and mixed dentition phases, interincisive diastemas are considered normal [11–13, 16]. However, in the permanent dentures, diastema is frequently associated with several occlusal problems, which include missing teeth, dental anomalies, abnormal bone structures, and excessive horizontal and/or vertical trespass [24]. It should be remembered that the diastema of racial and genetic etiologies are considered normal and the treatment will be dispensable, unless the patient considers the diastema an esthetic problem [24].

Patients' perception of the need for treatment for anterosuperior diastemas is influenced by the epoch and culture in which they live [29]. There is also a great contribution of the media to the opinion of people. In the 1960s, Gardiner [20] referred to a famous movie actor who presented a medium diastema and suggested, between the lines, that this feature, when smooth, may be well accepted for those individuals with a rather pleasant facial appearance. However, this cannot be considered for the majority of the population. The author's opinion was retracted through the following statement:

It was demonstrated [30] that when patients self-evaluate, they perceive a greater need for orthodontic treatment, when the problem is located in the anterior region, compromising aesthetics, as is the case of the anterosuperior diastema and anteroinferior crowding.

4.1. Treatment of diastemas in the mixed dentition

In the majority of cases, the central interincisive diastemas in the mixed dentition period are a temporary physiological feature of the "ugly duckling phase" [12, 13], which will be closed gradually with the eruption of the permanent lateral incisors and then with the eruption of the permanent canines. However, orthodontic interception is indicated in exceptional cases, where the diastema is preventing normal eruption of permanent teeth, stimulating the appearance or maintenance of deleterious habits, or compromising the child's self-esteem [16].

4.2. Treatment of diastemas in permanent dentition

There are several approaches used in the treatment of anterosuperior diastema, which vary according to the present etiologic factor [2, 16, 17]. The success of such treatment will depend on the elimination of these factors [17].

4.2.1. Orthodontic treatment

The orthodontic approach can be performed with the following objective: close the diastema or redistribute the spaces for a posterior reanatomization of the anterior teeth. Orthodontic treatment also has the function of treating, if present, any other associated occlusal problem and helping in the elimination of parafunctional habits. In cases where there is discrepancy of dental size, orthodontic treatment alone is not able to offer the best results. Therefore, these diastemas must be closed by means of composites, facets, or prosthetic crowns. However, for a better esthetic result of these restorations, orthodontic movement is indicated to redistribute the spaces before the cosmetic procedure [31].

Proffit, in the new volume of his book [32], divides the protocol of treatment of anteroposterior diastema according to two basic groups: (1) incisors with diastema and vestibular inclination and (2) diastema in the upper midline. In the first group, the diastema is usually caused by deleterious habit, which must be removed before the space closes, which can only be performed with a removable device, retracting the incisors. In the second group, the author recommends the closure of the space, followed by frenectomy, in case there is excess tissue pressed in the midline.

In cases where there is a deep overbite, it is interesting that it is corrected previously. This usually increases the horizontal overpass, making it possible to close spaces together with an anterior retraction [24].

4.2.2. Frenectomies

Labial frenulum is considered abnormal when it is enlarged and/or inserted near the gingival margin [15]. Some authors [16, 33] recommend frenectomy to be performed after orthodontic closure of space, since diastema closure and interdental papilla compression may act as a stimulus to promote atrophy of the fibrous tissue interposed between the incisors.

4.2.3. Restorative treatment

Peck and Peck [34] stated that teeth are, by nature, perfect structures. However, a tooth with altered anatomy can often form a malocclusion. For the authors, the orthodontist should increase their understanding of the limitations of orthodontic therapy, and know the value of procedures to change dental forms. Only in this way can treatment success be achieved.

Andrews [35] cited in his book "Straight Wire: Concept and Apparatus" that when there are spaces between teeth due to discrepancy of tooth size, where there are small teeth, orthodontic correction is contraindicated, and recommend the restoration of these teeth with composites or prosthetic crowns.

However, even if there is a discrepancy of dental size, orthodontic treatment may be an auxiliary tool to redistribute the spaces between the teeth before the restorative procedure. This allows the dentition in the anterior teeth to be performed according to the golden ratio, obtaining a better esthetic result [24, 31].

4.2.4. Other types of treatments

Bell [36] argued for the immediate closure of diastema by subapical and interdental osteotomy, justifying that there is a great unpredictability of diastole orthodontic closure stability and that this approach is difficult and takes a long time. In addition, the author believes that the alveolar bone is the major factor responsible for the difficulty in the orthodontic movement of the teeth and for the final stability, as opposed to the majority of authors who consider the labial frenulum and adjacent soft tissues as the main factor for relapse.

5. Stability of diastema treatment

Concern over the stability of results obtained with treatment has existed for more than a century [37].

Riedel [38], in reviewing the problem of containment in the literature, proposed nine theorems that should be considered for greater stability of treatment results. In the first, the author mentioned that orthodontically moved teeth tend to return to their original positions. In Theorem 3, it is reported that the etiological factors of malocclusion should be eliminated for greater stability. Theorem 6 states that the bone and adjacent tissues should have a time for reorganization around the new tooth position, so some type of holding device should be used. And finally, in Theorem 9, it is ensured that the higher the tooth movement, the less recurrence.

The work of Ormiston et al. [39] observed that the greater the severity of malocclusion, the greater the recurrence. This means that the greater the severity of malocclusion, the greater the movement required and the greater the relapse. In this way, they oppose Riedel's Theorem 9 [38].

There are few scientific studies that evaluate the diastema recurrence after orthodontic closure [15, 28, 40, 41].

Orthodontic corrections in the growth and eruption phases of the teeth are considered more stable by some authors. According to Reitan [37], there will be little or no recurrence after orthodontic movement of an erupting tooth due to the fact that the supporting tissues are in a proliferation stage as a result of the eruption process. New fibers will be formed as the root develops, and these new fibers will help maintain the new tooth position.

Almeida et al. [16] have speculated that the closure of diastema in the mixed denture phase is more stable than if treated in the permanent denture. Therefore, it does not require definitive containment, as long as the habit is removed and, in case of interincisive gingival hypertrophy, surgical correction is performed before removal of the device.

Edwards [15] cited several factors responsible for the reopening of the diastema: incorrect axial inclination of the central incisor roots, tooth size discrepancies, deleterious habits, deleterious occlusal patterns, such as displacement from centric relation to maximal habitual intercuspation or other mandible position, which generate lateral forces on the central incisors, anatomy of the teeth (wider cervical region than the incisal region), and possibly some muscular imbalance in the oral cavity. But in addition to these, the labial frenulum, along with associated tissues, is cited as the most frequent etiological factor in relapsing interincisal diastemas.

The influence of muscular imbalances on the maintenance of bad dental positions varies according to three factors: duration, frequency, and intensity. Studies [10, 22] emphasized that when an etiological factor, such as atypical lingual pressure, cannot be eliminated, it is very difficult to keep the space closed, without the use of permanent retention, especially in adult patients. Attia [10] mentioned that in these patients, the chances of success of improving the lingual posture with only exercises are minimal and indicates the glossectomy.

Shashua and Ärtun [28] evaluated the proportion of diastema recurrence and the possible variables that may have contributed to this recurrence in a sample of 96 patients 4–9 years after the end of treatment. Diastemas varied from 0.5 to 5.6 mm in the pre-treatment stage. The following variables were analyzed: initial diastema size, tooth size discrepancy, overbite, upper incisor inclination, maxillary incisor mobility, labial frenulum, intermaxillary septal cleft, root parallelism, anterior maxillary spacing, periodontal bone loss and heredity. Pre- and posttreatment data were obtained from the available documentation (models, radiographs, photographs, and clinical records). Post-retention data were collected from a follow-up visit of 37 patients (group A) and a telephone interview of 59 patients (group B). The incidence was 49% in the total, and 46% in group A, considering the patients with the diastema observed, or already portrayed by restoration or orthodontically, and still those who make continuous use of the retention by perceiving a tendency to reopen of space. However, in group A, the space in patients with recurrence ranged from 0.3 to 0.6 mm, but the mean was 0.1 mm. Logistic regression analysis revealed that the initial width of the diastema and the family tendency were risk factors for relapse. Although patients with abnormal braking had earlier initial diameters than those with a normal brake, no association was found between recurrence and the presence of an abnormal or crevice brake in the intermaxillary bone crest. The mobility of the upper incisors was the only parameter found in the postretention period that could be associated with the reopening of the space.

Surbeck et al. [41] evaluated the influence of occlusal changes on the stability in the anterior region of the maxilla. The sample was selected from study models for the posttreatment stage and was divided into three groups: (1) with anterosuperior spaces in this phase; (2) with crowding in the anterosuperior region; and (3) with perfect alignment. In group 1, it was found that the presence of spaces before treatment, as well as at the end of the treatment, increases the risk of increased spaces after treatment is finished. The authors suggest that the contention strategy should be altered according to the presence of spaces before treatment and their severity. Also, an association was observed between the increase of the spaces in the post-containment period and the reduction of the intercanine distance during the treatment. It was also found that reopening of spaces was associated with increased arch length and intercanine and intermolar distances in the posttreatment period.

5.1. The upper lip frenulum and its relation to the recurrence of diastema

Some authors [15, 21] agree that orthodontic closure of diastemas caused by an abnormal labial frenulum, without subsequent brake removal surgery, greatly increases the frequency of relapse in the post-retention period.

Edwards [15] evaluated the relation of the abnormal labial frenulum with both the etiology of diastema and the stability of its treatment. In this study, the author concluded that frenectomy had a great contribution to increase the stability of the orthodontic treatment of the median diastema and commented, citing that the upper labial frenulum is one of the most relevant factors for the reopening of orthodontically closed diastema.

On the contrary, Shashua and Ärtun [28] did not consider the central labial cleft lip and fissure in the central interincisive bone crest as risk factors for diastema recurrence, after evaluation of diastema relapse 4–9 years after the end of treatment. The authors [28] observed that the presence of the abnormal brake at the beginning of the treatment influenced the initial width of diastema. However, they emphasized that this type of brake can remodel spontaneously with the closing of the space.

5.2. Relation between periodontium and recurrence of diastema

It is believed that alveolar bone played the most important role in reopening orthodontically closed spaces [36]. However, several authors [15, 42] consider supra-alveolar gingival tissues as a primary factor in the relapse of dental positions.

Transseptal fibers are part of the supra-alveolar fibers group of the periodontal ligament and are composed mainly of collagen fibers. They are firmly inserted into the cementum, close to the cementum-enamel junction, and are responsible for holding together the adjacent teeth. They do not have elastic fibers, but their elastic characteristic is due to their structural form of tiny springs, which form as the fibers mature [25]. It is believed that their role in medial diastema recurrence is due to this elastic property, pressing the incisors mesially and pulling them incisively distally to the initial position [25, 42].

When they examined microscopically the interdental papilla of patients with median diastema, Campbell, Moore, and Matthews [42] observed that the insertion fibers of the brake had continuity with the gingival fibers of that area. The authors also verified an excess of accumulated and compressed gingival tissue in this area after the orthodontic closure of the space, which would act to reopen the spaces. In conclusion, it was suggested that the fibrous network of interincisive supra-alveolar tissues may be one of the main factors responsible for median diastema recurrence.

Similar situation, where a compression of gingival tissues was observed in orthodontically closed dental extraction sites, had already been observed by Edwards [15] and Parker [43]. In the aforementioned study, Edwards [15] noticed that the transseptal fibers, especially those near the alveolar ridge, reorganized and appeared normal after 10–14 days with retention of space closure. The author suggested that this was caused by the heavy forces applied during the final closure of space and by the approximation of the roots (parallelism), causing ischemia at the site and subsequent destruction of the compressed transseptal fibers. These, in turn, would be completely replaced by new fibers. Ten Cate et al. [44] have mentioned that it would be possible to remodel the transseptal fibers by a process called fibroblastic activity, where the fibroblasts are able to synthesize and degrade the collagen simultaneously, controlling its remodeling in the periodontal ligament and in the deeper transseptal areas.

In addition, Parker's findings [43] demonstrated that transseptal fibers within 60 days did not readapt to the new tooth position and were responsible for the reopening of the space. In this study, the effect of transseptal fibers on the stability of space closure was histologically evaluated, where the first permanent molar was extracted and the second premolar was retracted. In addition, the authors observed that the parallelism of the roots at the end of the closure increased stability and concluded that the fibrotomy of these fibers together with the containment had a positive effect on the stability of the retraction.

Bell [36] believed that the interdental septum was responsible for the instability of diastema closure and advocated subapical osteotomy in the space to be closed to facilitate movement and increase the stability of space closure.

5.3. Mesiodistal angulation of maxillary incisors

It has been mentioned in the literature that there is a greater stability of extraction space closure if the roots end up parallel, because when the roots also follow, the roots are also accompanied, a compression is generated in the place, causing ischemia and consequent destruction of the fibers transseptals. Subsequently, new fibers are formed and configured according to the new tooth position [33, 43].

Mulligan [45] stated that divergent roots are more conducive to keeping the space closed. He believes that when the roots are parallel, the vector of functional forces goes through the long axis of the tooth. However, when the roots are divergent, there is a space between the force vector and the tooth resistance center. This creates a moment that favors the approach of the crowns. The author also added that each patient has a moment of stability. And if within a period of up to 6 weeks without orthodontic treatment, the space remains closed, the ideal moment has been reached. But if there is a recurrence of the diastema, it would be necessary to further diverge the roots.

According to Reitan [37], the stability of the tooth position is greatly influenced by the direction in which the tooth was moved. The vestibular and lingual inclination of teeth has great chances of relapse. However, the mesial and distal movements, with a period of containment, are stable movements, except in cases of extrabuccal force for Class II correction.

Morais et al. reported no association between relapse of interincisor diastema and root parallelism. While midline diastema relapse occurred in 60% of the sample, lateral diastemas closure remained stable after treatment. Only initial diastema width and overjet relapse showed association with relapse of midline diastema [46].

5.4. Retention

In a study by Edwards [15], a recurrence rate of 88% was found in patients with abnormal labial frenulums who used retention for 16–22 months. In another similar group, but with a retention time of 8–10 months, this proportion was similar, 91% of cases with reopening of diastema. This may suggest that, in patients with abnormal labial frenulum, stability is not influenced by retention time, but rather by labial frenulum surgery.

Depending on the type of initial malocclusion, the use of retention throughout life is recommended [38].

Fixed retention is often cited as the only satisfactory method to promote stability at the closure of the previous diastema [32, 47]. However, the commonly available fixed retention present undesirable characteristics for long-term use, since they restrict access to gingival tissues, making their hygiene difficult. Currently, there is a type of fixed retention through small magnets attached to the lingual surface of the incisors, in previously diastematic areas [48].

Removable retention is not considered a good choice in cases of interincisive diastema because, soon after removal, the teeth already begin to move away [32, 45]. In addition, prolonged use of this retainer category would generate back-and-forth movements, which are potentially damaging.

6. Conclusions

The origin of the anterosuperior diastemas is multifactorial. In this sense, the clinician has several approaches for its treatment, which must be selected according to the etiological factor.

The etiology of the diastemas is associated to: abnormal labial frenulum microdontia, agenesis of maxillary incisors, dental discrepancy, shape of the anterior teeth, brachyfacial pattern, a positive tooth-bone discrepancy, supernumerary teeth, cysts, tumors, macroglossia, neuromuscular imbalance of the tongue, and orthodontic treatment.

Orthodontic treatment is a good alternative for diastemas closure, because it can also treat any other associated occlusal problem and help to eliminate parafunctional habits, if any.

When the width of the initial diastemas is very pronounced, the use of retainers can be considered throughout life. Fixed retention is often cited as the only satisfactory method to promote stability in the closure of previous anterosuperior diastemas, while removable retention is not considered a good option.

Acknowledgements

I would like to thank Juliana Fernandes de Morais for her previous contribution to this work.

Author details

Marcos Jimmy Carruitero Honores

Address all correspondence to: m_carruitero@usp.br; m_carruitero@hotmail.com

Department of Orthodontics, Bauru Dental School, University of São Paulo, Brazil

References

[1] Angle EH. Treatment of Malocclusion of the Teeth. 7th ed. Philadelphia: S.S. White Company; 1907

[2] Bishara SE. Management of diastemas in orthodontics. American Journal of Orthodontics. 1972;**61**(1):55-63

[3] Andrews LF. The six keys to normal occlusion. American Journal of Orthodontics. 1972; **62**(3):296-309

[4] Lavelle CL. Crowding and spacing within the human dental arch of different racial groups. Archives of Oral Biology. 1970;**15**(11):1101-1103

[5] McVay TJ, Latta GH. Incidence of the maxillary midline diastema in adults. The Journal of Prosthetic Dentistry. 1984;**52**(6):809-811

[6] Richardson ER, Malhotra SK, Henry M, Little RG, Coleman HT. Biracial study of the maxillary midline diastema. The Angle Orthodontist. 1973;**43**(4):438-443

[7] Bergström K, Jensen R, Martensson B. The effect of superior labial frenectomy in cases with midline diastema. American Journal of Orthodontics. 1973;**63**(6):633-638

[8] Steigman S, Weissberg Y. Spaced dentition. An epidemiologic study. The Angle Orthodontist. 1985;**55**(2):167-176

[9] Steigman S, Gershkovitz E, Harari D. Characteristics and stability of spaced dentition. The Angle Orthodontist. 1985;**55**(4):321-328

[10] Attia Y. Midline diastemas: Closure and stability. The Angle Orthodontist. 1993; **63**(3):209-212

[11] Baume LJ. Physiological tooth migration and its significance for the development of occlusion. I. The biogenetic course of the deciduous dentition. Journal of Dental Research. 1950;**29**(2):123-132

[12] Broadbent BH. Ontogenic development of occlusion. The Angle Orthodontist. 1941; **11**(4):223-241

[13] Burstone CJ. Distinguish developing malocclusion from normal occlusion. Dental Clinics of North America. 1964:479-491

[14] Moyers RE. Ortodontia. Rio de Janeiro: Guanabara Koogan; 1991

[15] Edwards JG. The diastema, the frenum, the frenectomy: A clinical study. American Journal of Orthodontics. 1977;**71**(5):489-508

[16] Almeida RR, Garib DG, Almeida-Pedrin RR, Almeida MR, Pinzan A, Junqueira MHZ. Diastema interincisivos centrais superiores: Quando e como intervir? Revista Dental Press de Ortodontia e Ortopedia Facial. 2004;**9**(3):137-156

[17] Baum AT. The midline diastema. Journal of Oral Medicine. 1966;**21**(1):30-39

[18] Gass JR, Valiathan M, Tiwari HK, Hans MG, Elston RC. Familial correlations and herita bility of maxillary midline diastema. American Journal of Orthodontics and Dentofacial Orthopedics. 2003;**123**(1):35-39

[19] Goodman NR. Treatment of diastema: Not always frenectomy. Dental Survey. 1975; **51**(4):28-29

[20] Gardiner JH. Midline spaces. Dental Practitioner. 1967;**17**(8):287-298

[21] Graber TM. Ortodoncia: Teoria y Práctica. 3rd ed. México, DC: Interamericana; 1980

[22] Graber TM. The "three M's": Muscles, malformation and malocclusion. American Journal of Orthodontics. 1963;**49**(6):418-450

[23] Bolton WA. The clinical application of tooth-size analysis. American Journal of Orthodontics. 1962;**48**(7):504-529

[24] Mondelli J, Pereira MA, Mondelli RFL. Etiologia e tratamento dos diastemas dentários. Biodonto. 2003;**1**(3):11-111

[25] Stubley R. The influence of transseptal fibers on incisor position and diastema formation. American Journal of Orthodontics. 1976;**70**(6):645-662

[26] Brown EE. Interdental separation in subclinical acromegaly caused by sinusitis. American Journal of Orthodontics. 1953;**39**(12):932-941

[27] Oesterle LJ, Shellhart WC. Maxillary midline diastemas: A look at the causes. Journal of the American Dental Association. 1999;**130**(1):85-94

[28] Shashua D, Ärtun J. Relapse after orthodontic correction of maxillary median diastema: A follow-up evaluation of consecutive cases. The Angle Orthodontist. 1999;**69**(3):257-263

[29] Offerman RE. A simple diastema closing device. Oral Health. 1986;**76**(9):21-22

[30] Peres KG, Traebert ESA, Marcenes A. Diferenças entre autopercepção e critérios normativos na identificação das oclusopatias. Revista de Saúde Pública. 2002;**36**(2):230-236

[31] Furuse AY, Franco EJ, Mondelli J. Esthetic and functional restoration for an anterior open occlusal relationship with multiple diastemata: A multidisciplinary approach. The Journal of Prosthetic Dentistry. 2008;**99**(2):91-94

[32] Proffit WR. Contenção. In: Proffit WR, Fields HW, Sarver DM, editors. Ortodontia Contemporânea. Rio de Janeiro: Elsevier Editora; 2008. pp. 575-588

[33] Edwards JG. The prevention of relapse in extraction cases. American Journal of Orthodontics. 1971;**60**(2):128-144

[34] Peck S, Peck H. Orthodontic aspects of dental anthropology. The Angle Orthodontist. 1975;**45**(2):95-102

[35] Andrews LF. Straight Wire. The Concept and Appliance. San Diego: L. A. Wells Co.; 1989

[36] Bell WH. Surgical-orthodontic treatment of interincisal diastemas. American Journal of Orthodontics. 1970;**57**(2):158-163

[37] Reitan K. Principles of retention and avoidance of posttreatment relapse. American Journal of Orthodontics. 1969;**55**(6):776-790

[38] Riedel RA. A review of the retention problem. The Angle Orthodontist. 1960;**30**:179-199

[39] Ormiston JP, Huang GJ, Little RM, Decker JD, Seuk GD. Retrospective analysis of long-term stable and unstable orthodontic treatment outcomes. American Journal of Orthodontics and Dentofacial Orthopedics. 2005;**128**(5):568-574

[40] Sullivan TC, Turpin DL, Artun J. A postretention study of patients presenting with a maxillary median diastema. The Angle Orthodontist. 1996;**66**(2):131-138

[41] Surbeck BT, Artun J, Hawkins NR, Leroux B. Associations between initial, posttreatment, and postretention alignment of maxillary anterior teeth. American Journal of Orthodontics and Dentofacial Orthopedics. 1998;**113**(2):186-195

[42] Campbell PM, Moore JW, Matthews JL. Orthodontically corrected midline diastemas. A histologic study and surgical procedure. American Journal of Orthodontics. 1975;**67**(2):139-158

[43] Parker GR. Transseptal fibers and relapse following bodily retration of teeth: A histologic study. American Journal of Orthodontics. 1972;**61**(4):331-344

[44] Ten Cate AR, Deporter DA, Freeman E. The role of fibroblasts in the remodeling of periodontal ligament during physiologic tooth movement. American Journal of Orthodontics 1976;**69**(2):155-168

[45] Mulligan TF. Diastema closure and long-term stability. Journal of Clinical Orthodontics. 2003;**37**(10):560-574

[46] Morais JF, Freitas MR, Freitas KM, Janson G, Castello Branco N. Postretention stability after orthodontic closure of maxillary interincisor diastemas. Journal of Applied Oral Science. 2014;**22**(5):409-415

[47] Hunt NP. Hypodontia—Problems of permanent space closure. British Journal of Orthodontics. 1985;**12**(3):149-152

[48] Springate SD, Sandler PJ. Micro-magnetic retainers: An attractive solution to fixed retention. British Journal of Orthodontics. 1991;**18**(2):139-141

5

The Role of Cytokines in Orthodontic Tooth Movement

Amila Vujacic, Jasna Pavlovic and

Aleksandra Konic-Ristic

Abstract

One of the most important breakthroughs in the understanding of biological features of bones is the explanation of the role of cytokine in reshaping of the bone (remodeling) including the alveolar tooth bone exposed to the effect of the mechanical force during the orthodontic treatment. Since remodeling of the bone initiated by orthodontic forces is connected during its early stage with the inflammation of the surrounding tissue, the assumption was presented about the role of the pro-inflammation cytokine in the process of remodeling of the bone, primarily *IL-1β, IL-6,* and *TNF*. These cytokines are mediators in the reactions of the acute stage of inflammation, as well as in the processes of metabolism, stimulation of resorption, and inhibition of bone creation. In this chapter, we aimed to review the existing knowledge about the roles and dynamics of the change in these three cytokines simultaneously during the early stage of the orthodontic tooth movement.

Keywords: orthodontic tooth movement, reshaping of bones, cytokines

1. Introduction

When more than 100 years ago the world knew about the theory about the regulation of the tooth movement, cytokines were unknown to science [1]. The first experimental evidence that supported the assumption about cytokines being the potential regulators of the reshaping process (remodeling) of bones during the orthodontic treatment was obtained approximately 20 years ago [2]. Since then, until today, the efforts of researchers last in order to clarify molecular events with cytokines as mediators, which follow the orthodontic tooth movement.

The role of cytokines in the orthodontic tooth movement is considered in the context of inflammation, which occurs at the very beginning of this process as a reaction to the mechanical pressure and represents necessary precondition for the realization of all its subsequent levels. In the conjunction of mechanical and biological mechanisms, which move the teeth during the orthodontic treatment, cytokines are given great importance for their feature of transmission of biochemical signals among numerous cells of various kinds reacting to orthodontic forces. Binding themselves to specific receptors at membranes of these cells, cytokines cause in them the biochemical changes responsible for the signal transmission to corresponding genes in these cells and, consequently, to the change of gene expression in them. This orthodontic tooth movement causes the features of unusually complex processes, whose different degrees—each individually and all together—are regulated by the network of positive and negative feedbacks, in which cytokine molecules act as mutual activators or inhibitors [3].

2. Orthodontic tooth movement and force effect

Orthodontic tooth movement is a biomechanical process initiated by the effect of mechanical forces, which overpower the bio-elasticity of the support tissue [4].

The process of orthodontic movement of teeth is based on the transformation (remodeling) of periodontal tissues and is initiated by external forces and differs from the processes that occur during normal jaw function (dentition, chewing) [5]. On the basis of remodeling of periodontium, there are mechanisms, which transform the physical effort into various cell responses within the periodontal system, which primarily leads to the disturbance and then to the establishment of the periodontal homeostasis on a different basis [6]. These mechanisms provide the adaptation of the biological system of periodontium to the changed conditions emerged as a result of the effect of orthodontic forces.

Biomechanical mechanisms of the orthodontic tooth movement, because of their complexity, have been explained by various, but not mutually exclusive theories. Orthodontic dogma is considered to be the one according to which the movement of the tooth in the periodontal space occurs by the effect of two dominant forces: pressure force (compression) and tensile strength (tension) [7]. As a result of the pressure, there is resorption (suction), whereas as a result of tension to apposition (addition) of alveolar bone, the movement of the tooth occurs as a direct outcome of the reshaping of the tissue around the tooth root caused by forces. On basis of this, processes are vascular, and consequently, cellular changes of the dental tissue are caused by chemical mediators, which are created and released under the influence of orthodontic forces. Even though, in the context of this, we must not neglect the theory, which emphasizes bending of the bones as the basis of the orthodontic tooth movement [8], as well as the theory of bioelectrical signals, which emphasizes the importance of electric potentials, which are created in the tissue as a response to the application of the mechanical force [9].

Orthodontic forces lead to the change of the structural features of dental tissues at the level of cells, molecules, and genes. Mutual activities of tooth cells, periodontal ligament, bone, and bioactive substances (cytokine, chemokine, hormone, growth factor, enzymes, neuropeptides, and ligands) are necessary because they provide that during these changes, the tooth and periodontal ligament remain clinically intact and surrounding bone is reorganized. The final outcome of these activities (the speed of orthodontic movement of teeth) may be defined as a phenotypic expression of numerous gene-controlled mechanisms, which connects the orthodontic tooth movement with hereditary basis, i.e., hereditary variations of factors which participate in this process [10].

3. Orthodontic tooth movement and biological mechanisms of reshaping of the mechanic-sensitive dental tissue

The cells of alveolar bones and periodontal ligament, gingiva, and tooth pulp react to the effect of orthodontic forces after the remodeling of extracellular matrix (ECM), which surrounds them [11]. Dental and periodontal cell responses to the applied mechanical force comprise interactions of intracellular and extracellular structural elements and mutual influences of the effects of various biochemical structures. The nature of changes in the process of reshaping is determined by the combinatory of interactions, which is different at different levels of the tooth movement [12]. The scheme no. 1 presents the main events in dental tissues, which follow orthodontic movement of the tooth.

4. Orthodontic tooth movement and the change in the structure of cytoskeleton

The function of all cells in mechanic-sensitive dental tissues is closely related to the ECM, which surrounds them and makes the corresponding microenvironment for cell activities, which emerge after the application of orthodontic force. The orthodontic treatment leads primarily to ECM periodontium deflection, which results in the changes of cytoskeleton structure of cells anchored in ECM. ECM is multicomponent tissue, which enables the transmission of mechanical signals to the corresponding cells and thus the occurrence of changes in the structure and function of a certain tissue [11]. The structural components of ECM (collagen, fibronectin, laminin, elastin, proteoglycans, hyaluronic acid, etc.) bind with the adhesive receptors at cells called integrins, via which the mechanical stimuli are transmitted into the cell causing the changes of cytoskeleton structures. The application of mechanical force outside disturbs the integrin receptors at fiber areas of periodontal ligament and gingiva and bone cells (osteoblast, osteoclast, osteocytes), and their adaptive response may increase or decrease the creation of integral elements of ECM in them and thus influence the change of the mass and morphological appearance of the bone [13].

5. Orthodontic tooth movement and reorganization of blood vessels

Blood vessels in periodontal ligament actively participate in the remodeling of dental tissues, which is related to the orthodontic tooth movement. Under the influence of mechanical forces, the reshaping of existing and creation of new blood vessels at periodontal ligament occur. These processes occur via numerous signal paths, which are activated after the deflection of ECM, which surrounds the cells of endothelia of blood vessels. They are mostly established via integrin of endothelial cells and ECM structures, which surround the blood vessels [14] and lead to the organization of endothelial cells unto multicellular pre-capillary network [11]. The response of blood vessels of periodontal ligament to the effect of mechanical forces is expressed by increased permeability, which, on its side, increases the fluid outpouring from capillary into the interstitial space [15]. These blood vessels play an essentially important role in aseptic inflammatory reaction caused by mechanical forces, acting as a source of inflammation mediators (cytokine and neurotransmitters), which mutually react with endothelial cells of periodontal capillary network encouraging them to bind circulating leukocytes and influence their relocation into periodontal ECM.

6. Orthodontic movement of teeth and inflammation

The mechanical stimulus stemming from the orthodontic forces causes aseptic inflammatory reaction within periodontal tissues, which initiates biological processes, which are connected to the reshaping of the bone [16]. Even though in normal conditions the movement of teeth is a sterile process, the early stage of orthodontic tooth movement is observed as a type of tissue injury and it is accompanied by the acute inflammatory response.

Generally speaking, the acute inflammation is an initial stage of defense reaction of the mechanism to the tissue injury (mechanical, physical, chemical, nutritive, biological). It occurs fast and does not last long and it emerges as the result of numerous, complex, and mutually related processes via which certain proteins and cells are transmitted from blood to the damaged tissue and whose final result is the recovery of the tissue. The acute phase of the inflammation is characterized by vascular changes (vasodilatation and increased permeability of blood vessels) and consequently, plasma leakage (exudation) and relocation of leukocytes (extravasation) from blood into the injured tissue.

Immediately upon the application of orthodontic force, the disturbance of the microcirculation of periodontal ligament occurs, which results in the ischemia of local tissue, periodontal vasodilatation, and migration of leukocytes via capillaries of periodontal ligament. The changes are temporary and, by the rule, do not have pathological effects.

Even though inflammatory changes occurred during the orthodontic tooth movement are mostly the consequence of reactive processes in the support tissue, mechanical stimuli may be transmitted also to the tooth pulp and may initiate the inflammatory response within this dental tissue [17].

6.1. Orthodontic movement of teeth and inflammation mediators

Inflammatory response in orthodontic tooth movement is followed by the increased creation of inflammatory mediators (cytokines, prostaglandins, leukotrienes), enzymes (matrix metalloproteinase, lactate-dehydrogenase, alkaline phosphatase, aspartate-aminotransferase), growth factor (epidermal growth factor—EGF), and neuropeptides (P-SP substance, calcitonin gene-related peptide—CGRP), which indicates the participation and mutual communication of cells of immune, endocrine, and nervous system in the regulation of the bone remodeling [16, 18–22].

The primary role in the initiation of a series of biochemical processes that stimulate or inhibit cellular activities during the inflammatory changes, initiated by the effect of orthodontic

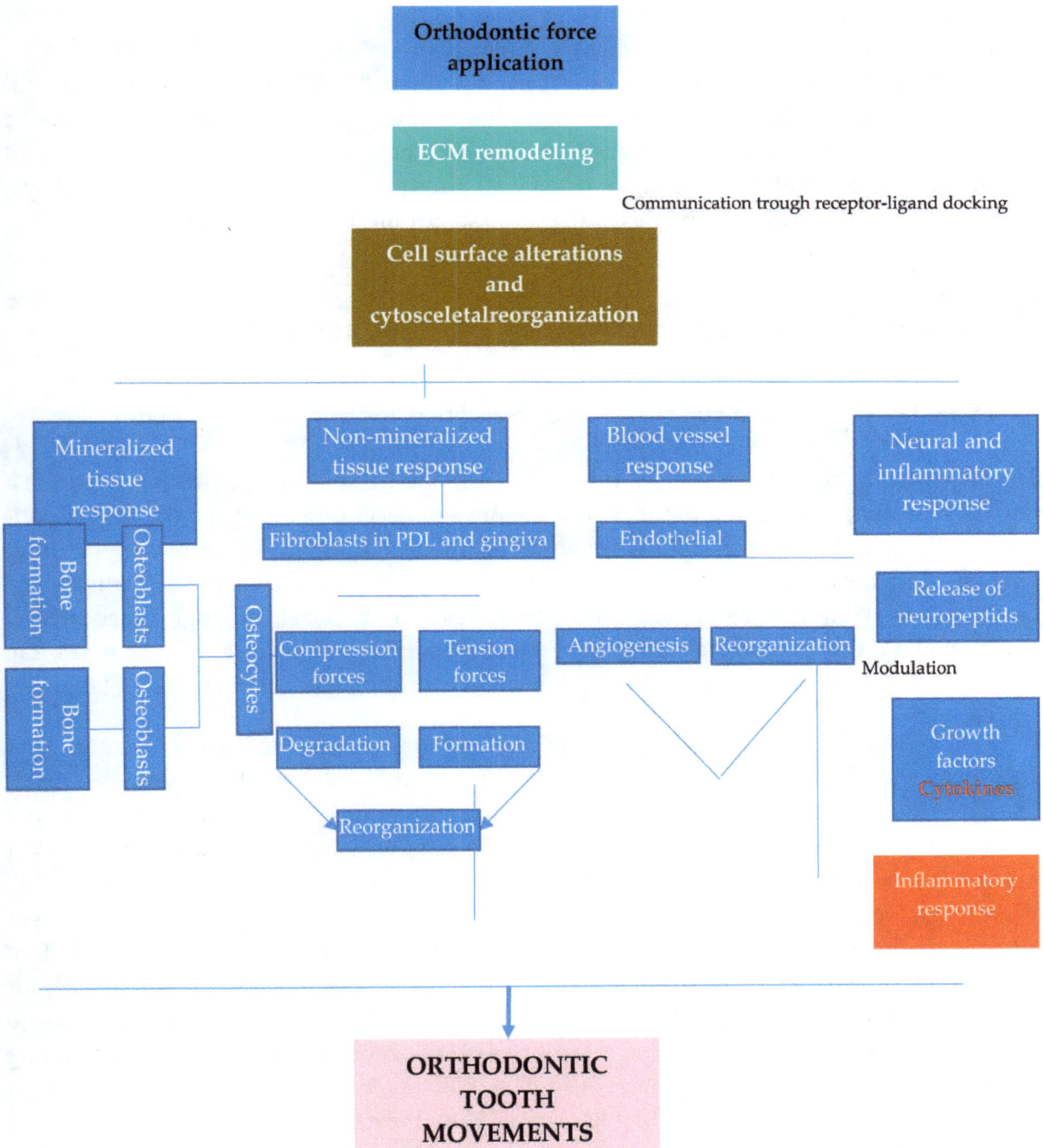

Figure 1. The sequence of events in dental tissues during orthodontic tooth movement. ECM—extracellular matrix; PDL—periodontal ligament.

forces, is attributed to cytokines [6]. Cytokines are small protein molecules, which transmit signals among cells. They are excreted by various cells as a response to external stimuli, and most frequently, they have a local effect. The effect of cytokines may be autocrine (to the cell which excretes it), paracrine (to other, adjacent cells), and endocrine (to distant cells). Cytokines express their effects by binding themselves to specific receptors at the cell membrane, which are affected by cytokines causing the biochemical changes responsible for the transmission of the signal to the corresponding genes in these cells and, consequently, to the change of the gene expression in them.

During the orthodontic tooth movement, cytokines are created by the inflammatory cells, which after the mechanical stimulus came outside widened capillaries of periodontal ligament [6, 18]. As the main regulators of the bone remodeling process during the orthodontic treatment, three cytokines are mentioned: interleukin 1 beta (IL-1β), interleukin 6 (IL-6), and tumor necrosis factor alpha (TNF-α) [6, 18, 23]. All three cytokines cause many local and systemic changes, which are the features of the acute stage of inflammation (**Figure 1**).

7. Orthodontic tooth movement and *IL-1β, IL–6,* and *TNF-α* effects

7.1. *IL-1β, IL–6,* and *TNF-α* and remodeling (resorption and apposition) of bones

The effects of *IL-1β, IL–6,* and *TNF-α* during the orthodontic tooth movement are going in a few connected directions and occur within the physiological process of remodeling of periodontal tissue after the application of mechanical forces. Judging by their concentration in gingival fluid, the creation of all three interleukins is already increased at the beginning stage of this process (12th and 24th hour) when leukocytes and fibroblasts of gingiva, periodontal ligament and alveolar bone make them as mediators of inflammation due to forces [6, 18, 23]. The maximum level is reached on the third day after the application of these forces [23].

IL-1β, IL–6, and *TNF-α* are osteotropic cytokines. They are released at the inflammatory spot and directly or indirectly (via substances whose synthesis and excretion they influenced) react with bone cells initiating the process of bone resorption [16]. Generally, it is believed that the bone resorption caused by inflammation is caused by local stimulation of osteoclast initiated by the effects of cytokines released from the infiltrated inflammatory cells [24, 25]. The process occurs in a complex signal manner via receptors of *TNF–α* (*TNF–R1*) at osteoblasts [24]. This receptor is activated by nuclear transcription factor *NF-κB,* so it is therefore called receptor activator of *NF-κB* ligand (*RANKL*) [26]. *RANKL* binds itself for the receptor at mature osteoclasts called *RANK*. Binding itself for *RANK, RANKL* may activate mature osteoclast and their precursors in the direction of oclastogenesis. It is prevented from doing so by natural antagonist osteoprotegerin (OPG), soluble receptor bait for RANKL, which prevents its binding for *RANK,* acting as a natural inhibitor of maturation and activation of osteoclast [27, 28]. For *TNF–α* and IL-*1β*, it is shown that together or independently from one another, *IL-1β* via *IL-1RI* receptors at osteoblasts may regulate the balance between *RANKL* and *OPG* in microenvironment of bones and mesenchymal tissue along the bone [29], not only intensifying the expression of *RANKL* and contributing to the resorption of bones, but also that they may activate osteoclasts at RANKL independently [30]. There is evidence that *IL-1β* and *IL-6* released by osteoclasts themselves may cooperate with pro-inflammatory *IL-1β* and IL-6 in osteoclastogenesis [31].

The termination of the resorption of bones and initiation of its reformation comprises inhibition of the osteoclast function and stimulation of the activity of osteoblasts. The termination of resorption cycle includes the inhibition factors, which are created not only by surrounding cells but also by the osteoclasts themselves. They regulate negatively the activity of these cells causing their apoptosis and preventing their creation and simultaneously increasing the function of osteoblasts. This stage of normal bone remodeling is followed by lowering of the level of pro-inflammatory cytokines. The number of cells of inflammation, which are created by *IL-1β*, *IL–6*, and *TNF–α*, as well as the level of these cytokines in gingival fluid is decreased after 7–10 days since the beginning of the effect of mechanical forces [18, 23], which overlaps with the initial phase of reparation of periodontal tissue, which lasts for approximately 9 days [31]. During this stage, blood vessels are no longer excessively permeable [32]. In this stage the creation of transforming growth factor beta is intensified (TFG-β), insulin-like growth factor (IFG I and II), fibroblast growth factor (FGF), IL-10, etc. [33], which modulate the reactivity of osteoblasts and prevent the bone resorption [31]. Complicated interactions among these factors, with many of them still not being explained entirely, create the basis of the coordinated formation of a new bone at the resorption location.

7.2. *IL-1β*, *IL-6*, and *TNF-α* and orthodontic forces

Although the causal relationship of cytokine expression and orthodontic force is not entirely explained, it is believed that the direction and the nature of these forces affect the level of changes in the blood flow and thus the relationship of inflammatory mediators, which are expressed in periodontal tissues and gingival sulcus. The blood flow is decreased at the spot of compression (ligament compression) and increased at the spot of tension (ligament stretching); therefore, the response of the tissue at this location is greatly determined by the opposing forces that affect them. The inflammatory reaction occurs in both spots and the content of *IL-1β*, *IL–6*, and *TNF-α* is increased both in the zone of compression and in the zone of tension (in comparison with the control teeth), but the level of some of them in either of these zones is different [34, 35]. It is believed that these differences are the reflection of specificity of the process, which occurs at the location of effect of certain force during the orthodontic treatment [34]. Even though they are not completely harmonized, the data so far show that the level of pro-inflammatory cytokines in comparison with control teeth is generally higher in the compression zone than in the tension zone, which is connected to the role of these cytokines in the regulation of osteoclastogenesis mediated by RANKL (vide supra) and the process of bone resorption at the compression spot [34, 35]. Simultaneously, it is shown that the expression of anti-inflammatory cytokine *TGF-β* is greater at the tension spot than at the compression spot, which is attributed to its role in the process of inhibition of osteoclastogenesis and bone formation at the tension spot [35]. However, the balance between pro-inflammatory and anti-inflammatory mediators at the spots of compression and tension is still not studied enough.

The effects of cytokine in the response of the tissue to orthodontic forces are connected to the creation of nitrogen oxide (NO), which is known to be one of the important regulators of bone remodeling. For the creation of NO, the activity of two enzymes is necessary: inducible nitrogen-oxide synthesis (iNOS) and endothelial nitrogen-oxide synthesis (eNOS). The gene expression of these two enzymes is activated by pro-inflammatory (*IL-1β, TNF-α*) and anti-inflammatory (*IL-4, IL-10, TGF-β*) cytokines, which are created during the resorption and reparation of bones [36]. At the experimental model (rat), it was noticed that after the application of the orthodontic force iONS is the mediator in the bone resorption caused by the inflammation at the compression zone and eNOS in the bone creation at the tension zone [37].

Orthodontic forces express their effect to the dental pulp initiating the responses of fibroblast in it. Even though it is considered that the reactions of the pulp to the orthodontic treatment are very small, they still bring about changes in the blood flow and releasing of *IL-1β, IL-6,* and *TNF-α* from the pulp fibroblast, which results in its inflammation [17]. The process is specifically related to the pulp innervations and neurogenic mechanisms [38], and in the case of more expressed effect of mechanical forces may lead to the resorption of the tooth root [39].

7.3. *IL-1β, IL-6,* and *TNF-α* and "neurogenic inflammation"

The orthodontic tooth movement is accompanied by releasing neuropeptides from peripheral endings of sensor nerves, which permeate the dental pulp and periodontium, as well as from the inflammatory cells localized in the periodontal tissue. Released neuropeptides regulate the microcirculation of the pulp and mediate in inflammatory processes during remodeling of bones, characteristic for orthodontic tooth movement [19]. Such neural effect, which is generally called "neurogenic inflammation," is connected to the pain, which partially occurs during stretching and pressing of the tissue under the influence of mechanical forces and partially because of the interaction of numerous inflammatory mediators with local pain receptors [38, 40].

The main mediators of neutrogenic inflammation are neuropeptides, SP and CGRP, which are proven to have vasodilatation effect, increase vascular permeability and participate in the inflammatory processes related to the damage, and recovery of the tissue [41]. The increase of the level of these neuropeptides is recorded in gingival fluid immediately after the effect of orthodontic forces, which occurs simultaneously with the increase of the level of pro-inflammatory cytokines *IL-1β, IL-6, TNF-α* in this liquid [42]. Although the ratio of neuropeptides and cytokines included in the process of inflammation, which occurs during the orthodontic tooth movement, is still not entirely clear, the data show that SP and CGRP stimulate the excretion of *IL-1β, IL-6,* and *TNF-α* from fibroblast of human dental pulp, but they do not work synergistically [16, 42]. The neuropeptide SP is included in the resorption phase of the reshaping of the bone during the orthodontic tooth movement by stimulating the creation of RANKL in the cells of human dental pulp similar to fibroblasts [43]. The SP expression may be prevented by *TGF-β* [44], whose excretion overlaps with the initial stage of reparation of periodontal tissue.

The effects of neuropeptides to cytokines are not unidirectional [19, 38]. *IL-1β* and *TNF-α* secreted from inflammatory cells after the stimulation with SP lead to the creation of nerve growth factor (NFG), which then leads to the increased production of SP and CGRP, which establishes the mechanisms of positive feedback during the inflammatory response [41].

7.4. *IL-1β, IL-6,* and *TNF-α* and other inflammatory mediators in periodontium

Apart from mutual interactive effects in the processes of inflammatory responses and bone remodeling during the orthodontic tooth movement, *IL-1β, IL-6,* and *TNF-α* frequently have effects in the combination with various other bioactive structures included in these processes.

After the primary inflow to the inflammation location and the initiation of an early stage of periodontal remodeling, these cytokines start the second tide of cytokine regulation of this process by "introducing" other relevant cytokines. It is shown that an early but not initial phase of the orthodontic tooth movement is followed by the increase of the level of *IL-8* in gingival fluid [6, 45], which is known to regulate inflammatory responses in periodontium in combination with other cytokines [46]. *IL-1β, IL-6,* and *TNF-α* stimulate the creation of *IL-8* in monocytes, macrophages, epithelial cells, and fibroblasts of periodontium, so that the IL-8 mechanism of feedback could initiate the creation of *IL-1β, IL-6,* and *TNF-α* [6], when periodontal system moves from resorptive to formative stage of bone remodeling. With IL-8 during the orthodontic treatment, the level of IL-2 also increases and it is considered to be the indicator of inflammatory activities in periodontium [47].

The increased expression of pro-inflammatory cytokines in human periodontium, due to orthodontic forces, is followed by prominent increase in the level of prostaglandin E_2 (PGE_2). This prostaglandin, which is created in various cells of mammals as one of the intermediary products of metabolism and arachidonic acid, is the mediator in the sustaining of local homeostasis, modulating numerous physiological processes including the inflammation. During the resorptive phase of bone remodeling caused by mechanical stress and initiated by acute inflammatory response, PGE_2 is created in cells of periodontal ligament (mechanically deformed osteoblasts and gingival fibroblasts), stimulating the creation of osteoclasts, which intensifies the bone resorption [16]. In this process, *IL-1β* and *TNF-α* express synergistic effects to the creation of PGE_2 stimulating the fibroblasts to the synthesis of this prostaglandin. The increased level of PGE_2 in the reaction results in the decrease of the expression of pro-inflammatory cytokines [48] and, consequently, the inhibition of the inflammatory response and stimulation of the bone formation. This dual role of PGE_2 (resorption on the one hand and bone formation on the other) is interpreted by the possibility of prostaglandin directing in different manners the bone cells: for resorption those in bone marrow and for the bone formation those at their surface.

The inflammatory response, which occurs during the orthodontic tooth movement, is followed by the increase of β_2 expression, microglobulin (β_2-*MG*), glycoproteins, which together with the pro-inflammatory cytokines initiate the process of bone remodeling [18]. β_2-*MG* occurs in soluble form in different bodily fluids of organisms including the gingival fluid and also is in the composition of the main histocompatible locus of I class (MHC class I), which is expressed at the surface of various cells, mostly lymphocytes and monocytes. In the process of bone remodeling, after a mechanical stress, β_2-*MG* is included as a regulatory factor of the bone metabolism, with the function of a stimulator of the osteoclast activity in the resorption stage and the function of the increase of the binding for bone cells *IGF-I* in the stage of bone formation [49].

Apart from pro-inflammatory cytokines and other pro-inflammatory substances, during the orthodontic tooth movement to gingival fluid, various metabolites are released, too. For lactate-dehydrogenase (*LDH*) [21] and metalloproteinase 8 [20], it is shown that they increase their level or the activity simultaneously with pro-inflammatory cytokines, in approximately the same time, so it is considered that their existence reflects the increased periodontal remodeling caused by orthodontic forces primarily at early stages of this process. *LDH* is intracellular, cytoplasmic enzyme, which is released outside the cell under conditions of cellular necrosis or tissue degradation. It is believed that the increase of the *LDH* level at gingival fluid during the orthodontic tooth movement follows the process of bone resorption [21]; metalloproteinase 8 is the isoform of the enzyme of collagenase, which is released from periodontal fibroblasts due to the effects of mechanical forces. In the increased level in gingival fluid, it emerges during the initial stage of the orthodontic tooth movement, expressing the increased periodontal remodeling caused by these forces [20].

The damage of dental tissues caused by inflammation and its reparation are based on many elements and their coordination inside and outside cells. Even though there are differences between pathological inflammatory changes and those which accompany mechanically caused reshaping of tissues, the basic cellular responses to stimuli, regardless of their nature, express essentially the same properties [50]. Our researches of changes of individual integral parts of the immune system and ECM in normal and inflammatory gingiva [51–53] were the basis for the examination of the expression of IL-*1β*, *IL-6*, and *TNF-α* and their mutual relation in gingival fluid and tissue of gingiva of children and adults who underwent the orthodontic treatment. Analyzing the causes of gingival fluid and tissue of free gingiva of orthodontically treated teeth (experimental teeth) and their nontreated antagonists (control teeth) in four different moments in time ("zero" hour, 24th hour, 72nd hour, and 168th hour after the application of the separator), we have reached the knowledge about the dynamics of the change in the local cytokine network during the initial stage of orthodontic tooth movement and differences existing in the amplitude of these changes between children and adult examinees [54]. The results led us to assume that in the first moments of orthodontic treatment, the constitutive creation of pro-inflammatory cytokines is created and then it is overcome in the following time intervals by more expressive reaction of cells to the effects of mechanical force. The time coincidence of quantitative changes of *IL-1β*, *IL-6*, and *TNF-α* in gingival fluid and tissue expression of orthodontically treated teeth indicate that these three cytokines could be in specific interdependence during the early stage of the orthodontic tooth movement. Put into the context of the concept about the pharmacological modulation of the tooth movement, especially the aspect which leads the acceleration of the process of tooth movement in the connection with the local application of cytokine, the results could be very useful.

8. Conclusion

The early stage of the tooth movement is followed by the inflammatory response of the tissue to the effects of the mechanical force, which are conducted and regulated by pro-inflammatory cytokines *IL-1β, IL-6,* and *TNF-α*, acting as mutual activators and inhibitors.

Note

The execution of this chapter was financially supported by the Ministry for Science and Technological Development of the Republic of Serbia (project no. OI175061).

Author details

Amila Vujacic[1*], Jasna Pavlovic[2] and Aleksandra Konic-Ristic[3]

Address all correspondence to: amilavujacic@gmail.com

1 The Faculty of Medicine, The University of Pristina, Kosovska Mitrovica, Serbia

2 School of Medicine, University of Pristina, Kosovska Mitrovica, Serbia

3 School of Agriculture and Food Science, Dublin, Ireland

References

[1] Sandstedt C. Einige Bettrage zur Theorie der Zahnregulierung. Nordisk Tandläkare Tidskrift. 1904;**5**:236-256

[2] Davidovitch Z, Nicolay O, Ngan PW, Shanfeld JL. Neurotransmitters, cytokines and control of alveolar bone remodeling in orthodontics. Dental Clinics of North America. 1988;**32**:411-435

[3] Callard R, George AJT, Stark J. Cytokines, chaos, and complexity. Immunity. 1999;**11**: 507-513

[4] Storey E. The nature of tooth movement. American Journal of Orthodontics. 1973;**63**: 292-314

[5] Wise GE, King GJ. Mechanisms of tooth eruption and orthodontic tooth movement. Journal of Dental Research. 2008;**87**:414-434

[6] Ren Y, Vissink A. Cytokines in crevicular fluid and orthodontic tooth movement. European Journal of Oral Sciences. 2008;**116**:89-97

[7] Schwartz AM. Tissue changes incident to orthodontic tooth movement. International Journal of Orthodontics. 1932;**18**:331-352

[8] Grimm FM. Bone bending, a feature of orthodontic tooth movement. American Journal of Orthodontics. 1972;**62**:384-393

[9] Basset CAL, Becker RO. Generation of electric potentials by bone in response to mechanical stress. Science. 1962;**137**:1063-1065

[10] Iwasaki LR, Crouch LD, Nickel JC. Genetic factors and tooth movement. Seminars in Orthodontics. 2008;**14**:135-145

[11] Krishnan V, Davidovitch Z. On a path to unfolding the biological mechanisms of orthodontic tooth movement. Journal of Dental Research. 2009;**88**:597-608

[12] Massella RS, Meister M. Current concepts in the biology of orthodontic tooth movement. American Journal of Orthodontics and Dentofacial Orthopedics. 2006;**129**:458-468

[13] Chiquet M, Renedo AS, Huber F, Fluck M. How do fibroblasts translate mechanical signals into changes in extracellular matrix production? Matrix Biology. 2003;**22**:73-80

[14] Chien S. Role of shear stress direction in endothelial mechanotransduction. Molecular & Cellular Biomechanics. 2008;**5**:1-8

[15] Lew KK. Orthodontically induced microvascular injuries in the tension zone of the periodontal ligament. The Journal of Nihon University School of Dentistry. 1989;**31**:493-501

[16] Yamaguchi M, Kasal K. Inflammation in periodontal tissues in response to mechanical forces. Archivum Immunologiae et Therapiae Experimentalis. 2005;**53**:388-398

[17] Yamaguchi M, Kasai K. The effects of orthodontic mechanics on the dental pulp. Seminars in Orthodontics. 2007;**13**:272-280

[18] Uematsu S, Mogi M, Deguchi T. Interleukin (lL)-1β, tumor necrosis factor-α epidermal growth factor, and β2-microglobulin levels are elevated in gingival crevicular fluid during human orthodontic tooth movement. Journal of Dental Research. 1996;**75**:562-567

[19] Vandevska-Radunovic V. Neural modulation of inflammatory reactions in dental tissues incident to orthodontic tooth movement. A review of literature. European Journal of Orthodontics. 1999;**21**:231-247

[20] Apajalahti S, Sorsa T, Railavo S, Ingman T. The In vivo levels of matrix metalloproteinase-1 and -8 in gingival crevicular fluid during initial orthodontic tooth movement. Journal of Dental Research. 2003;**82**:1018-1022

[21] Perinetti G, Serra E, Paolantonio M, Brue C, Di Meo S, Filippi MR, et al. Lactate dehydrogenase activity in gingival crevicular fluid during orthodontic treatment: A controlled, short-term longitudinal study. Journal of Periodontology. 2005;**76**:411-417

[22] Yamaguchi M, Yoshii M, Kasai K. Relationship between substance P and interteukin-1β in gingival crevicular fluid during orthodontic tooth movement in adults. European Journal of Orthodontics. 2006;**28**:241-246

[23] Alhashimi N, Frithlof L, Brudvik P, Bakhiet M. Orthodontic tooth movement and de novo synthesis of pro-inflammatory cytokines. American Journal of Orthodontics and Dentofacial Orthopedics. 2001;**119**:307-312

[24] Azuma Y, Kaji K, Katogi R, Takeshita S, Kudo A. Tumor necrosis factor-α induces differentiation of and bone resorption by osteoclasts. Journal of Biological Chemistry. 2000;**275**:4858-4864

[25] Palmquist P, Lundberg P, Lundberg I, Hanstrom L, Lerner UH. 11-1β and TNF-a regulate IL-6-type cytokines in gingival fibroblasts. Journal of Dental Research. 2008;**87**:558-563

[26] Li H, Lin X. Positive and negative signaling components involved in TNF-a-induced NF-kB activation. Cytokine. 2008;**41**:1-8

[27] Lacey DL, Timms E, Tan HL, Kelley MJ, Dunstan CR, Burgess T, et al. Osteoprotegerin ligand is a cytokine that regulates osteoclast differentiation and activation. Cell. 1998; **93**:357-368

[28] Kong VY, Yoshida H, Sarosi I, Hong-Lin T, Timms E, Capparelli C, et al. OPRLG is a key regulator of osteoclastogenesis, lymphocyte development and lymph-node organogenesis. Nature. 1999;**397**:315-323

[29] Wei S, Kitaura H, Zhou P, Ross FP, Teitelbaum SL. IL-1 mediates TNF-induced osteodastogenesis. The Journal of Clinical Investigation. 2005;**115**:282-290

[30] Katagiri T, Takahashi N. Regulatory mechanisms of osteblast and osteoclast differentiation. Oral Diseases. 2002;**8**:147-159

[31] Hill PA, Orth M. Bone remodeling. British Journal of Orthodontics. 1998;**25**:101-107

[32] Meikle MC. The tissue, cellular, and molecular regulation of orthodontic tooth movement: 100 years after Cart Sandstedt. European Journal of Orthodontics. 2006;**28**:221-240

[33] Martin TJ, Ng K. Mechanisms by which cells of the osteoblast lineage control osteoclast formation and function. Journal of Cell Biology. 1994;**56**:357-366

[34] Dudic A, Kiliaridis S, Mombelli A, Glannopoulou C. Composition changes in gingival crevicular fluid during orthodontic tooth movement: Comparisons between tension and compression sides. European Journal of Oral Sciences. 2006;**114**:416-422

[35] Garlet TP, Coelho U, Silva JS, Garlet GP. Cytokine expression pattern in compression and tension sides of the periodontal ligament during orthodontic tooth movement in humans. European Journal of Oral Sciences. 2007;**115**:355-362

[36] van't Hof RJ, Armour KJ, Smith LM, Armour KE, Wei XQ, Liew FY, et al. Requirement of the inducible nitric oxide synthase pathway for IL-1-induced osteoclastic bone resorption. Proceedings of the National Academy of Sciences of the United States of America. 2000;**97**:7993-7998

[37] Tan SD, Xie R, Klein-Nulend J, van Rheden RE, Bronckers ALJJ, Kuijpers-Jagtman AM, et al. Orthodontic force stimulates eNOAS and iNos in rat osteocytes. Journal of Dental Research. 2009;**88**:255-260

[38] Lundi FT, Linden GJ. Neuropeptides and neurogenic mechanisms in oral and periodon tal inflammation. Critical Reviews in Oral Biology and Medicine. 2004;**15**:82-98

[39] Rezniak N, Wasserstein A. Orthodontically induced inflammatory root resorption. Part II: The clinical aspects. The Angle Orthodontist. 2002;**72**:180-184

[40] Giannopoulou C, Dudic A, Kiliaridis S. Pain discomfort and crevicular fluid changes induced by orthodontic elastic separators in children. The Journal of Pain. 2006;**7**:367-376

[41] Schaffer M, Beiter T, Dieter Becker H, Hunt TK. Neuropeptides. Mediators of inflammation and tissue repair? Archives of Surgery. 1998;**133**:1107-1116

[42] Yamaguchi M, Kojima T, Kanekava M, Aihara N, Nogimura A, Kasai K. Neuropeptides stimulate production of interteukin-1β, IL-6, and tumor necrosis factor-a in human dental pulp cells. Inflammation Research. 2004;**53**:199-204

[43] Kojima T, Yamaguchi M, Kasai K. Substance P stimulates release of RANKL via COX-2 expression in human dental pulp cells. Inflammation Research. 2006;**55**:78-84

[44] Blum A, Setiawan T, Hang L, Stoyanoff K, Weinstock JV. Interleukin-12 (lL-12) and IL-23 induction of supstance P synthesis in murine T cells and macrophages is subject to IL-10 and transforming growth factor β regulation. Infection and Immunity. 2008;**76**:3651-3656

[45] Tuncer BB, Ozmeric N, Tuncer C, Teoman I, Caklici B, Yucel A, et al. Levels of interleukin-8 during tooth movement. The Angle Orthodontist. 2005;**75**:631-636

[46] Maeda A, Soejima K, Bandow K, Kuroe K, Kakimoto K, Miyawaki S, et al. Force induced IL-8 from periodontal ligament cells requires IL-1β. Journal of Dental Research. 2007;**86**:629-634

[47] Başaran G, Ozer T, Kaya FA, Hamamci O. Interleukins 2, 6, and 8 levels in human gingival sulcus during orthodontic treatment. American Journal of Orthodontics and Dentofacial Orthopedics. 2006;**130**:7.e1-7.e6

[48] Lee K-J, Park Y-C, Yu H-S, Choi S-H, Yoo Y-J. Effects of continuous and interrupted orthodontic force on interleukin-1β and prostaglandin E2 production in gingival crevicular fluid. American Journal of Orthodontics and Dentofacial Orthopedics. 2004;**125**:168-177

[49] Centrella M, McCarthy TL, Canalis M. β2-Microglobulin enhances insulin-like growth factor I receptor levels and synthesis in bone cell cultures. The Journal of Biological Chemistry. 1989;**264**:18268-18271

[50] Todorović V, Marković D, Milošević-Jovčić N, Petakov M, Balint B, Čolić M, et al. Matične ćelije zubne pulpe i njihov potencijalni značaj u regenerativnoj medicini. Stomatološki Glasnik Srbije. 2008;**55**:170-179

[51] Stefanović G, Marković D, Ilić V, Brajović G, Petrović S, Milošević-Jovčić N. Hypogalactosylation of salivary and gingival fluid IgG in patients with advanced periodontitis. Journal of Periodontology. 2006;**77**:1887-1893

[52] Stefanović G, Ćirić D, Ilić V, Brajović G, Petrović S, Milošević-Jovčić N. Hipogalaktozilacija imunoglobulina G (IgG) gingivalne tečnosti i pljuvačke u parodontitisu. Stomatološki Glasnik Srbije. 2006;**53**:7-16

[53] Brajović G, Stefanović G, Ilić V, Petrović S, Stefanović N, Nikolić-Jakoba N, et al. Association of fibronectin with hypogalactosylated IgG, in gingival crevicular fluid in periodontitis. Journal of Periodontology. 2010;**81**:1472-1480

[54] Vujačić A. Ortodontsko pomeranje zuba i sinteza proinflamatornih citokina [doktorska disertacija]. Kosovska Mitrovica: Medicinski fakultet Univerziteta u Prištini; 2011

6

Advances in Orthodontic Tooth Movement: Gene Therapy and Molecular Biology Aspect

Phimon Atsawasuwan and Sajjad Shirazi

Abstract

Accelerated orthodontic tooth movement has been recently the topic of interest for orthodontic practitioners. Increased numbers of both clinical and research articles associated with the accelerated orthodontic treatment have been published in peer-reviewed journals in the last couple of years. Biochemical approaches such as administration of drugs, vitamins, and proteins and/or physical approaches such as surgery, vibration, and photobiomodulation have been widely reported and demonstrated the predicted outcome; however, the results are controversial. Very few reports addressed on genetic background of patients or utilization of molecular biological approach on the accelerated orthodontic treatment. In this chapter, we will discuss about biology of tooth movement and how the advances in gene therapy and molecular biology technology would shape the future of orthodontic treatment.

Keywords: gene therapy, molecular biology, orthodontic, accelerated tooth movement

1. Introduction

Orthodontic tooth movement is a biological process that requires the relay of mechanical loading to biological signals by periodontal ligament (PDL) and alveolar bone (AB) cells such as osteoblasts, osteocytes and osteoclasts. The mechanotransduction of signals involves dynamic cellular communication which allows for coordinated cellular response of alveolar bone remodeling and periodontal tissue homeostasis that occurs in response to orthodontic force. This complex process depends on adaptive tissue remodeling of periodontium for both anabolic and catabolic events. Compression and tension forces from orthodontic treatment create stress and strain to the PDL and AB cells and their surrounding extracellular matrices (ECM), which respond to the stress and strain from orthodontic forces by expressing and secreting biologic mediators and inflammatory cytokines, osteoclast differentiation factors and ECM proteins such as collagen I, III, V and their modifying enzymes and proteases. These biomolecules, in turn, initiate the activation of fibroblasts, osteoblasts, osteocytes and recruitment and differentiation of osteoclasts leading to anabolic activities on the tension side and increased osteoclastic activity and low bone density on the compression side of tooth movement. These cellular and molecular events are strictly controlled at transcriptional, posttranscriptional and translational levels and the interference of these events affects the rate of tooth movement. Therefore, understanding the mechanism of cellular and molecular events of tooth movement will allow us to apply the cutting edge knowledge to improve clinical orthodontic practice using gene therapy or molecular biology approaches.

2. Orthodontic tooth movement models

Several models have been proposed for mechanism of initiation of orthodontic tooth movement as below.

1. Pressure-tension model: it was derived from the observation of experiments from animal models, in which a force of a given direction was applied to a tooth to create the tension and compression areas in periodontal tissues [1–4]. The histological studies demonstrated that bone was deposited on the alveolar wall on the tension side of the tooth in the presence of both heavy and light forces, with newly formed bone spicules followed the orientation of the periodontal fiber bundles. On the compression side, with the light forces, alveolar bone was resorbed directly by numerous multinucleated osteoclasts in Howship's lacunae (frontal resorption). In contrast, the periodontal tissues were compressed with heavy forces, leading to capillary thrombosis, cell death and the production of localized cell-free areas (hyalinization). Hyalinization phenomenon was later supported by several investigators [5–7]. At the hyalinization sites, osteoclastic resorption of the adjacent alveolar wall did not take place directly, but was initiated from the neighboring marrow spaces referred as 'undermining resorption' [8].

2. Bone bending/piezoelectric current model: it was observed that the deformation that occurred when an external load was applied to a long bone produced electrical current in the surface curvature of the bone. Increased bone concavity was shown to be associated with electronegativity and bone formation; while increased bone convexity was associated with electropositivity and bone resorption [9]. This model has major flaws given the fact that piezoelectricity does not require the presence of living cells. Dead bone produces the same effects, which appear to be generated by shearing forces acting on the collagen fibers of the bone matrix. Therefore, the stress-generated electrical potentials could be a by-product of deformation. In addition, the magnitude of the current is small and may not be sufficient to induce cellular changes [8, 10].

3. Neurogenic inflammation model: it was based on the assumption that orthodontic tooth movement was the result of inflammatory processes triggered by peripheral nerve fibers referred as neurogenic inflammation. This inflammation is characterized by the release of neuropeptides such as calcitonin gene-related peptide (CGRP) and substance P upon the stimulation of

afferent nerve endings [11]. A report showed that the nerve ending released the neuropeptides after periodontal ligament had been strained by the force applied to the tooth [12].

4. Fluid flow shear stress model: it was based on the concept that osteocytes respond to mechanical forces. Locally strain derived from the displacement of fluid in bony canaliculi of osteocytes is very important [13]. When loading occurs, interstitial fluid squeezes through the thin layer of the non-mineralized matrix surrounding the cell bodies and cell processes, resulting in local strain at the cell membrane and activation of the affected osteocytes [14]. With regard to orthodontic force, the force on the side of the tooth receiving orthodontic pressure creates shear stress and activates responses on osteocytes [15]. The shear stress on the osteocytes induces increased secretion of biological mediators from the osteocytes leading to activation of osteoclasts [16, 17]. At the same time, on the tension side, the increased pulling force on the periodontal ligament is transferred to the bone. The resulting deformation drives the fluid flow shear stress on the network of osteocytes. This shear stress induces osteocyte activation, and osteocytes respond by secreting signaling molecules that contribute to osteoclast recruitment and differentiation.

In addition, it has been shown that compressive force induces bone matrix deformation and microcracks; and the accumulation of microscopic cracks in the bone matrix may induce additional damage to osteocytes in the microcrack region [18]. Microcracks are more prevalent on the pressure-side than on the tension-side of the tooth, and it has been hypothesized that microcracks were the first damage induced by the orthodontic force to induce osteocyte apoptosis and bone remodeling. Osteocyte apoptosis has been observed at the pressure side in an experimental tooth movement model in animal models, which may be associated with the subsequent bone resorption [19, 20]. Therefore, the microcracks may play a role in the initiation of bone resorption on the pressure side of the tooth under the compressive force of orthodontic loading [21].

3. Molecular mechanism of orthodontic tooth movement

Although there are several models proposed to explain the events of orthodontic tooth movement, no single model could directly and comprehensively explain this process. The evidence from histological and animal studies has shown that this complex biological process is initiated from the application of mechanical forces onto the orthodontic appliances, which converts into the biological signals to stimulate mechanosensitive cells. (**Figure 1**) [22] Literatures showed that orthodontic force application induced physiologic adaptation of alveolar bone with small magnitude of reversible injury to periodontium [23]. Significant evidence suggests that when mechanical loading forces are relayed from the orthodontic appliances to the PDL and bone tissues, the mechanoreceptor cells percept the loading forces as shear stress and strain [24] as the tooth shifts its position in the PDL space resulting in compression and tension areas in PDL and bone tissues [25].

The sequence of biological events after loading of orthodontic force occurs as (1) fluid flow changes and matrix strain (**Figure 2**); (2) strain on mechanoreceptor cells (**Figure 2**); (3) cell activation (**Figure 3**); and (4) tissue remodeling leading to tooth movement (**Figure 4**) [15].

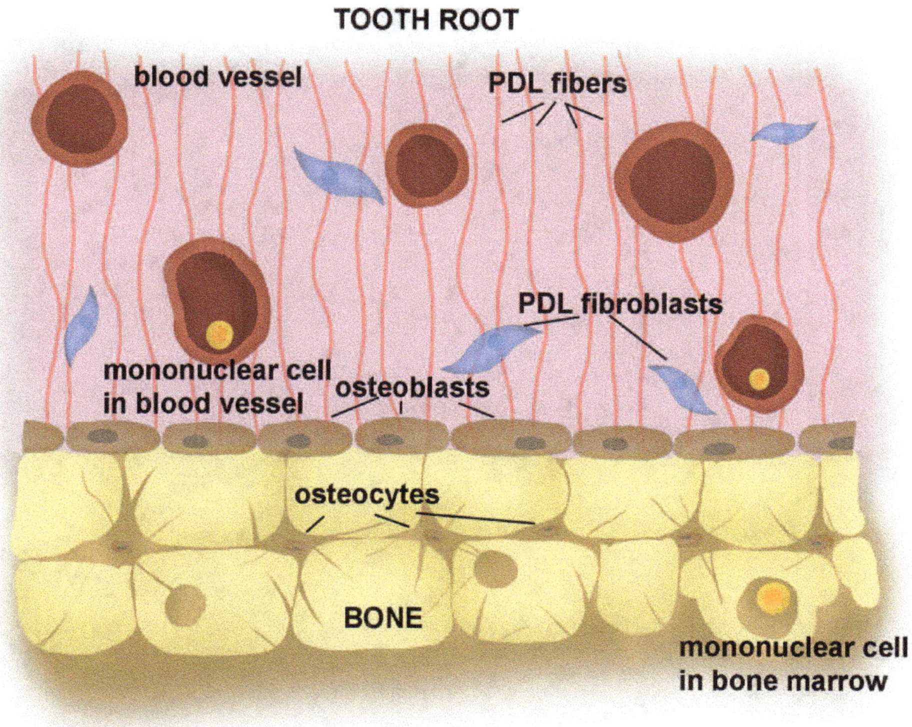

Figure 1. Illustration of cellular events of periodontal ligament and alveolar bone at non-loading state. Blood vessels and periodontal fibroblasts reside in between the periodontal ligament collagen fibers. Inactive osteoblasts line along the alveolar bone surface and quiescent osteocytes reside in their bony lacunae. Modified from Hatch [25].

The mechanoreceptor cells in periodontal tissue include osteocytes and bone lining osteoblasts in alveolar bone and fibroblasts in PDL. The final result as tissue remodeling occurs in both mineralized and non-mineralized ECM during the tooth movement [26]. Recent studies have indicated that osteocytes are capable of sensing strain in their bone lacunae following mechanical loading of the bone [21]. The mechanism of how osteocytes sense, transfer, and respond to mechanical strain remains unclear. Osteocyte processes have been shown to utilize integrins, gap junctions and ion channels to respond to mechanosensing external physical stimuli [27, 28]. Fluid flow-induced shear stress is the strain resulted from an immediate change in fluid flow in the lacunar-canalicular system leading to an increasing strain on the osteocytes. This shear stress can amplify the mechanical signals to the osteocytes [14, 29]. Several proteins such as integrins, connexin 43, osteopontin, and vitronectin, and several transcriptional factors such as c-Fos expression in the osteocytes are affected by loading forces [30–32]. In addition, the reduced number of primary cilia of osteocytes could affect their secretion of prostaglandins (PGs) and increased cyclooxygenase-2 (COX2) and RANKL/OPG ratio in osteocytes in response to fluid flow shear stress [33, 34]. Recent studies showed that osteocytes can induce both anabolic and catabolic bone signals in response to loading [35–37], yet the mechanism of how osteocytes switch from catabolic activity to anabolic activity is unclear. Under compression, osteocytes undergo apoptosis and are coupled with bone resorption [19, 38]. However, fluid flow shear stress may induce osteocytes to secrete anabolic bone proteins such as prostaglandin-E2 (PGE2) or nitric oxide (NO) [39, 40]. Several recent evidence demonstrated the significance of osteocytes during osteoclast differentiation and

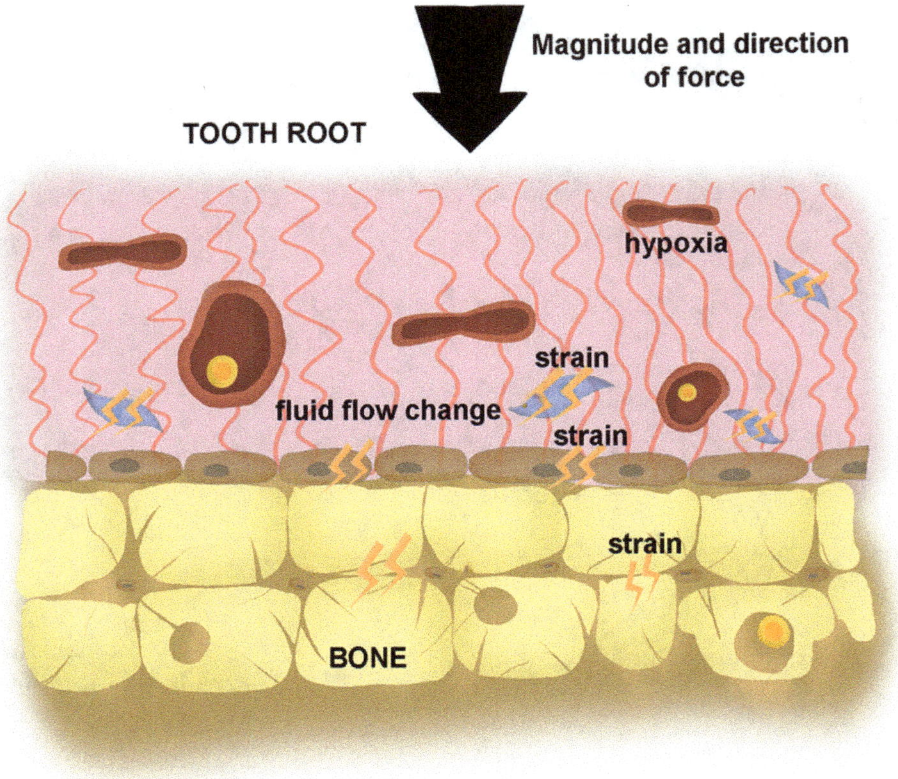

Figure 2. Initial cellular events in periodontal ligament after force loading during tooth movement. The blood vessels are squeezed then local hypoxia and fluid flow change are initiated from the loading force. The mechanical strain affects the periodontal fibroblasts and osteoblasts in the periodontal ligament space. The strain creates fluid flow shear stress and strain on the osteocytes in their bone lacunae. The mechanical strain induces secretion of inflammatory cytokines and biological signaling mediators including interleukins, prostaglandins, tumor necrosis factors, nitric oxide, growth factors, proteinases and cell differentiation factors. These mediators, in turn, activate the periodontal fibroblasts, osteoblasts and osteocytes. Modified from Hatch [25].

activation [41–43]. The osteocyte ablation *in vivo* caused a significant reduction in osteoclastogenesis and osteoclastic activity under loading forces, suggesting the important roles of osteocytes during orthodontic tooth movement [44]. Increased evidence supported the close association between osteocytes and osteoclasts during tooth movement. Experimental tooth movement in mice demonstrated increased expression of osteopontin [45], matrix extracellular phosphoglycoprotein (MEPE) [46], and receptor activator of nuclear factor-kB ligand (RANKL) [43, 47] in osteocytes. These proteins play important roles in osteoclastic activity and osteoclastogenesis because deficiency of these proteins results in significant reduction or absence of the osteoclasts and increased bone mass in the animals [43, 48]. Osteocyte apoptosis occurred abundantly on the compression side of tooth movement in 1 day after loading, and then an increased number of osteoclasts were observed until day 3, resulting increased tooth movement by day 10 [49]. It is speculated that apoptotic osteocytes may release signaling proteins such as RANKL and interleukin (IL), to osteoclast precursors, and initiate osteoclastogenesis. In contrast, when subjected to fluid flow sheer stress, osteocytes secrete NO and PGE2, which these proteins have potent, anabolic, and direct effects on osteoblasts [40, 50, 51]. PGE2 expression increased in loaded bone tissue [52]. NO secreted from osteocytes promotes osteoblast differentiation, and

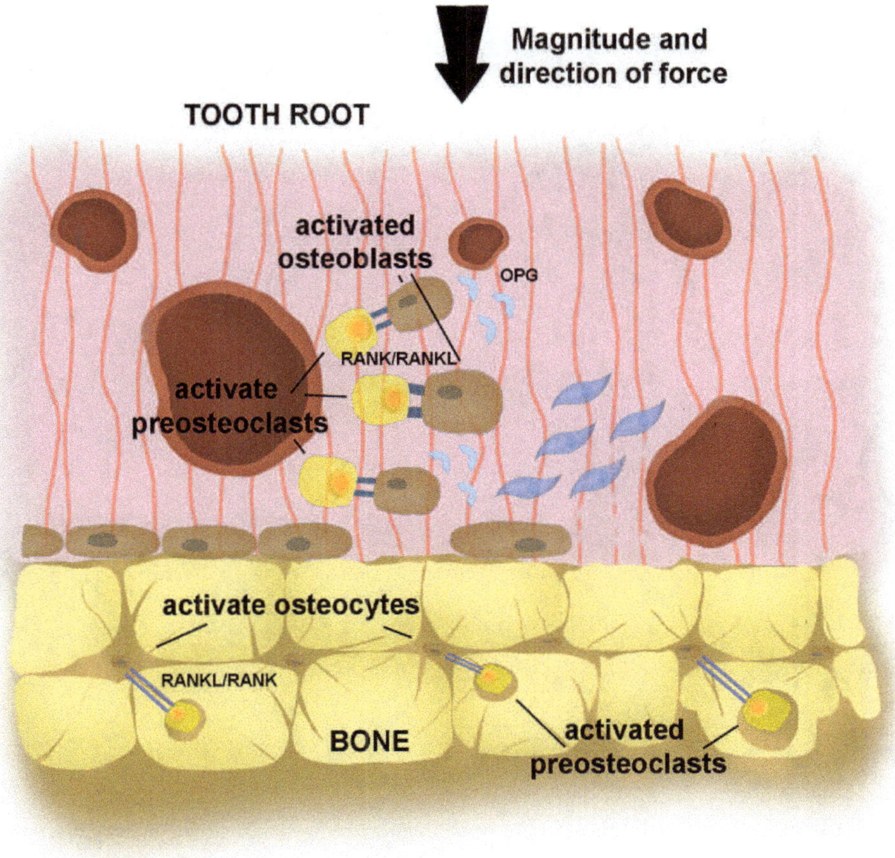

Figure 3. Intermediate cellular events in periodontal ligament during tooth movement. The blood vessels dilate due to the response to the released mediators and cytokines. The activated fibroblasts, osteoblasts and osteocytes are ready to secrete M-CSF and RANKL to activate preosteoclasts from blood and bone marrow. In addition, the activated osteoblasts release OPG to act as competitive decoys for RANKL. The PDL fibroblasts release MMPs to degrade collagen fibers in the periodontal ligaments. Modified from Hatch [25].

plays an important role in bone formation during loading [40, 53]. NO can influence bone mass and simultaneously inhibit osteoclast activity [54]. Increased NO production by osteocytes after mechanical stimulation by fluid flow modulates apoptosis-related gene expression suggesting that NO maintains osteocyte viability [55].

Beside osteocytes, preosteoblasts are also responsive to mechanical force. Mechanical force loading triggers several cell signaling pathways in osteoblasts such as calcium (Ca^{2+}), NO, IL1β and adenosine triphosphate (ATP) in a short period of time [24, 56, 57]. NO and IL are potent mediators secreted during orthodontic tooth movement [58, 59]. Preosteoblast differentiation can be induced on the tension side of tooth movement via integrin/focal adhesion kinase signaling and Ca^{2+} channels [60, 61]. Fluid shear stress can trigger Ca^{2+} signaling pathway and promotes ATP release, PGE2 secretion and proliferation of osteoblasts [24, 57]. While on the compression side, reduced blood flow in PDL and localized hypoxia occurs. The reduction in O_2 tension stabilizes hypoxia inducible factor-1 (HIF-1), a transcription factor that activates vascular endothelial growth factor (VEGF) and RANKL expression in PDL fibroblasts and osteoblasts leading to osteoclast differentiation and favoring bone resorption in areas of compression [62–64]. As mentioned above, inflammatory cascade is important for orthodontic

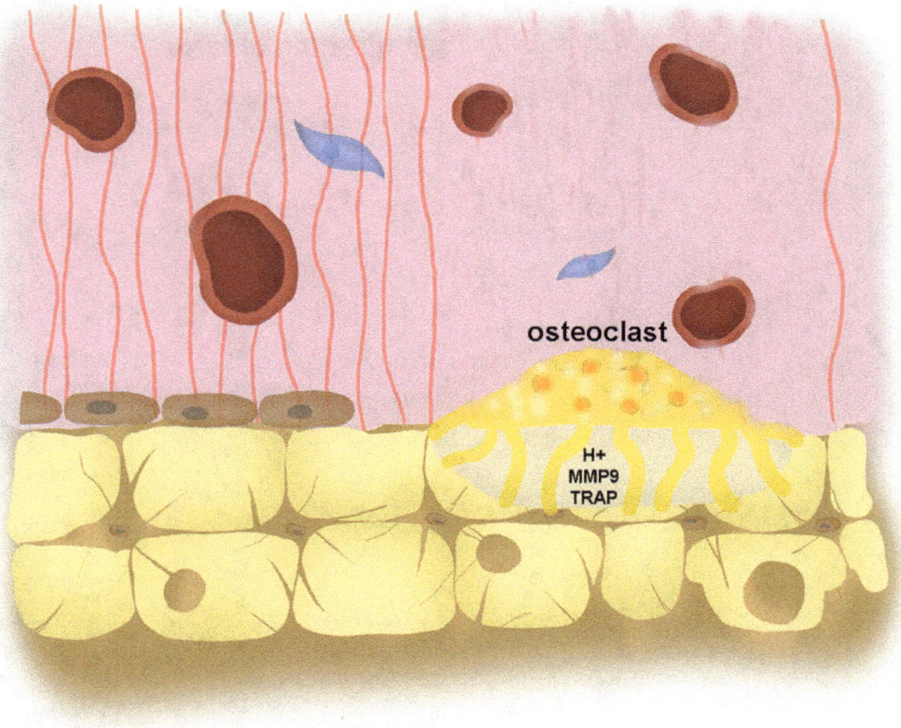

Figure 4. Late cellular events in periodontal ligament and alveolar bone front during tooth movement. The activated osteoclast is derived from the fusion of preosteoclasts, creates ruffle border to seal the bone surface area and releases MMP9, TRAP and acid to resorb bone matrix and minerals. Apoptotic osteocytes also release the biomolecules and mediators to activate osteoclast recruitment for bone resorption leading to tooth movement. Modified from Hatch [25].

tooth movement. During the process, inflammatory cytokine such as IL-1β, PGE2, tumor necrosis factor-alpha (TNF-α) and NO are secreted from preosteoblast in PDL and osteocytes in bone lacunae during the orthodontic tooth movement [59, 65, 66]. Compression is associated with elevated COX-2 which catalyzes production of PG, including PGE2, from arachidonic acid [67, 68]. Administration of PGE2 into alveolar bone of mice induces both osteoclasts and osteoblasts [26]. During orthodontic tooth movement, pain sensation occurs and, coincidentally, substance P and calcitonin gene related peptide (CGRP) are induced to be secreted during the tooth movement. These neuropeptides can enhance cellular secretion of inflammatory cytokine and in turn increase vasodilation and permeability of surrounding blood vessels [69–72]. Several evidence showed that the inhibition of inflammation hindered tooth movement [73, 74], while inflammation in the alveolar bone promoted tooth movement [75, 76].

Osteoclasts are the major key cells that play significant roles during tooth movement. Osteoclasts are multinucleated giant cells which are formed by the fusion of mononucleated osteoclast precursors derived from hematopoietic origin and function to resorb the alveolar bone during tooth movement. The osteoclast progenitor cells require macrophage colony stimulating factors (M-CSF) for their proliferation and survival. M-CSF is a secreted cytokine by osteoblasts and affects osteoclast progenitors. The RANK/RANKL/OPG system has been a crucial mechanism in osteoclastogenesis during bone resorption and tooth movement [77–79]. Receptor activator for nuclear factor κB (RANK) is a transmembrane protein and a member of tumor necrosis factor receptor family that is expressed on osteoclastic precursors, preosteoclasts and osteoclasts. Receptor activator for nuclear factor κB ligand (RANKL) is a transmembrane protein and is a member of the tumor necrosis factor superfamily that is expressed on preosteoblasts, osteoblasts and osteocytes [80]. RANK is the receptor for RANKL and the binding between both of them stimulates the differentiation of preosteoclasts into mature osteoclasts. Osteoprotegerin (OPG) is a soluble extracellular tumor necrosis receptor protein that is secreted by preosteoblasts and osteoblasts. OPG is a decoy receptor for RANKL in regulating bone metabolism and inhibiting osteoclastogenesis and bone resorption. RANKL/OPG ratio is an important determinant of bone mass and skeletal integrity and also an indicator for the osteoclast function [78, 79]. Increased evidence demonstrated the direct association of tooth movement and activities of osteoclasts. Accelerated osteoclast resorption in alveolar bone of OPG deficient mice was observed during tooth movement [81] while inhibition of RANKL or deletion of RANKL in mice resulted in suppression of tooth movement [47]. In addition, local administration of M-CSF resulted in modulation of rate of tooth movement in animals [82].

Overall, the mechanism of tooth movement is complex and need strictly coordinated regulation of PDL, osteoclasts, osteocytes and osteoblasts. It is very challenging clinically to apply optimal force onto the tooth to avoid hyalinization. Clinically, tooth movement in patients is a result of combination of undermining and frontal resorption [83]. Compression sides involve increased expression of PGE2, TNF-α and IL-1β. PGE2 promotes osteoblast and osteoclast differentiation and activity. Activated osteoblasts secrete RANKL and OPG to trigger osteoclast differentiation and activity. TNF-α and IL-1β promote osteoclast differentiation and activity. In addition, matrix metalloproteinases (MMPs) expression is increased as well as the expression of M-CSF [84]. Loading compressive force affects osteocytes to upregulate the expression of connexin 43 [85], endothelial nitric oxide synthase (iNOS) [50], osteopontin [45], SOST [86] and RANKL [47]. These molecules recruit osteoclast precursors and activate osteoclasts to resorb the alveolar bone on the compression side. While on the tension side, increased expression of transforming growth factor-β (TGF-β), a potent ECM growth factor, was detected [87]. Several anabolic molecules such as bone sialoprotein (BSP) [88], collagen I (ColI) [89], vascular endothelial growth factor (VEGF) [84, 90], tissue inhibitors of metalloproteinases (TIMPs) [91], insulin-like growth factor (IGF) and its related receptor [92], heat shock protein 27 (HSP 27) [93] and ATP [94] were increasingly expressed on tension side during tooth movement. IL-6 around the osteocytes under loading can promote its signaling toward osteoblast pathway [53]. The presence of TIMPs around tension side is speculated to control the activity of MMP and remodeling pattern in alveolar bone. The anabolic events such as increased osteoblast activity and decreased osteoclast activity occur on the tension side of tooth movement.

4. Studies on genetic manipulation of tooth movement

Administration of proteins that affect or activate osteoclasts could be a direct approach to modulate tooth movement though the dosage and side effects such as root resorption are factors of consideration. With modern advanced technology, the manufacturer can generate a large amount of human recombinant proteins for therapeutic purposes. However, the life span of these proteins once administered in human body is short and may not reach therapeutic level [95]. Gene therapy is a therapeutic approach that uses genes to treat or prevent diseases. Gene therapy is designed to introduce nucleotides into the cells to compensate for mutated genes or to restore the normal protein. If a mutation causes a crucial protein to be defective or missing, gene therapy may be able to introduce a normal copy of the gene to restore the function of the protein. After integration of the genes that encoded the target protein into the patient's genetic machinery, gene therapy can allow the body to produce the required protein constantly so the level of protein will be constantly high at therapeutic level [96]. The concept of gene therapy includes cloning of selected DNA/RNA fragments into a delivery system in order to administer into the host or patient. The delivery system could be viral vectors or non-viral vectors such as liposomes, peptides, polymer particles, gene gun and electric perforation [97]. The clinical application of gene therapy can be achieved with *in vivo* or *ex vivo* approaches. The *in vivo* gene therapy will include injection of vectors into the patient directly while the *ex vivo* approach includes the introduction of vector into the cells then the transfected cells are transplanted back into the patient [98–100].

Recently gene therapy has been approved to be implemented in medicine. The U.S. Food and Drug Administration (FDA) regulates all gene therapy products in the United States and oversees research in this area. In medicine, the FDA recently approved gene therapy for the treatment of some types of leukemia and inherited blindness [101]. Several experiments of gene therapy in dentistry involved orofacial pain, squamous cell carcinoma, tooth and bone regeneration, salivary gland disease and orthodontic treatment [102].

The gene therapy experiments in orthodontic treatment are still limited to cell cultures or animal experiments [103]. The purposes of previous gene therapy in orthodontic treatment were to investigate the possibility of acceleration of tooth movement or reduction of root resorption by modification of osteoclast differentiation factors such as RANKL or OPG [104–109]. The first attempt for gene therapy in orthodontic treatment aimed to transfer OPG gene into periodontal tissue to reduce osteoclast activity and inhibit tooth movement. The gene transfer approach using a hemagglutinating virus of Japan (HVJ) envelope vector carrying mouse OPG messenger RNA (mRNA) was performed in rats for 21 days of tooth movement. The vector solution was administered into rat's palatal gingiva by infiltration injection. The result showed that local OPG gene transfer reduced the number of osteoclasts and decreased tooth movement by 50% in rats in the experimental group compared to the ones in the control group. The effect of OPG gene transfer was local and did not affect bone mineral density of tibia of the animals [105]. The same group of investigators performed another experiment using the same system to transfer mouse RANKL mRNA to periodontal tissue to activate osteoclastogenesis and accelerate tooth movement in rats. The results showed that local RANKL gene transfer induced increased numbers of osteoclasts and accelerated tooth movement by approximately 150% in the rats in the experimental group compared to the control group. The effect of RANKL gene transfer was local and did not elicit any systemic effects. Interestingly, the number of osteoclasts was reduced time dependently after gene transfer [104]. Another group of investigators compared corticotomy with gene therapy using a hemagglutinating virus of Japan envelope vector containing mouse RANKL mRNA in rats for 32 days. The results showed increased level of RANKL protein 3 folds in the gene therapy group and 2 folds in the corticotomy group after 10 days; however, the level of RANKL protein was maintained in the gene therapy group but not in the corticotomy group. The number of osteoclasts in the RANKL gene therapy group was significantly higher at day 10 with or without tooth movement compared to the tooth movement only group. The tooth movement distance was 2 times more in the RANKL gene therapy group and 1.5 times in the corticotomy group; however, the rate of tooth movement slowed down in the corticotomy and controls groups but was constant in the RANKL gene therapy group. It was concluded that gene therapy was an alternative treatment for corticotomy to accelerate tooth movement and the efficacy of treatment was higher than corticotomy to accelerate tooth movement [106]. The OPG gene transfer experiment was performed by another group of investigators using the same viral envelope packaging and delivery system to investigate the inhibition of orthodontic relapse in rats. The first molars in the rats were moved mesially for 3 weeks then the springs were removed to generate orthodontic relapse in the rats. The rats received OPG gene therapy then were observed for 2 weeks. The results showed that relapse was significantly inhibited 2 times compared to the mock and control groups. The bone mineral density and bone volume fraction of alveolar bone were significantly increased in the gene therapy group compared to the mock and control groups. No difference of bone mineral density and bone volume fraction of tibia was found among groups. The investigators stated that local OPG gene therapy to periodontal tissues could inhibit relapse after orthodontic tooth movement via osteoclastogenesis inhibition [110]. The same group of investigators further investigated the effect of local OPG gene therapy on orthodontic root resorption with the same design of experiment. They utilized a microcomputed tomogram and histological analyses. The result showed no difference between root resorption at the beginning and the end of tooth movement in the OPG gene therapy group. However, the repair of root resorption in the gene therapy group was higher than other control groups [107]. Another study investigated the effect of local OPG gene therapy using mesenchymal stem cells as carriers for plasmid containing OPG mRNA. This cell mediated OPG gene transfer was generated by insertion of plasmid containing OPG mRNA into the mesenchymal stem cells and the cells were injected into the animals. The result showed that the cells containing OPG package grew in the animals' PDL and the number of osteoclasts, level of RANKL and bone resorption were reduced significantly after single injection. The level of OPG was highest in the gene therapy group [108].

Gene therapy is a promising treatment option for a number of diseases (including inherited disorders, some types of cancer, and certain viral infections). This approach is still in the developing process as an alternative approach to treat deformity or disease that conventional method could not achieved. Although many clinical trials have shown the efficacy of the treatment, the technique remains risky and is still under processes of investigation to make sure that it will be safe and do not elicit any systemic or hereditary effects for the patients.

5. Future of genetic manipulation of tooth movement

With the rise of advanced technology in biomedical engineering and medicine, gene therapy is no longer a science fiction. Several gene therapies have been approved to treat many conditions and deformities not only in the United States but worldwide [111]. In the past decade, gene targeting using endogenous microRNA (miRNA) has emerged as a powerful tool for targeted gene delivery. miRNAs are short, noncoding and highly conserved RNA sequences that tightly regulate the expression of genes by binding to their target sequence in the corresponding mRNAs [112, 113]. Majority of miRNA biogenesis involves transcription by RNA polymerase II to generate primary microRNA (pri-miRNA) followed by Drosha (RNase III enzyme) processing, which produces precursor miRNA (pre-miRNA). The pre-miRNA is transported to the cytoplasm via exportins/RanGTP complex. In the cytoplasm, the pre-miRNA is cleaved by another RNase III enzyme called Dicer to generate mature miRNA. The mature miRNA then forms a microRNA associated RNA-induced silencing complex (miRISC) with Argonaute proteins. The complex is steered to the target mRNA via base pairing with the target sequence of the miRNA. The degree of perfect complementarity at nucleotides 2–8 (binding sequence) in the 5′-end of the miRNA is essential for a successful action of the RISC complex. Depending on the extent of complementarity with the target sequence, gene expression is repressed either by inhibition of translation or by cleavage of the corresponding mRNA [114]. The process of gene therapy using endogenous miRNAs involves selection process of miRNA candidates, design of expression cassettes if constant expression is needed, selection of delivery carrier, and evaluation of system in cells, animal models and clinical trials [114]. Several miRNAs have been reported for their expression and roles in PDL and alveolar bones [115–118]. Under loading, several miRNAs in PDL and alveolar bone respond to the loading force and orientation of forces in different pattern of expression [119–121]. miRNA-21 has been shown to have critical roles in PDL, osteoblasts and osteoclasts [120, 122–127]. In addition, miRNA-21 deficient mouse demonstrated delayed tooth movement compared to the control mice via inhibition of osteoclastogenesis [127]. miRNA-29 was reported as a crucial miRNA for alveolar bone remodeling during tooth movement due to its expression under different orientation of loading forces and its expression profile in crevicular fluid during tooth movement in human [121, 128]. miRNA-29 expression in human PDL was up-regulated under compression but down-regulated under stretch force orientation [121] and its expression on crevicular fluid increased along the course of tooth movement [128]. Moreover, miRNA-29 sponge transgenic mice demonstrated delayed tooth movement due to the decreased numbers of osteoclasts [129]. These microRNAs could be a target candidate for gene therapy for orthodontic tooth movement. There are viral and nonviral delivery systems in clinical trials for gene therapy. Among viral vector system, lentiviral vector-based system has been developed and tested for its safety for more than 10 years. Non-integrating lentiviral vector have been investigated as a means of avoiding insertional mutagenesis. However, there is a disadvantage of this approach regarding the short-lived of the vectors in dividing cells [130]. Nonviral gene delivery systems (nVGDS) have great potential for therapeutic purposes and have several advantages over viral delivery including lower immunogenicity and toxicity, better cell specificity, better modifiability, and higher productivity. However, there is no ideal nVGDS; hence, there is widespread research to improve their properties [97]. The nVGDS system includes chemicals, peptides, liposomes, and polymers [97]. Exosomes are small (30–150 nm in diameter) extracellular vesicles that are formed in multivesicular bodies and are released from cells as the multivesicular bodies fuse with the plasma membrane. The exosomes were proposed to be used for delivery of miRNAs, protein and oligonucleotide complex [131], and were found to be cell secreted from osteoclasts [131] and in gingival crevicular fluid during the course of tooth movement [128].

Another genome editing system that has recently gained attention in research and clinical application is CRISPR/Cas9 system. The CRISPR/Cas9 system is based on CRISPR (clustered regularly interspaced short palindromic repeats) sequence and CRISPR associated (Cas) gene mechanism that are crucial for innate defense mechanism in bacteria and archaea enabling the organisms to respond to and eliminate invading genetic materials from their phages [132]. The CRISPR/Cas9 system consists of two key molecules that introduce a mutation into the DNA. First, Cas9 is an enzyme that acts as a pair of DNA scissor. It cuts the two strands of DNA at a specific location in the genome so the genome editing could be performed either addition or removal. The other molecule is guide RNA (gRNA) which consists of a small piece of predesigned RNA sequence (~20 bases long) located within a long RNA scaffold. The long RNA scaffold binds to DNA and the gRNA sequence guides Cas9 to edit the specific part of genome. gRNA sequence is designed to be complementary to the target DNA sequence in the target gene in the genome. gRNA sequence consists of short palindromic repeats and the sequences that complement with the target genes. The target sequences should be present close to protospacer adjacent motif (PAM) sequence which increases the specificity of Cas9. After Cas9 nuclease enzyme site specifically cleaves double stranded DNA activating double-strand break repair machinery. If the DNA repair template is provided, the piece of DNA repair template will be inserted into the sequence of target genes [133, 134]. With this mechanism, the plasmid containing gRNA, Cas9 sequences, TracrRNA (transactivating CRISP RNA) and DNA repair template sequence can be introduced into cells or embryo of the animals by viral or nonviral delivery system [135]. Until now, there is no CRISPR/Cas9 experiment involving orthodontic tooth movement, however, this technology has been implemented in recent mineralized tissue research [136–139]. Future directions of gene therapy include the enhancement of the lentiviral vector-based approaches, fine tuning of the conditioning regimen, and the design of safer vectors or nonviral vector delivery system. In orthodontic field, the gene therapy approach will need several fundamental cell culture and animal experiments to demonstrate the safety and efficacy of the treatment concept. Clinical trials are required as the next step to ascertain the clinicians and patients for efficacy of the treatments.

Acknowledgements

We would like to acknowledge Ms. Pornpasdchanok Asawasuwan for all artworks in the manuscript. This manuscript was supported by ROAAP fund, the University of Illinois at Chicago, Brodie Craniofacial Endowment fund, and the National Institute of Dental and Craniofacial Research (DE024531).

Author details

Phimon Atsawasuwan[1]* and Sajjad Shirazi[2,3]

*Address all correspondence to: patsawas@uic.edu

1 Department of Orthodontics, University of Illinois at Chicago, Chicago, Illinois, United States

2 Department of Oral Biology, University of Illinois at Chicago, Chicago, Illinois, United States

3 Dental and Periodontal Research Center, Tabriz University of Medical Sciences, Iran

References

[1] Sandstedt C. Einige Beitrage zur Theorie der Zahnregulierung. Nordisk Tandlakare Tidskrift. 1904;**5**:236-256

[2] Sandstedt C. Einige Beitrage zur Theorie der Zahjnregulioerung. Nordisk Tandlakare Tidskrift. 1905;**6**:141-168

[3] Schwarz AM. Tissue changes incidental to orthodontic tooth movement. International Journal of Orthodontia, Oral Surgery and Radio. 1932;**18**:331-352

[4] Oppenheim A. Biologic orthodontic theory and reality: A theoretical and practical treatise. The Angle Orthodontist. 1935;**5**:159-211

[5] Reitan K. Clinical and histologic observations on tooth movement during and after orthodontic treatment. American Journal of Orthodontics. 1967;**53**(10):721-745

[6] Rygh P. Ultrastructural cellular reactions in pressure zones of rat molar periodontium incident to orthodontic tooth movement. Acta Odontologica Scandinavica. 1972;**30**(5): 575-593

[7] Rygh P. Ultrastructural vascular changes in pressure zones of rat molar periodontium incident to orthodontic movement. Scandinavian Journal of Dental Research. 1972;**80**(4): 307-321

[8] Parinetti G, Contardo L, Franchi L, Bacceti T. The biology of orthodontic tooth movement and the impact of anti-inflammatory drugs. In: McNamara JA, Hatch N, Kapila SD, editors. Effective and Efficient Orthodontic Tooth Movement. Vol. 48. Ann Arbor, Michigan: The University of Michigan; 2011. pp. 117-140

[9] Bassett CA, Becker RO. Generation of electric potentials by bone in response to mechanical stress. Science. 1962;**137**(3535):1063-1064

[10] McDonald F. Electrical effects at the bone surface. European Journal of Orthodontics. 1993;**15**(3):175-183

[11] Brain SD. Sensory neuropeptides: Their role in inflammation and wound healing. Immunopharmacology. 1997;**37**(2–3):133-152

[12] Kvinnsland I, Kvinnsland S. Changes in CGRP-immunoreactive nerve fibres during experimental tooth movement in rats. European Journal of Orthodontics. 1990;**12**(3):320-329

[13] Goulet GC, Cooper DM, Coombe D, Zernicke RF. Influence of cortical canal architecture on lacunocanalicular pore pressure and fluid flow. Computer Methods in Biomechanics and Biomedical Engineering. 2008;**11**(4):379-387

[14] Weinbaum S, Cowin SC, Zeng Y. A model for the excitation of osteocytes by mechanical loading-induced bone fluid shear stresses. Journal of Biomechanics. 1994;**27**(3):339-360

[15] Henneman S, Von den Hoff JW, Maltha JC. Mechanobiology of tooth movement. European Journal of Orthodontics. 2008;**30**(3):299-306

[16] Burger EH, Klein-Nulend J, Smit TH. Strain-derived canalicular fluid flow regulates osteoclast activity in a remodelling osteon—A proposal. Journal of Biomechanics. 2003;**36**(10): 1453-1459

[17] Tan SD, de Vries TJ, Kuijpers-Jagtman AM, Semeins CM, Everts V, Klein-Nulend J. Osteocytes subjected to fluid flow inhibit osteoclast formation and bone resorption. Bone. 2007; **41**(5):745-751

[18] Verna C, Dalstra M, Lee TC, Cattaneo PM, Melsen B. Microcracks in the alveolar bone following orthodontic tooth movement: A morphological and morphometric study. European Journal of Orthodontics. 2004;**26**(5):459-467

[19] Hamaya M, Mizoguchi I, Sakakura Y, Yajima T, Abiko Y. Cell death of osteocytes occurs in rat alveolar bone during experimental tooth movement. Calcified Tissue International. 2002;**70**(2):117-126

[20] Meikle MC. The tissue, cellular, and molecular regulation of orthodontic tooth movement: 100 years after Carl Sandstedt. European Journal of Orthodontics. 2006;**28**(3):221-240

[21] Murshid SA. The role of osteocytes during experimental orthodontic tooth movement: A review. Archives of Oral Biology. 2017;**73**:25-33

[22] King GJ, Keeling SD, Wronski TJ. Histomorphometric study of alveolar bone turnover in orthodontic tooth movement. Bone. 1991;**12**(6):401-409

[23] Wise GE, King GJ. Mechanisms of tooth eruption and orthodontic tooth movement. Journal of Dental Research. 2008;**87**(5):414-434

[24] Riddle RC, Donahue HJ. From streaming-potentials to shear stress: 25 years of bone cell mechanotransduction. Journal of Orthopaedic Research. 2009;**27**(2):143-149

[25] Hatch N. The biology of tooth movement: Current concept on and applications to clinical practice. In: McNamara JH, Hatch N, Kapila SD, editors. Effective and Efficient Orthodontic Tooth Movement. Vol. 48. Ann Arbor, Michigan: The University of Michigan; 2011. pp. 73-91

[26] Krishnan V, Davidovitch Z. On a path to unfolding the biological mechanisms of orthodontic tooth movement. Journal of Dental Research. 2009;**88**(7):597-608

[27] Wang Y, McNamara LM, Schaffler MB, Weinbaum S. Strain amplification and integrin based signaling in osteocytes. Journal of Musculoskeletal & Neuronal Interactions. 2008; **8**(4):332-334

[28] Komori T. Functions of the osteocyte network in the regulation of bone mass. Cell and Tissue Research. 2013;**352**(2):191-198

[29] Kamioka H, Kameo Y, Imai Y, Bakker AD, Bacabac RG, Yamada N, et al. Microscale fluid flow analysis in a human osteocyte canaliculus using a realistic high-resolution image-based three-dimensional model. Integrative Biology (Camb). 2012;**4**(10):1198-1206

[30] Gluhak-Heinrich J, Gu S, Pavlin D, Jiang JX. Mechanical loading stimulates expression of connexin 43 in alveolar bone cells in the tooth movement model. Cell Communication & Adhesion. 2006;**13**(1–2):115-125

[31] Miyauchi A, Gotoh M, Kamioka H, Notoya K, Sekiya H, Takagi Y, et al. AlphaVbeta3 integrin ligands enhance volume-sensitive calcium influx in mechanically stretched osteocytes. Journal of Bone and Mineral Metabolism. 2006;**24**(6):498-504

[32] Hoshi K, Kawaki H, Takahashi I, Takeshita N, Seiryu M, Murshid SA, et al. Compressive force-produced CCN2 induces osteocyte apoptosis through ERK1/2 pathway. Journal of Bone and Mineral Research. 2014;**29**(5):1244-1257

[33] You L, Temiyasathit S, Lee P, Kim CH, Tummala P, Yao W, et al. Osteocytes as mechanosensors in the inhibition of bone resorption due to mechanical loading. Bone. 2008;**42**(1):172-179

[34] Malone AM, Anderson CT, Tummala P, Kwon RY, Johnston TR, Stearns T, et al. Primary cilia mediate mechanosensing in bone cells by a calcium-independent mechanism. Proceedings of the National Academy of Sciences of the United States of America. 2007; **104**(33):13325-13330

[35] Jacobs CR, Temiyasathit S, Castillo AB. Osteocyte mechanobiology and pericellular mechanics. Annual Review of Biomedical Engineering. 2010;**12**:369-400

[36] Bonewald LF. Mechanosensation and transduction in osteocytes. Bonekey Osteovision. 2006;**3**(10):7-15

[37] Bonewald L. Osteocytes as multifunctional cells. Journal of Musculoskeletal & Neuronal Interactions. 2006;**6**(4):331-333

[38] Verborgt O, Gibson GJ, Schaffler MB. Loss of osteocyte integrity in association with microdamage and bone remodeling after fatigue in vivo. Journal of Bone and Mineral Research. 2000;**15**(1):60-67

[39] Bakker AD, Soejima K, Klein-Nulend J, Burger EH. The production of nitric oxide and prostaglandin E(2) by primary bone cells is shear stress dependent. Journal of Biomechanics. 2001;**34**(5):671-677

[40] Klein-Nulend J, Semeins CM, Ajubi NE, Nijweide PJ, Burger EH. Pulsating fluid flow increases nitric oxide (NO) synthesis by osteocytes but not periosteal fibroblasts—Correlation with prostaglandin upregulation. Biochemical and Biophysical Research Communications. 1995;**217**(2):640-648

[41] O'Brien CA, Nakashima T, Takayanagi H. Osteocyte control of osteoclastogenesis. Bone. 2013;**54**(2):258-263

[42] Xiong J, Onal M, Jilka RL, Weinstein RS, Manolagas SC, O'Brien CA. Matrix-embedded cells control osteoclast formation. Nature Medicine. 2011;**17**(10):1235-1241

[43] Nakashima T, Hayashi M, Fukunaga T, Kurata K, Oh-Hora M, Feng JQ, et al. Evidence for osteocyte regulation of bone homeostasis through RANKL expression. Nature Medicine. 2011;**17**(10):1231-1234

[44] Matsumoto T, Iimura T, Ogura K, Moriyama K, Yamaguchi A. The role of osteocytes in bone resorption during orthodontic tooth movement. Journal of Dental Research. 2013; **92**(4):340-345

[45] Terai K, Takano-Yamamoto T, Ohba Y, Hiura K, Sugimoto M, Sato M, et al. Role of osteopontin in bone remodeling caused by mechanical stress. Journal of Bone and Mineral Research. 1999;**14**(6):839-849

[46] Gluhak-Heinrich J, Pavlin D, Yang W, MacDougall M, Harris SE. MEPE expression in osteocytes during orthodontic tooth movement. Archives of Oral Biology. 2007;**52**(7):684-690

[47] Shoji-Matsunaga A, Ono T, Hayashi M, Takayanagi H, Moriyama K, Nakashima T. Osteocyte regulation of orthodontic force-mediated tooth movement via RANKL expression. Scientific Reports. 2017;**7**(1):8753

[48] Gowen LC, Petersen DN, Mansolf AL, Qi H, Stock JL, Tkalcevic GT, et al. Targeted disruption of the osteoblast/osteocyte factor 45 gene (OF45) results in increased bone formation and bone mass. The Journal of Biological Chemistry. 2003;**278**(3):1998-2007

[49] Sakai Y, Balam TA, Kuroda S, Tamamura N, Fukunaga T, Takigawa M, et al. CTGF and apoptosis in mouse osteocytes induced by tooth movement. Journal of Dental Research. 2009;**88**(4):345-350

[50] Tan SD, Xie R, Klein-Nulend J, van Rheden RE, Bronckers AL, Kuijpers-Jagtman AM, et al. Orthodontic force stimulates eNOS and iNOS in rat osteocytes. Journal of Dental Research. 2009;**88**(3):255-260

[51] Klein-Nulend J, Burger EH, Semeins CM, Raisz LG, Pilbeam CC. Pulsating fluid flow stimulates prostaglandin release and inducible prostaglandin G/H synthase mRNA expression in primary mouse bone cells. Journal of Bone and Mineral Research. 1997;**12**(1):45-51

[52] Thorsen K, Kristoffersson AO, Lerner UH, Lorentzon RP. In situ microdialysis in bone tissue. Stimulation of prostaglandin E2 release by weight-bearing mechanical loading. The Journal of Clinical Investigation. 1996;**98**(11):2446-2449

[53] Bakker AD, Kulkarni RN, Klein-Nulend J, Lems WF. IL-6 alters osteocyte signaling toward osteoblasts but not osteoclasts. Journal of Dental Research. 2014;**93**(4):394-399

[54] Yoo SK, Warita H, Soma K. Duration of orthodontic force affecting initial response of nitric oxide synthase in rat periodontal ligaments. Journal of Medical and Dental Sciences. 2004;**51**(1):83-88

[55] Tan SD, Kuijpers-Jagtman AM, Semeins CM, Bronckers AL, Maltha JC, Von den Hoff JW, et al. Fluid shear stress inhibits TNFalpha-induced osteocyte apoptosis. Journal of Dental Research. 2006;**85**(10):905-909

[56] Salter DM, Wallace WH, Robb JE, Caldwell H, Wright MO. Human bone cell hyperpolarization response to cyclical mechanical strain is mediated by an interleukin-1beta autocrine/paracrine loop. Journal of Bone and Mineral Research. 2000;**15**(9):1746-1755

[57] Genetos DC, Geist DJ, Liu D, Donahue HJ, Duncan RL. Fluid shear-induced ATP secretion mediates prostaglandin release in MC3T3-E1 osteoblasts. Journal of Bone and Mineral Research. 2005;**20**(1):41-49

[58] Hayashi K, Igarashi K, Miyoshi K, Shinoda H, Mitani H. Involvement of nitric oxide in orthodontic tooth movement in rats. American Journal of Orthodontics and Dentofacial Orthopedics. 2002;**122**(3):306-309

[59] Iwasaki LR, Chandler JR, Marx DB, Pandey JP, Nickel JC. IL-1 gene polymorphisms, secretion in gingival crevicular fluid, and speed of human orthodontic tooth movement. Orthodontics & Craniofacial Research. 2009;**12**(2):129-140

[60] Ward DF Jr, Salasznyk RM, Klees RF, Backiel J, Agius P, Bennett K, et al. Mechanical strain enhances extracellular matrix-induced gene focusing and promotes osteogenic differentiation of human mesenchymal stem cells through an extracellular-related kinase-dependent pathway. Stem Cells and Development. 2007;**16**(3):467-480

[61] Ward DF Jr, Williams WA, Schapiro NE, Weber GL, Christy SR, Salt M, et al. Focal adhesion kinase signaling controls cyclic tensile strain enhanced collagen I-induced osteogenic differentiation of human mesenchymal stem cells. Molecular & Cellular Biomechanics. 2007;**4**(4):177-188

[62] Park HJ, Baek KH, Lee HL, Kwon A, Hwang HR, Qadir AS, et al. Hypoxia inducible factor-1alpha directly induces the expression of receptor activator of nuclear factor-kappaB ligand in periodontal ligament fibroblasts. Molecules and Cells. 2011;**31**(6):573-578

[63] Dandajena TC, Ihnat MA, Disch B, Thorpe J, Currier GF. Hypoxia triggers a HIF-mediated differentiation of peripheral blood mononuclear cells into osteoclasts. Orthodontics & Craniofacial Research. 2012;**15**(1):1-9

[64] Li Y, Jacox LA, Little SH, Ko CC. Orthodontic tooth movement: The biology and clinical implications. The Kaohsiung Journal of Medical Sciences. 2018;**34**(4):207-214

[65] Grieve WG 3rd, Johnson GK, Moore RN, Reinhardt RA, LM DB, Prostaglandin E. (PGE) and interleukin-1 beta (IL-1 beta) levels in gingival crevicular fluid during human orthodontic tooth movement. American Journal of Orthodontics and Dentofacial Orthopedics. 1994;**105**(4):369-374

[66] Grant M, Wilson J, Rock P, Chapple I. Induction of cytokines, MMP9, TIMPs, RANKL and OPG during orthodontic tooth movement. European Journal of Orthodontics. 2013;**35**(5):644-651

[67] Chao CF, Shih C, Wang TM, Lo TH. Effects of prostaglandin E2 on alveolar bone resorption during orthodontic tooth movement. Acta Anatomica (Basel). 1988;**132**(4):304-309

[68] Sanuki R, Mitsui N, Suzuki N, Koyama Y, Yamaguchi A, Isokawa K, et al. Effect of compressive force on the production of prostaglandin E(2) and its receptors in osteoblastic Saos-2 cells. Connective Tissue Research. 2007;**48**(5):246-253

[69] Hall M, Masella R, Meister M. PDL neuron-associated neurotransmitters in orthodontic tooth movement: Identification and proposed mechanism of action. Today's FDA. 2001; **13**(2):24-25

[70] Yamaguchi M, Kojima T, Kanekawa M, Aihara N, Nogimura A, Kasai K. Neuropeptides stimulate production of interleukin-1 beta, interleukin-6, and tumor necrosis factor-alpha in human dental pulp cells. Inflammation Research. 2004;**53**(5):199-204

[71] Kyrkanides S, Huang H, Faber RD. Neurologic regulation and orthodontic tooth movement. Frontiers of Oral Biology. 2016;**18**:64-74

[72] Kobayashi M, Horinuki E. Neural mechanisms of nociception during orthodontic treatment. Journal of Oral Science. 2017;**59**(2):167-171

[73] Kirschneck C, Meier M, Bauer K, Proff P, Fanghanel J. Meloxicam medication reduces orthodontically induced dental root resorption and tooth movement velocity: A combined in vivo and in vitro study of dental-periodontal cells and tissue. Cell and Tissue Research. 2017;**368**(1):61-78

[74] Liu Y, Zhang T, Zhang C, Jin SS, Yang RL, Wang XD, et al. Aspirin blocks orthodontic relapse via inhibition of CD4(+) T lymphocytes. Journal of Dental Research. 2017;**96**(5):586-594

[75] Kavoli S, Mirzaie M, Feizi F, Rakhshan V, Arash V, Bijani A. Local injection of carrageenan accelerates orthodontic tooth movement: A preliminary experimental animal study. International Orthodontics. 2017;**15**(4):588-599

[76] Pu H, Hua Y. Hydrogen sulfide regulates bone remodeling and promotes orthodontic tooth movement. Molecular Medicine Reports. 2017;**16**(6):9415-9422

[77] Yamaguchi M. RANK/RANKL/OPG during orthodontic tooth movement. Orthodontics & Craniofacial Research. 2009;**12**(2):113-119

[78] Boyce BF, Xing L. The RANKL/RANK/OPG pathway. Current Osteoporosis Reports. 2007;**5**(3):98-104

[79] Boyce BF, Xing L. Biology of RANK, RANKL, and osteoprotegerin. Arthritis Research & Therapy. 2007;**9**(Suppl 1):S1

[80] Xiong J, Piemontese M, Onal M, Campbell J, Goellner JJ, Dusevich V, et al. Osteocytes, not osteoblasts or lining cells, are the main source of the RANKL required for osteoclast formation in remodeling bone. PLoS One. 2015;**10**(9):e0138189

[81] Oshiro T, Shiotani A, Shibasaki Y, Sasaki T. Osteoclast induction in periodontal tissue during experimental movement of incisors in osteoprotegerin-deficient mice. The Anatomical Record. 2002;**266**(4):218-225

[82] Brooks PJ, Heckler AF, Wei K, Gong SG. M-CSF accelerates orthodontic tooth movement by targeting preosteoclasts in mice. The Angle Orthodontist. 2011;**81**(2):277-283

[83] Proffit WR, Fields HW, Sarver DM, Ackerman JL. Comtemporary Orthodontics. 5th ed. St. Louis, MO: Mosby Elsevier; 2013

[84] Kaku M, Motokawa M, Tohma Y, Tsuka N, Koseki H, Sunagawa H, et al. VEGF and M-CSF levels in periodontal tissue during tooth movement. Biomedical Research. 2008;**29**(4):181-187

[85] Su M, Borke JL, Donahue HJ, Li Z, Warshawsky NM, Russell CM, et al. Expression of connexin 43 in rat mandibular bone and periodontal ligament (PDL) cells during experimental tooth movement. Journal of Dental Research. 1997;**76**(7):1357-1366

[86] Shu R, Bai D, Sheu T, He Y, Yang X, Xue C, et al. Sclerostin promotes bone remodeling in the process of tooth movement. PLoS One. 2017;**12**(1):e0167312

[87] Wang LL, Zhu H, Liang T. Changes of transforming growth factor beta 1 in rat periodontal tissue during orthodontic tooth movement. The Chinese Journal of Dental Research. 2000;**3**(1):19-22

[88] Olson C, Uribe F, Kalajzic Z, Utreja A, Nanda R, Rowe D, et al. Orthodontic tooth movement causes decreased promoter expression of collagen type 1, bone sialoprotein and alpha-smooth muscle actin in the periodontal ligament. Orthodontics & Craniofacial Research. 2012;**15**(1):52-61

[89] Domon S, Shimokawa H, Yamaguchi S, Soma K. Temporal and spatial mRNA expression of bone sialoprotein and type I collagen during rodent tooth movement. European Journal of Orthodontics. 2001;**23**(4):339-348

[90] Kohno S, Kaku M, Tsutsui K, Motokawa M, Ohtani J, Tenjo K, et al. Expression of vascular endothelial growth factor and the effects on bone remodeling during experimental tooth movement. Journal of Dental Research. 2003;**82**(3):177-182

[91] Takahashi I, Onodera K, Nishimura M, Mitnai H, Sasano Y, Mitani H. Expression of genes for gelatinases and tissue inhibitors of metalloproteinases in periodontal tissues during orthodontic tooth movement. Journal of Molecular Histology. 2006;**37**(8–9):333-342

[92] Kheralla Y, Gotz W, Kawarizadeh A, Rath-Deschner B, Jager A. IGF-I, IGF-IR and IRS1 expression as an early reaction of PDL cells to experimental tooth movement in the rat. Archives of Oral Biology. 2010;**55**(3):215-222

[93] Muraoka R, Nakano K, Kurihara S, Yamada K, Kawakami T. Immunohistochemical expression of heat shock proteins in the mouse periodontal tissues due to orthodontic mechanical stress. European Journal of Medical Research. 2010;**15**(11):475-482

[94] Kariya T, Tanabe N, Shionome C, Manaka S, Kawato T, Zhao N, et al. Tension force-induced ATP promotes osteogenesis through P2X7 receptor in osteoblasts. Journal of Cellular Biochemistry. 2015;**116**(1):12-21

[95] Makarov SS, Olsen JC, Johnston WN, Anderle SK, Brown RR, Baldwin AS Jr, et al. Suppression of experimental arthritis by gene transfer of interleukin 1 receptor

antagonist cDNA. Proceedings of the National Academy of Sciences of the United States of America. 1996;**93**(1):402-406

[96] Wirth T, Parker N, Yla-Herttuala S. History of gene therapy. Gene. 2013;**525**(2):162-169

[97] Wu P, Chen H, Jin R, Weng T, Ho JK, You C, et al. Non-viral gene delivery systems for tissue repair and regeneration. Journal of Translational Medicine. 2018;**16**(1):29

[98] Karthikeyan BV, Pradeep AR. Gene therapy in periodontics: A review and future implications. The Journal of Contemporary Dental Practice. 2006;**7**(3):83-91

[99] Prabhakar AR, Paul JM, Basappa N. Gene therapy and its implications in dentistry. International Journal of Clinical Pediatric Dentistry. 2011;**4**(2):85-92

[100] Grol MW, Lee BH. Gene therapy for repair and regeneration of bone and cartilage. Current Opinion in Pharmacology. 2018;**40**:59-66

[101] https://www.fda.gov/biologicsbloodvaccines/cellulargenetherapyproducts/approved products/default.html [Accessed: Jun 28, 2018]

[102] Siddique N, Raza H, Ahmed S, Khurshid Z, Zafar MS. Gene therapy: A paradigm shift in dentistry. Genes (Basel). 2016;**7**(11):5-12

[103] Abraham P, Maliekal TT. Single cell biology beyond the era of antibodies: Relevance, challenges, and promises in biomedical research. Cellular and Molecular Life Sciences. 2017;**74**(7):1177-1189

[104] Kanzaki H, Chiba M, Arai K, Takahashi I, Haruyama N, Nishimura M, et al. Local RANKL gene transfer to the periodontal tissue accelerates orthodontic tooth movement. Gene Therapy. 2006;**13**(8):678-685

[105] Kanzaki H, Chiba M, Takahashi I, Haruyama N, Nishimura M, Mitani H. Local OPG gene transfer to periodontal tissue inhibits orthodontic tooth movement. Journal of Dental Research. 2004;**83**(12):920-925

[106] Iglesias-Linares A, Moreno-Fernandez AM, Yanez-Vico R, Mendoza-Mendoza A, Gonzalez-Moles M, Solano-Reina E. The use of gene therapy vs. corticotomy surgery in accelerating orthodontic tooth movement. Orthodontics & Craniofacial Research. 2011; **14**(3):138-148

[107] Zhao N, Liu Y, Kanzaki H, Liang W, Ni J, Lin J. Effects of local osteoprotegerin gene transfection on orthodontic root resorption during retention: An in vivo micro-CT analysis. Orthodontics & Craniofacial Research. 2012;**15**(1):10-20

[108] Amuk NG, Kurt G, Baran Y, Seyrantepe V, Yandim MK, Adan A, et al. Effects of cell-mediated osteoprotegerin gene transfer and mesenchymal stem cell applications on orthodontically induced root resorption of rat teeth. European Journal of Orthodontics. 2017;**39**(3): 235-242

[109] Andrade I Jr, Sousa AB, da Silva GG. New therapeutic modalities to modulate orthodontic tooth movement. Dental Press Journal of Orthodontics. 2014;**19**(6):123-133

[110] Zhao N, Lin J, Kanzaki H, Ni J, Chen Z, Liang W, et al. Local osteoprotegerin gene transfer inhibits relapse of orthodontic tooth movement. American Journal of Orthodontics and Dentofacial Orthopedics. 2012;**141**(1):30-40

[111] Doostparast Torshizi A, Wang K. Next-generation sequencing in drug development: Target identification and genetically stratified clinical trials. Drug Discovery Today. 2018. DOI: 10.1016/j.drudis.2018.05.015 in press

[112] Fabian MR, Sonenberg N. The mechanics of miRNA-mediated gene silencing: A look under the hood of miRISC. Nature Structural & Molecular Biology. 2012;**19**(6):586-593

[113] Bartel DP. MicroRNAs: Target recognition and regulatory functions. Cell. 2009;**136**(2): 215-233

[114] Dhungel B, Ramlogan-Steel CA, Steel JC. MicroRNA-regulated gene delivery systems for research and therapeutic purposes. Molecules. 2018;**23**(7):1-14

[115] Irwandi RA, Vacharaksa A. The role of microRNA in periodontal tissue: A review of the literature. Archives of Oral Biology. 2016;**72**:66-74

[116] Zhou X, Luan X, Chen Z, Francis M, Gopinathan G, Li W, et al. MicroRNA-138 inhibits periodontal progenitor differentiation under inflammatory conditions. Journal of Dental Research. 2016;**95**(2):230-237

[117] Luan X, Zhou X, Trombetta-eSilva J, Francis M, Gaharwar AK, Atsawasuwan P, et al. MicroRNAs and periodontal homeostasis. Journal of Dental Research. 2017;**96**(5):491-500

[118] Wang Y, Jia L, Zheng Y, Li W. Bone remodeling induced by mechanical forces is regulated by miRNAs. Bioscience Reports. 2018;**38**(4):1-12

[119] Yuan Y, Zhang L, Tong X, Zhang M, Zhao Y, Guo J, et al. Mechanical stress regulates bone metabolism through microRNAs. Journal of Cellular Physiology. 2017;**232**(6): 1239-1245

[120] Wei FL, Wang JH, Ding G, Yang SY, Li Y, Hu YJ, et al. Mechanical force-induced specific MicroRNA expression in human periodontal ligament stem cells. Cells, Tissues, Organs. 2014;**199**(5–6):353-363

[121] Chen Y, Mohammed A, Oubaidin M, Evans CA, Zhou X, Luan X, et al. Cyclic stretch and compression forces alter microRNA-29 expression of human periodontal ligament cells. Gene. 2015;**566**(1):13-17

[122] Li H, Yang F, Wang Z, Fu Q, Liang A. MicroRNA-21 promotes osteogenic differentiation by targeting small mothers against decapentaplegic 7. Molecular Medicine Reports. 2015; **12**(1):1561-1567

[123] Wei F, Liu D, Feng C, Zhang F, Yang S, Hu Y, et al. MicroRNA-21 mediates stretch-induced osteogenic differentiation in human periodontal ligament stem cells. Stem Cells and Development. 2015;**24**(3):312-319

[124] Wei F, Yang S, Guo Q, Zhang X, Ren D, Lv T, et al. MicroRNA-21 regulates osteogenic differentiation of periodontal ligament stem cells by targeting Smad5. Scientific Reports. 2017;**7**(1):16608

[125] Li C, Li C, Yue J, Huang X, Chen M, Gao J, et al. miR-21 and miR-101 regulate PLAP-1 expression in periodontal ligament cells. Molecular Medicine Reports. 2012;**5**(5):1340-1346

[126] Sugatani T, Vacher J, Hruska KA. A microRNA expression signature of osteoclastogenesis. Blood. 2011;**117**(13):3648-3657

[127] Chen N, Sui BD, Hu CH, Cao J, Zheng CX, Hou R, et al. microRNA-21 contributes to orthodontic tooth movement. Journal of Dental Research. 2016;**95**(12):1425-1433

[128] Atsawasuwan P, Lazari P, Chen Y, Zhou X, Viana G, Evans CA. Secretory microRNA-29 expression in gingival crevicular fluid during orthodontic tooth movement. PLoS One. 2018;**13**(3):e0194238

[129] Dong Y, Lu A, Patel P, Qian Y, Al-Qaysi A, Zhou X, Viana G, Nares S, Atsawasuwan P. Delayed tooth movement in miRNA-29 sponge transgenic mice. Journal of Dental Research. 2018;**97**(Spec Iss A):429

[130] Milone MC, O'Doherty U. Clinical use of lentiviral vectors. Leukemia. 2018;**32**(7):1529-1541

[131] Holliday LS, McHugh KP, Zuo J, Aguirre JI, Neubert JK, Rody WJ Jr. Exosomes: Novel regulators of bone remodelling and potential therapeutic agents for orthodontics. Orthodontics & Craniofacial Research. 2017;**20**(Suppl 1):95-99

[132] Makarova KS, Wolf YI, Alkhnbashi OS, Costa F, Shah SA, Saunders SJ, et al. An updated evolutionary classification of CRISPR-Cas systems. Nature Reviews. Microbiology. 2015; **13**(11):722-736

[133] Doudna JA, Charpentier E. Genome editing. The new frontier of genome engineering with CRISPR-Cas9. Science. 2014;**346**(6213):1258096

[134] Hsu PD, Lander ES, Zhang F. Development and applications of CRISPR-Cas9 for genome engineering. Cell. 2014;**157**(6):1262-1278

[135] Khan S, Mahmood MS, Rahman SU, Zafar H, Habibullah S, Khan Z, et al. CRISPR/Cas9: The Jedi against the dark empire of diseases. Journal of Biomedical Science. 2018;**25**(1):29

[136] Lambert LJ, Challa AK, Niu A, Zhou L, Tucholski J, Johnson MS, et al. Increased trabecular bone and improved biomechanics in an osteocalcin-null rat model created by CRISPR/Cas9 technology. Disease Models & Mechanisms. 2016;**9**(10):1169-1179

[137] Subramaniam M, Pitel KS, Bruinsma ES, Monroe DG, Hawse JR. TIEG and estrogen modulate SOST expression in the murine skeleton. Journal of Cellular Physiology. 2018; **233**(4):3540-3551

[138] Sakaguchi Y, Nishikawa K, Seno S, Matsuda H, Takayanagi H, Ishii M. Roles of enhancer RNAs in RANKL-induced osteoclast differentiation identified by genome-wide cap-analysis of gene expression using CRISPR/Cas9. Scientific Reports. 2018;**8**(1):7504

[139] Farr JN, Weivoda MM, Nicks KM, Fraser DG, Negley BA, Onken JL, et al. Osteoprotection through the deletion of the transcription factor Rorbeta in mice. Journal of Bone and Mineral Research. 2018;**33**(4):720-731

7

Contemporary Treatment Approaches to Obstructive Sleep Apnea Syndrome

Handan Tuğçe Oğuz

Abstract

Upper airway diseases decrease sleep time and/or quality, which leads to excessive day time sleepiness, fatigue, and lack of concentration. Upper airway diseases can be classified into two groups: upper airway resistance syndrome and sleep apnea syndrome. Sleep apnea syndrome is a disease, which occurs during sleeping, characterized by apneic and hypopneic events, low oxygen levels in lungs, blood oxygen desaturation, sleep arousal, and/or awakening. It increases morbidity and mortality of the patients. Sleep apnea syn drome has three types: central, mixed, and obstructive. Central and mixed apnea can be treated only by medical practitioners. But in the treatment of obstructive sleep apnea, orthodontists and maxillofacial surgeons have an important role. The aim of this chapter is to present current information about etiology, diagnostic tools, and treatment alternatives of obstructive sleep apnea and to introduce dental sleep medicine to orthodontists.

Keywords: dental sleep medicine, obstructive sleep apnea, dental treatment approaches for obstructive sleep apnea, pediatric obstructive sleep apnea

1. Introduction

Sleep-related breathing disorders are pathological changes in respiratory pattern during sleep. They increase morbidity and mortality, decreasing the life quality of patients. The patients complaining about waking up restless and headache, daytime sleepiness, lack of concentration, emotional changes, and unbalanced blood pressure may probably have a secret sleep-related breathing disorder.

Dental sleep medicine is an area of dental practice that focuses on dental therapy to treat sleep-disordered breathing, including snoring and obstructive sleep apnea. Dentists who are specialized in dental sleep medicine can diagnose the early signs and symptoms of potential obstructive sleep apnea.

2. Upper airway diseases

Upper airway diseases decrease sleep time and/or quality, which leads to excessive daytime sleepiness, fatigue, and lack of concentration. Upper airway diseases can be classified into two groups: upper airway resistance syndrome and sleep apnea syndrome.

Snoring is the most evident symptom of these syndromes, but it is not a disease. Snoring is just a sound resulting from soft tissues in the upper airway vibrating during inspiration, due to the increased velocity of air, caused by the decrease in size of airway space. Almost all patients with upper airway resistance syndrome and sleep apnea syndrome snore. However, snoring patients may or may not also have sleep apnea or upper airway resistance syndromes. Prevalence of snoring is estimated in 35–40% of the population. Snoring is a sign that some type of resistance is occurring in the upper respiratory system.

Upper airway resistance syndrome (UARS) occurs when resistance of upper respiratory system increases and breathing effort crosses over from harmless snoring. The transformation of snoring to UARS can be caused by aging (muscle tone in the throat decreases in time) and weight gain. In upper airway resistance syndrome, breathing needs much effort due to the narrow upper airway, and this extra effort leads to sleep arousal, frequent nocturnal awakenings, chronic insomnia, and excessive daytime sleepiness. Apnea and hypopnea are not symptoms of this disease.

UARS and obstructive sleep apnea syndrome (OSAS) have similar etiologies and symptoms, so differential diagnosis is very important. The key differences between UARS and OSAS consist of apnea-hypopnea existence, gender, and weight differences. In UARS apnea and hypopnea are either absent or very low. UARS patients are often in average weight, but OSAS patients are generally overweight or obese. UARS affects two genders equally, but OSAS affects men more than women.

UARS treatment consists of behavior and lifestyle changes, oral-dental appliances, and continuous positive airway pressure (CPAP) therapy. When UARS is untreated or treatment is unsuccessful, it can end up developing sleep apnea syndrome.

Sleep apnea syndrome is a chronic, progressive, and life-threatening disorder which occurs during sleeping and characterized by apneic and hypopneic events, hypoxia, blood oxygen desaturation, sleep arousal, and/or awakening. Sleep apnea has three types: central, obstructive, and mixed. In central apnea respiratory muscles need extra effort because breathing is limited or completely blocked due to the obstruction in the upper airway. Mixed apnea is the combination of central and obstructive apnea. Central and mixed apnea can be treated only by medical practitioners. But in the treatment of obstructive sleep apnea, dentists have an important role [1–4].

3. Obstructive Sleep Apnea Syndrome (OSAS)

Obstructive sleep apnea syndrome is a sleep-related breathing disorder that increases morbidity and mortality in patients, which is characterized by recurrent episodes of partial or complete upper airway obstructions and blood oxygen desaturation during sleep. This syndrome leads to severe long-term health problems as a result of the decrease in blood pressure during apnea and hypopnea episodes. Increased risk of high blood pressure, heart disease, heart arrhythmias, heart failure, and stroke can be seen in OSA patients.

OSAS prevalence is estimated at 3–7% in men and 2–5% in women. People from all ages, even pediatric and adolescent ages, can be affected from OSAS, but middle ages have the highest prevalence.

There are some definitions and indexes in order to define and classify the syndrome:

Apnea is the arousal of breathing for 10 seconds or more. It is a full obstruction of the airway when a person is asleep.

Hypopnea is a reduction in ventilation of at least 50% that results in a decrease in arterial saturation of 4% or more. It occurs due to partial airway obstruction.

Apnea index (AI) shows the average number of apneas and hypopneas per hour of sleep. The term respiratory disturbance index (RDI) can be used instead of AHI.

Arousal is a sudden change from a deeper sleep stage to a superficial sleep stage. It ends up in apnea and hypopnea.

Arousal index shows the average number of arousals per hour of sleep.

Minimum oxygen saturation is the minimum oxygen saturation level recorded in the whole sleep time [5–9].

4. Pathogenesis of obstructive sleep apnea

Upper airway has a great tendency to obstruction. Any pathological change that narrows the airway leads to OSAS. The pharynx is the site of upper airway obstruction during sleep. The size of the pharyngeal lumen depends on the balance between the forces that narrows and dilates the airway. The force that narrows the upper airway is the suction type, negative air pressure occurring during inspiration, and personal anatomical factors. The force that dilates the upper airway is the tension of the genioglossus and tensor veli palatini muscles surrounding the airway and tension of other small muscles attached to the pharynx. The difference between the narrowing and dilating forces are called transmural pressure. During sleep the tension of the muscles surrounding the airway decreases. The tongue and soft palate displace to the posterior wall of the oropharynx and narrows the upper airway. The airflow rate increases due to the narrowing airway dimension. The increased airflow applies more negative, suction-type pressure to the airway lumen. The increased negative airway pressure, decreased muscle activity, and airway lumen diameter lead to upper airway obstruction and apnea. During apnea the blood oxygen desaturation decreases, carbon dioxide saturation increases, and pH decreases. This change leads to the stimulation of central nervous system chemoreceptors, and awakening occurs to end up in apneic process. When the patient awakens, the tension of the muscles increases, which ends up in the obstruction of the upper airway. Blood oxygen saturation increases, carbon dioxide saturation decreases, pH increases, and the patient falls asleep again. This sleeping, apnea, awakening cycle continues during total sleep time [3, 5, 6, 8].

5. Etiology of obstructive sleep apnea

The etiology of OSAS is multifaceted. The factors that lead to OSA can change in adults and pediatric and adolescent patients.

5.1. Adult OSAS etiology

General factors: Age, gender, obesity, alcohol consumption, sedative medicine consumption.

Anatomical factors: Lesions and anatomical variations, nasal obstruction, neck circumference, head and neck position, airway shape, and dimension.

Mechanical factors: Supine position, upper airway resistance, upper airway compliance, intraluminal pressure, extraluminal pressure, thoracic caudal traction, mucosal adhesive affects, vascular factors.

Neuromuscular factors: Upper airway dilator muscles, upper airway reflexes, dilator muscle, and diaphragm relations.

Central factors: Hypocapnic apneic threshold, periodical breathing, arousal, and cytokines.

5.2. General factors

1. Age: OSA can be seen in all ages but mostly seen in middle ages. The tissue elasticity, ventilation on central, and pulmonary and cardiovascular functions decrease with age, and those factors lead to OSAS.
2. Gender: Men are affected more than women because of testosterone hormone inhibits respiration and men have more pharyngeal and supraglottic airway resistance than women.
3. Obesity: There is a close correlation between obesity and apnea. Obese patients have more fat deposits around soft palate. The fat infiltration from lateral to upper airway decreases the airway area and leads to apnea.
4. Alcohol and sedative medicine consumption: Investigations indicate that the activity of genioglossus and tensor veli palatini muscles decreases when the patient is asleep in a supine position. Alcohol and sedative medicine consumption can exaggerate this condition; the airway area decreases leading to apnea.

5.3. Anatomical factors

1. Lesions and anatomical variations: Changes in craniofacial form, inadequate muscle activity, soft tissue anomalies, micrognathia, retrognathia, macroglossia, enlarged soft palate, steep mandibular plane angle, nasal obstruction, adenotonsillar hypertrophy, reduced airway lumen, vocal cord dysfunction, edema of the epiglottis, polyps, tumors, acromegaly, nasal obstruction, juvenile temporomandibular ankylosis, and syndromes (Franceschetti-Treacher Collins, Apert, Crouzon, Pierre Robin, and Down syndromes) may cause OSA.

2. Neck circumference: Neck circumference is a significant predictor of OSA. Men and women have a greater risk for OSA if they have neck circumferences of 17 and 16 inch or greater, respectively.

3. Head and neck position: When a patient changes from upright to supine position, the thickness of the soft palate increases, and the anteroposterior oropharyngeal cross-sectional area decreases. The decrease in cross-sectional area is most evident in posterior of the soft palate.

4. Airway lumen diameter and shape: The investigations have shown that the OSAS patients have narrower airway area even they are awake and upright position. The airway has an anteroposterior configuration in normal people, but OSAS patients' airway has horizontal configuration [1–12].

6. Symptoms of obstructive sleep apnea

Major symptoms: Snoring, apnea, excessive daytime sleepiness.

Cardiopulmonary symptoms: Systemic hypertension, pulmonary hypertension, nocturnal arrhythmia, atypical breath ache, acute pulmonary edema, reversible proteinuria.

Neurobehavioral and social: Restlessness and headache in the morning, insomnia, depression, anxiety, mood disturbances, tendency to accidents, nervousness, forgetfulness.

Other symptoms: Dry mouth, night transpiration, nocturnal cough, hearing loss, gastroesophageal reflux [1–21].

7. Classification of OSAS

The severity of OSAS can be classified into three groups according to the apnea-hypopnea index (AHI). An AHI score smaller than 5 is considered normal. An AHI score between 10 and 20 represents mild obstructive sleep apnea, AHI score of 21–40 represents moderate obstructive sleep apnea, and AHI score greater than 40 represents severe obstructive sleep apnea [10–12, 22].

8. Diagnostic methods of OSAS

OSAS is a life-threatening syndrome which affects cardiovascular, pulmonary, psychological, and neurological systems. Because of this reason, the diagnosis and treatment plan of this syndrome should be done by a multidisciplinary team. The team should consist of medical practitioners, sleep specialists, psychiatrists, and dentists. The diagnosis and treatment plan should be done after a comprehensive medical and dental history and examination [10, 12, 13, 22].

The diagnostic methods of OSAS can be done in steps:

1. Clinical examination
2. Endoscopical examination
3. Polysomnography (PSG)
4. Radiological examination

8.1. Clinical examination

a. Nose-ear-throat and head-neck inspection: Inspection of the tonsil, soft palate, and tongue; inspection of maxillofacial characteristics; inspection of craniofacial characteristics, neck circumference, and natural head position.

b. Dental inspection: Malocclusion, maxillar and mandibular deficiency, narrow maxilla and maxillar segment, and dry mouth.

c. Systemic examination: Weight and inspection of pulmonary, cardiac, and neurobehavioral functions.

8.2. Endoscopic examination

Endoscopic examination is frequently used for the inspection of upper airway from the nose to the glottis. The dynamic upper airway changes and the level of collapse in upper airway can be seen in this method. Especially before surgical treatments, the level and severity of collapse can be seen, and the operation can be planned according to these data.

8.3. Polysomnography (PSG)

Nocturnal, laboratory-based polysomnography is the gold standard diagnostic tool for obstructive sleep apnea syndrome. It is used for diagnosing, determining the severity of disease, and evaluating various other sleep disorders that can exist with or without OSAS. It is also used after OSAS treatment for the evaluation of the treatment effectiveness. A classical PSG consists of electroencephalogram (EEG), electromyogram (EMG), and electrooculogram (EOG) records. PSG measures sleep cycles and stages by recording airflow in and out of lungs during breathing, the level of oxygen in blood, breathing effort and rate, brain waves, electrical activity of muscles, eye movements, and heart rate. The most important parameters measured by PSG are apnea index (AI), hypopnea index (HI), apnea-hypopnea index (AHI), and minimum oxygen desaturation. PSG can be done either at a sleep center or in the patients at home. But home-based PSG records do not have the same reliability as sleep center-based PSG records.

8.4. Radiological inspection

Upper airway imaging should be performed in OSAS patients in order to examine the anatomy of the pharynx, surrounding the craniofacial and soft tissue structures. Lateral cephalometry, computerized tomography (CT), and MR imaging (MRI) are the most commonly used radiological inspection methods of OSAS.

8.4.1. Lateral cephalometry

It is the most commonly used radiological inspection method of OSAS. It allows to investigate the sagittal and vertical positions of the maxilla and mandible according to the cranial base, maxillomandibular relationships, the sagittal and vertical position of hyoid bone, soft palate anatomy, and head posture. It is cheap and noninvasive but documentation can be done in two dimensions.

Cephalometric analysis alone is insufficient to diagnose OSAS. But some cephalometric parameters can accept a signal for OSAS risk. Increased mandibular plane angle, steep occlusal plane, over-erupted posterior dentition, large gonial angle, anterior open bite, adipose tissue placed in the submental and parapharyngeal region, larger and wider soft palate, and increased linear distance from the mandibular plane to the hyoid bone (a distance bigger than 15.4 mm) create OSA risk [10, 13].

8.4.2. Computed tomography (CT)

The high-resolution and three-dimensional evaluation of the skeletal system and soft tissues in maxillofacial complex can be performed by computed tomography. CT imaging is done in supine position and can give us the opportunity of recording the changes in upper airway cross-sectional area in different phases of respiration and predicting the collapse area in OSAS patients. The disadvantages of this technique are as follows: being expensive, high radiation level, and the low-resolution images of fat tissues around upper airway according to MR imaging [14].

8.4.3. Magnetic resonance imaging (MRI)

Magnetic resonance imaging allows 3D imaging and accurate measurement of the upper airway, soft tissues, and skeletal structures. MRI is performed in supine position, it allows high-resolution visualization of soft tissues and fat deposits around pharyngeal airway, and the volume and area of the airway can be measured accurately. With ultrafast mode dynamic observation can be done. But it is expensive and cannot be used in patients who have claustrophobia, ferromagnetic clips, or pacemaker [15].

9. Treatment of adult obstructive sleep apnea syndrome

OSAS is a life-threatening disease. Because of this reason, early, accurate, and individualized treatment should be performed by a multidisciplinary team. The aim of OSAS treatment is to decrease the number of obstructive episodes and severity and the collapse tendency and increase the airway area, blood oxygen saturation, and life quality.

Treatment options in OSAS are:

1. Behavioral modification
2. Surgical treatments
3. Use of nasal continuous positive airway pressure device (nCPAP)
4. Use of oral appliances

9.1. Behavioral modification

Weight loss, quitting smoking and alcohol, changing sleep positions and head posture, and avoidance of central nervous system depressors may be beneficial for some patients. Weight loss may decrease OSA symptoms by reducing the size of the tongue and soft palate. Quitting alcohol and depressor drugs prevents the relaxation of upper airway muscles. Alteration of sleeping position can prevent the tongue and mandible moving backward and narrowing the airway. The patients are instructed to sleep on their sides rather than their backs.

9.2. Surgical treatment

OSA resulted from anatomic obstruction of the upper airway, unsuccessful behavioral therapies, and inability to tolerate CPAP or oral appliances, which are inclusion criteria for surgical treatment. Tracheostomy, tonsillectomy and adenoidectomy, genial advancement with or without hyoid myotomy, uvulopalatopharyngoplasty, laser glossectomy and lingualplasty, maxillomandibular advancement, and epiglottoplasty are the surgical techniques used for the treatment of OSAS.

9.3. Nasal continuous positive airway pressure (nCPAP) device treatment

It is a device which has a small air pump connected to either a sealed face or nose mask. The device opens the pharyngeal airway and prevents the soft tissues from collapsing and blocking the airway. It is the gold standard treatment option for moderate to severe OSAS cases, and the success rate is about 75%. However, patient compliance is poor because of the pump noise, the irritation of nasal mucosa because of the airflow to the nose, xerostomia, and poor retention. The patient non-compliance ratio was reported to range from 46 to 83%. The ordinary usage of nCPAP device for 4–6 weeks decreases the volume of the tongue and increases the pharyngeal volume. Inclusion criteria for nCPAP therapy are moderate and severe OSAS patients with AHI score greater than 20, mild OSAS patients with AHI scores between 10 and 20 but has excessive daytime sleepiness and cardiopulmonary or cerebrovascular risks, anatomical-based OSAS patients whose medical health condition is inappropriate to surgical treatment, and mild-to-moderate OSA patients who have failed behavioral modification therapy and unable to tolerate oral appliances [1–10, 16, 17].

10. Oral appliance therapy

Oral appliance treatment was first introduced in the 1980s and is a very effective treatment option for mild-to-moderate OSAS and seven patients with severe OSA who cannot tolerate CPAP or refuse surgical therapy. The American Sleep Disorders Association reported that oral appliance therapy is the primary treatment for patients with mild OSA and a secondary treatment option for moderate to severe OSA. For severe OSA patients, reduction in AHI score occurs, but it cannot turn into the normal range. If the AHI score cannot be decreased to 20, long-term health risks will continue. Oral appliances can be successful if only they are used after the etiological factors are eliminated. Only obstructive sleep apnea can be treated with oral devices; they are not indicated for central and mixed apneas [10–12, 16–21, 23–32].

10.1. Oral appliance therapy indications

1. Snoring patients
2. Upper airway resistance syndrome
3. Mild OSAS patients who have failed behavioral modification therapy
4. Moderate to severe OSAS patients who refused or failed CPAP therapy or surgery

10.2. Oral appliance therapy contraindications

1. Central or mixed obstructive sleep apnea
2. TMJ diseases
3. Periodontal diseases
4. Insufficient oral hygiene
5. Anatomical based OSAS

11. Types of oral appliances

Oral appliances can be classified into four groups according to their affect mechanisms:

1. Mandibular advancement devices (MADs)
2. Tongue retaining devices (TRDs)
3. Palate lifting appliances (PLA)
4. OPAP appliances (oral appliances + CPAP device)

12. Mandibular advancement devices (MADs)

MADs were first described by Pierre Robin in 1934 in the treatment of a patient with micrognathia as a modified monobloc in order to reposition the mandible in a more forwarded position and open the airway. This advancement makes the attached soft tissues and tongue stretch and stabilize; by this way, oro- and hypopharyngeal airways enlarge.

MAD appliances can be divided into several groups: monobloc-style one-piece or twin block-style two-piece, available to activation or unavailable to activation, teeth-supported or teeth- and tissue-supported, and soft- or hard-materialed. All of these appliances increase the distance between soft palate and posterior wall of the pharynx and enlarge the space between tongue root and posterior region of the oropharynx.

Tooth- and tissue-supported, soft-materialed, activation-optioned MAD appliances are reported to be more successful in OSAS treatment. One-pieced or two-pieced appliance design does not affect the treatment success.

MAD-type oral appliances are found the most effective type of oral appliances in OSAS treatment [10–12, 17, 19, 23, 25–30].

12.1. MAD indications

Normal or reduced facial height, patients have at least eight teeth per arch, patients who have normal soft palate thickness and normal positioned soft palate, and obese patients.

12.2. MAD contraindications

The patients with thick and enlarged soft palate, periodontal disease, and TMJ problems.

MAD appliance construction:

a. Upper and lower dental impressions are taken.

b. Maximum opening, left and right lateral excursion, and maximum protrusion are measured.

c. The appliance is constructed using a position 75% of the patients' maximum protrusion. Vertical opening amount changes individually. But it is recommended to open the bite at least 5 or 6 millimeters.

d. Bite registrations in centric occlusion and advanced position are obtained. A George gauge and light-body impression material can be helpful in stabilizing the construction bite position.

e. The MAD appliance fabricated from soft acrylic, hard acrylic, silicone-based, or Essix-based materials according to the type of the chosen appliance.

12.3. MAD treatment mechanism

MADs displace the mandible, suprahyoid, and genioglossus muscles anteriorly. This anterior movement prevents oropharyngeal airway obstruction. The forward and downward displacement of the mandible also decreases the gravitational effect of the tongue in supine position and enlarges the velopharynx by stretching the palatoglossal and palatopharyngeal arches (**Figures 1** and **2**).

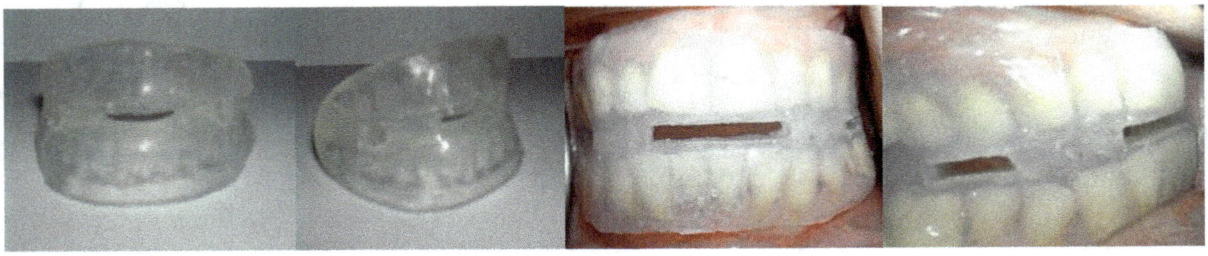

Figure 1. One-piece, non-activation MAD appliance.

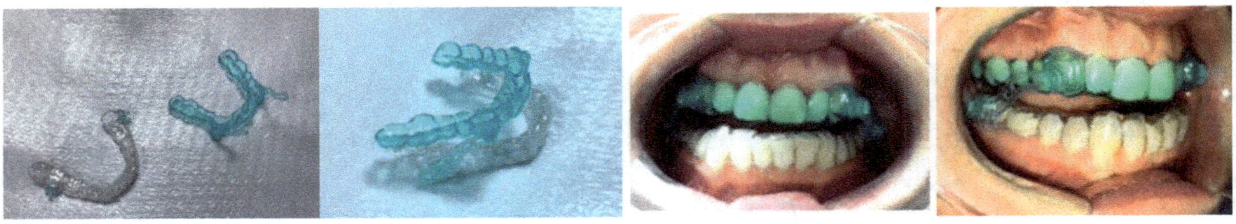

Figure 2. Two-piece, activation-optioned MAD appliance.

13. Tongue-retaining devices (TRDs)

Tongue-retaining devices were first described by Cartwright and Samelson in 1982 [28]. During sleeping and in supine position, the tongue and all gravity-dependent tissues tend to fall posteriorly. With TRDs, the tongue is prevented from dropping posteriorly by suction created when the patient forces the tongue into a hollow bulb built into the device. The forward position of the tongue increases the volume and decreases the resistance of upper airway. The superiority of TRDs over MADs is that they can be used for edentulous patients [10–12, 16, 17, 19, 20, 23, 25, 31].

13.1. TRD indications

Edentulous OSA patients, OSA patients who have TMJ disorders, OSA patients with big tonsils and large tongues, OSA patients who have less than six teeth per arch, hypothyroidism, and sleep position–related apnea-hypopnea occurrence.

13.2. TRD contraindications

Severe periodontal diseases, bruxism, chronic nasal obstruction, patients who are unable to move their tongue anteriorly, and obese OSA patients.

13.3. TRD appliance construction

The TRD appliance can be fabricated from soft copolymer materials by the technician to the OSA patient individually, or standard fabricated appliances can be used to the patient.

13.3.1. Individualized TRD appliance construction

a. Upper and lower dental impressions are taken.

b. Maximum opening, left and right lateral excursion, and maximum protrusion measured.

c. The appliance is constructed using a position 75% of the patients' maximum protrusion. Vertical opening amount differs patient to patient, but it is more than MAD vertical opening amount, in order to place the hollow bulb part.

d. The appliance is fabricated from soft copolymer material like a monobloc with a hollow bulb part to place the tongue.

13.3.2. Fabricated TRD appliance construction

a. The tongue is measured by wrapping a piece of dental floss around the tongue. Then, the floss is removed and measured.

b. The fabrication appliances have two types, edentulous and dentulous, and three sizes, small, medium, and large.

c. The correct type and size are chosen for the patient.

d. The bulb appliance is moistened and compressed and the tongue is inserted.

TRD-type appliances are found to be effective in mild to moderate OSA treatment. They decrease AI, HI, AHI, oxygen desaturation, and excessive daytime sleepiness and increase minimum oxygen desaturation and genioglossus muscle activity. But the patient compliance is low with TRDs because of the irritation in the tongue, hypersalivation, uncomfortable feeling, and non-esthetic appearance.

14. Palate lifting appliances (PLA)

They are used in patients who have a thick and enlarged soft palate. The appliance supports and stabilizes the soft palate, prevents soft palate blocking the airway, and reduces the vibration of soft palate leading to snoring. But they are uncomfortable appliances and the patient compliance rates are very low. Because of this reason, they are not frequently used in OSA treatment [10, 11].

15. OPAP appliances (oral appliance + CPAP device)

nCPAP device applies very high pressure and high airflow rate which leads to irritation of nasal, oral, and throat mucosa and decreases patient compliance. When MAD-type oral appliances are combined with CPAP device, the pressure given by nCPAP diminishes; irritation of nasal, oral, and throat mucosa decreases; and patient compliance and treatment success increase. The adaptation of CPAP and MAD appliance should be done by a dental sleep specialist [10, 18].

16. Side effects of oral appliance therapy

There are very few side effects of oral appliances when compared to other treatment alternatives. Researches have reported that patients prefer treatment with an OA over surgery or CPAP appliance, and compliance with OA has been reported to be 40–80%.

The side effects of OA therapy can be divided into two groups:

1. Short-term side effects of OA therapy: Excessive salivation or dry mouth, TMJ sounds and/or TMJ pain, tooth pain, odd bite feeling in the morning, gum irritation, tenderness in masticatory muscles, or myofascial pain. These complications are generally mild and transient [10, 11, 19, 20].
2. Long-term side effects of OA therapy: OA therapy for OSAS patients is a lifelong treatment. Skeletal, dental, and occlusal changes can occur from OA therapy in 2 or more years' time. Craniofacial changes related to long-term oral appliance use can be determined with cephalometric investigations. Skeletal changes generally occur after average treatment duration of 5 years. The changes can be summarized as more downward and forward position of the mandible, increased lower facial height, decreased overbite and overjet, retroclination of the maxillary incisors, proclination of the mandibular incisors, changes in molar relationship, and curve of Spee flattening. Long-term use of OA also makes differences in upper airway configuration. Palatal length decreases and pharyngeal area increases in time. These changes can be due to the loss of edema caused by snoring and repetitive apneas [10, 32–38].

17. Efficacy and success of oral appliance therapy

OA therapy is an effective and safe long-term therapy for patients with snoring, mild to moderate OSAS. However, the efficiency varies on many factors including the type of OA, materials used for fabrication, piece number of appliance (monobloc or bibloc), titration ability (titrable or untitrable), and degree of sagittal and vertical mandibular displacement.

The efficacy criteria of oral appliance therapy in OSA are:

a. Positive changes in PSG test: Decrease in AHI, AI, HI, arousal score, increase in blood oxygen saturation, sleep time, and efficiency

b. Positive subjective feedback of patients: Decrease or quitting snoring and decrease in daytime sleepiness

c. Enlargement of pharyngeal airway area [10–12, 25, 28, 31, 32]

17.1. To summarize

1. MADs are reported more effective than other types of OAs.
2. Monobloc-type one-piece and soft-materialed OAs are found to be more efficient in reducing AHI, AI, and snoring.
3. Forward and downward displacement of the mandible is recommended for enlargement in pharyngeal airway area. But this displacement amount should be assessed individually.
4. No definite conclusions can be drawn regarding which type or design of OA has a beneficial influence on subjective treatment efficacy. Individually determination of appliance is very important in OA treatment success [10–12, 16, 17, 19, 20, 23, 25–28, 30–32].

18. Intraoral appliance treatment guideline for OSAS patients

The American Sleep Disorders Association (ASDA) has prepared a protocol for OA treatment in OSAS patients. A dental sleep specialist should follow up the stages below in the treatment of an OSAS patient [21, 24]:

1. Detailed medical and dental history.
2. PSG and medical specialist's report investigation.
3. Dental investigation: Soft tissue and intraoral inspection, periodontal-occlusal-TMJ inspection, intraoral habits and parafunction inspection, teeth and restoration inspection, and radiological inspection.
4. Upper-lower dental impressions and bite registration are obtained.
5. Selection of OA type for the patient individually. (The success and compliance rate varies case to case, and choosing the right type of OA is the most important stage of OA treatment protocol.)
6. OA fabrication.
7. Adjustment of the OA. Appliance fit and comfort are controlled, and usage instructions are given to patient.
8. Follow-up PSG and lateral cephalogram are taken after appropriate appliance adjustment/titration and patient adaptation period. Objective determination of the treatment efficiency can only be observed by PSG test with the appliance in place. Nearly all patients report positive change subjectively; however, they should be proven with PSG reports.
9. If the treatment is found to be effective in the first year of the therapy, four follow-up appointments are recommended. After 1 year, two follow-up appointments per year are enough. At the follow-up appointments, appliance fit, comfort, effectiveness, and patient

compliance are investigated. If the OA is found to be less effective, the titration of OA or fabrication of a new OA should be done.

19. Pediatric and adolescent obstructive sleep apnea

Obstructive sleep apnea in pediatric and adolescent patients is characterized by episodic partial or complete upper airway obstruction during sleep. All children with OSAS snore. It has been estimated to occur in 5–6% of children. It is most seen in preschool children; the peak age is 3–6 years, which coincides with the growth of adenoids and tonsils. Pediatric OSAS is similar to adult OSAS, but there are differences. Sleep disruption occurred by respiratory pauses less than ten seconds. Hypopneic episodes can be seen, usually more than five to ten episodes per night with oxygen saturations less than 85%. Pediatric OSAS effects both gender at the same ratios, different from adult OSA. Seven percent to nine percent of children snore every night; 18% of them snore in nasal, ear, or throat infection periods. The prevalence of pediatric OSAS is estimated about 0.5–3%. AHI scores of pediatric sleep apnea is controversial. Some protocols of AHI score greater than 1 should be accepted as a pediatric OSA predictor; some protocols accepting AHI score greater than 5 is pathognomonic.

19.1. Pediatric and adolescent OSA etiology

Hypertrophic adenoids, hypertrophic tonsils, maxillary transverse deficiency, class 3 maxillary skeletal deficiency, class 2 mandibular skeletal deficiency, overweight and obesity, and craniofacial anomalies. (Pierre Robin Sequence, Goldenhar syndrome, Crouzon syndrome, Apert syndrome, cleft lip and/or palate, vertical face anomalies, Marfan syndrome, and associated 22q deletion syndromes).

19.2. OSA symptoms in children

Abnormal breathing during sleeping, frequent awakenings or restlessness, frequent nightmares, enuresis, difficult awakening, excessive daytime sleepiness, hyperactivity-behavior problems, daytime mouth breathing, poor or irregular sleep patterns, early recognition of mouth breathing and airway obstruction; symptoms of recurrent blocked nose; recurrent nasal, ear, and throat infections; parents concerned about snoring should alert the dental professional for definitive diagnosis for pediatric OSA.

19.3. Differences between pediatric and adult OSA

a. Pediatric OSAS effects both genders equally.

b. Snoring is irregular and interrupted with apneic-hypopneic events in adult OSAS. In pediatric OSAS snoring can be continuous.

c. Daytime sleepiness is mostly seen in adult OSA. In pediatric OSA behavioral changes and growth retardation are seen more than daytime sleepiness.

d. Mouth breathing is mostly seen in pediatric OSA [39–42].

e. Obesity is mostly seen in adult OSA; in pediatric OSA, the patient can be of normal weight or thin.

f. The etiology of pediatric OSA is mostly hypertrophic adenoids and tonsils. In adult OSA retropharyngeal and retrolingual pathologies are more effective.

g. The gold standard treatment protocol for adult OSA is CPAP appliance. In pediatric OSA adenotonsillectomy is advised rather than CPAP therapy.

19.4. Clinical inspection in pediatric sleep apnea syndrome

a. Nose-ear-throat and head-neck inspection: Craniofacial, orofacial, and maxillofacial characteristics are investigated. In craniofacial inspection symptoms of various syndromes are investigated. In orofacial inspection features of the tongue, soft palate, and tonsils are investigated. In maxillofacial inspection maxillofacial characteristics like facies adenoidalis, rhinolalia clausa, long-thin face, narrow maxilla and maxillary segment, overlenghtened teeth, hypoplastic mandible, and septum deviation are investigated.

b. Systemic inspection: Includes inspection of pulmonary, cardiac, physical, and mental condition functions and weight.

20. Pediatric OSA treatment protocol

1. Surgical approaches: In pediatric patients dentists should examine oropharynx carefully. Both the lingual and pharyngeal tonsils can be visible intraorally, but the adenoids will not. When hypertrophic tonsils are observed clinically or radiographically, referral for endoscopic evaluation and possible surgical removal by a pediatric otolaryngologist should be made. Early removal of these tissues can prevent the long-face growth pattern with narrow upper and lower dental arches and anterior open bite.

2. Weight loss and behavioral changes

3. Rapid maxillary expansion (RME): Cephalometric and acoustic rhinometry studies report that with RME maxilla, the palate and floor of nasal cavity expand, which leads to increase the volume and decrease the airflow resistance in nasal cavity. It also makes statistically significant changes in tongue size position and hyoid position. The expansion in maxillary dentition gives the tongue a greater space and more forward positioning to the tongue. The widened maxillary basal bone on the velum, the superior pharyngeal constrictor muscles, and the surrounding orofacial musculature can increase the muscle tonus.

4. Class 2 growth modification therapy: When the pediatric and adolescent patients have both mandibular deficiency and obstructive sleep apnea, mandibular advancement devices like Herbst, twin block, monobloc, bionator, Frankel 2, etc. can be used for the treatment.

5. Class 3 growth modification therapy: When the pediatric or adolescent patients have both class 3 maxillary deficiency and OSA, class 3 growth modification therapy is recommended. In this treatment maxilla is widened first with RPE, followed by orthopedic traction with protraction face mask (reverse pull headgear).

6. CPAP therapy: This therapy can be advised to severely affected adolescent OSAS patients. In pediatric and adolescent population, the long-term use of CPAP can cause craniofacial side effects. The force applied from the elastic strap of CPAP mask applies a restraining force on the maxilla. So, CPAP therapy can lead a class 3 skeletal deficiency in pediatric and adolescent OSA patients. But it is unclear how much of the malocclusion results from CPAP and how much results from an underlying adverse growth pattern.

21. Conclusion

Sleep-related breathing disorders are complicated problems, which decrease life quality and increase morbidity and mortality in patients.

Dentists, who are specialized in dental sleep medicine, can see the early symptoms of these diseases and can be frontline screeners for potential OSAS diagnosis. In the treatment of snoring and mild-to-moderate obstructive sleep apnea, the oral appliance therapy was found to be a very effective treatment option.

Author details

Handan Tuğçe Oğuz

Address all correspondence to: htugce@gmail.com

Private Orthodontics Clinic, Ankara, Turkey

References

[1] European Respiratory Society and European Lung Foundation. 2003. Lung health in Europe—Facts and figures. Available from: www.europeanlungfoundation.org/uploads/Document/WEB_CHEMIN_13411_1222853571.pdf

[2] Sleep-related Breathing Disorders in Adults. Recommendations for syndrome definition and measurement techniques in clinical research. The Report of an American Academy of Sleep Medicine Task Force. Sleep. 1999;**22**:667-689

[3] Young T, Palta M, Demsey J, Skotrud J, Weber S, Bodr S. The occurrence of sleep disordered breathing among middle aged adults. The New England Journal of Medicine. 1993;**328**:1230-1235

[4] Lowe AA. Orthodontists and sleep-disordered breathing. American Journal of Orthodontics and Dentofacial Orthopedics. 1996;**110**(1):28-35

[5] Krieger J. Clinical presentation of sleep apnea. The European Respiratory Journal. 1998;**10**:75-105

[6] Koenig SM, Suratt P. Obstructive sleep apnea: The syndrome. In: Johnson-Jones, editor. Obstructive Sleep Apnea. London, UK: Taylor; 2001. pp. 3-16

[7] Strohl KP, Redline S. Recognition of obstructive sleep apnea. American Journal of Respiratory and Critical Care Medicine. 1996;**154**:279-289

[8] Kryger MH. Fat, sleep and Charles Dickens: Literary and medical contributions to the understanding of sleep apnea. Clinics in Chest Medicine. 1985;**6**(4):555-562

[9] Kuhl W. History of clinical research on the sleep apnea syndrome. Respiration. 1997; **64**(1):5-10

[10] Oğuz HT, Üçüncü N. Orthodontic approach to obstructive sleep apnea syndrome cases. Turkish Journal of Orthodontics. 2005;**18**:175-187

[11] Oğuz HT, Üçüncü N. The treatment of obstructive sleep apnea syndrome with oral appliances. AOT. 2007;**24**(3):193-198

[12] Oğuz HT. Investigation of treatment efficiency with MA appliance on simple snoring and mild obstructive sleep apnea syndrome [thesis]. Ankara: Gazi University; 2007

[13] Kuo GP, Torok CM, Aygun N, Zincreich J. Diagnostic imaging of the upper airway. Proceedings of the American Thoracic Society. 2011;**8**:40-45

[14] Zinsy SR, Moraes LC, Moura P, Ursi W. Assessment of pharyngeal airway space using cone-beam computed tomography. Dental Press Journal of Orthodontics. 2010; **15**(5):150-158

[15] Welch KC, Foster GD, Christensen T, Ritter BA, Wadden TA, Arens R, et al. A novel volumetric magnetic resonance imaging paradigm to study upper airway anatomy. Sleep. 2002;**25**(5):532-542

[16] Fleisher KE, Krieger AC. Current trends in the treatment of obstructive sleep apnea. Journal of Oral and Maxillofacial Surgery. 2007;**65**:2056-2068

[17] Prabhat KC, Goyal L, Bey A, Maheshhwari S. Recent advances in the management of obstructive sleep apnea: The dental perspective. Journal of Natural Science, Biology and Medicine. 2012;**3**:13-17

[18] Thornton WK. Combined CPAP oral appliance therapy. Sleep. 2002;**6**(3):125-127

[19] Lowe AA, Schmidt-Novara WW. Oral appliance therapy for snoring and apnea. Sleep. 1995;**18**(6):501-510

[20] Pancer J. Oral appliance therapy for SDB. Sleep. 2003;**4**(4):24-36

[21] Schmidt-Nowara W, Lowe A, Wigand L, Cartwright R, Perez-Guerra F, Mean S. Practice parameters for the treatment of snoring and obstructive sleep apnea with oral appliances. Sleep and Breathing. 1995;**18**(6):511-513

[22] ASDA—Diagnostic Classification Steering Committee. The International Classification of Sleep Disorders Diagnostic and Coding Manual. 2nd ed. Lawrence, KS: Allen Press Inc; 1997

[23] Ahrens A, McGrath C, Hagg U. A systematic review of the efficacy of oral appliance design in the management of obstructive sleep apnoea. European Journal of Orthodontics. 2011;**33**:318-324

[24] Ngiam J, Balasubramaniam R, Darendeliler MA, Cheng AT, Waters K. Clinical guidelines for oral appliance therapy in the treatment of snoring and obstructive sleep apnoea. Australian Dental Journal. 2013;**58**:408-419

[25] Ahrens A, McGrath C, Hagg U. Subjective efficacy of oral appliance design features of oral appliance design features in the management of obstructive sleep apnea. American Journal of Orthodontics and Dentofacial Orthopedics. 2010;**138**:559-576

[26] Johnston CD, Gleadhil IC, Cinnamond MJ, Gabbey J, Burdan D. Mandibular advancement appliances and obstructive sleep apnea: A randomized clinical trial. European Journal of Orthodontics. 2002;**24**(3):251-262

[27] Johal A, Battagel J, Hector M. Controlled, prospective trial of psychosocial function before and after mandibular advancement splint therapy. American Journal of Orthodontics and Dentofacial Orthopedics. 2011;**139**:581-587

[28] Okuno K, Sato K, Arısaka T, Hosohoma K, Gotoh M, Taga M, et al. The effect of oral appliance that advanced the mandible forward and limited mouth opening in patients with obstructive sleep apnea: A systematic review and meta-analysis of randomised controlled trials. Journal of Oral Rehabilitation. 2014;**41**:542-554

[29] Seehra J, Sherriff M, Winchester L. Craniofacial characteristics of successful responders to mandibular advancement splint therapy: A pilot study. The British Journal of Oral & Maxillofacial Surgery. 2014;**52**:314-316

[30] Zhou J, Liu YH. A randomised crossover study comparing two oral appliances in the treatment for mild to moderate obstructive sleep apnoea/hypopnea syndrome. Journal of Oral Rehabilitation. 2012;**39**:914-922

[31] Ono T, Lowe AA, Ferguson KA, Pae EK, Fleetham JA. The effect of the tongue retaining device on awake genioglossus muscle activity in patients with obstructive sleep apnea. American Journal of Orthodontics and Dentofacial Orthopedics. 1996;**110**(1):28-35

[32] Rose EC, Barthlen GM, Staats R, Jonas IE. Therapeutic efficacy of an oral appliance in the treatment of an obstructive sleep apnea: A two year follow up. American Journal of Orthodontics and Dentofacial Orthopedics. 2002;**121**(3):273-279

[33] Marklund M. Predictors of long-term orthodontic side effects from mandibular advancement devices in patients with snoring and obstructive sleep apnea. American Journal of Orthodontics and Dentofacial Orthopedics. 2006;**129**(2):214-221

[34] Gong X, Zhang J, Zhao Y, Gao X. Long-term therapeutic efficacy of oral appliances in treatment of obstructive sleep apnea-hypopnea syndrome. The Angle Orthodontist. 2013;**83**:653-658

[35] Almeida FR, Lowe AA, Sung JO, Tsuki S, Otsuka R. Long-term sequellae of oral appliance therapy in obstructive sleep apnea patients: Part 1. Cephalometric analysis. American Journal of Orthodontics and Dentofacial Orthopedics. 2006;**129**:195-204

[36] Chen H, Lowe A, Almeida FR, Fleetham JA, Wang B. Three dimensional computer assisted study model analysis of long term oral appliance wear. Part 2. Side effects of of oral appliances in obstructive sleep apnea patients. American Journal of Orthodontics and Dentofacial Orthopedics. 2008;**134**:408-417

[37] Doff MHJ, Hoekema A, Pruim GJ, Slater Huddleston JJR, Stegenga B. Long-term oral appliance therapy in obstructive sleep apnea: A cephalometric study of craniofacial changes. Journal of Dentistry. 2010;**38**:1010-1018

[38] Doff MHJ, Finnema KJ, Hoekema A, Wijkstra PJ, Bont LGM, Stegenga B. Long-term oral appliance therapy in obstructive sleep apnea syndrome: A controlled study on dental side effects. Clinical Oral Investigations. 2013;**17**:475-482

[39] Conley RS. Evidence for dental and dental specialty treatment of obstructive sleep apnoea. Part 1: The adult OSA patient and Part 2: The paediatric and adolescent patient. Journal of Oral Rehabilitation. 2011;**38**:136-156

[40] Erişen L. Paediatric obstructive sleep apnea syndrome-contemporary approaches. Contemporary Paediatrics. 2005;**2**:7-17

[41] Verhulst SL, Schrauwen N, Haentjens D, Rooman RP, Van Gaal L, De Backer WA, et al. The prevelance, anatomical correlates and treatment of sleep-disordered breathing in obese children and adolescents. Sleep Medicine Reviews. 2008;**12**:139-146

[42] Narang I, Mathew JL. Childhood obesity and obstructive sleep apnea. Journal of Nutrition and Metabolism. 2012. Article ID: 134202. DOI: 10.1155/2012/134202. [Epub 2012 Aug 22]

8

Micro-Osteoperforations

Esra Bolat

Abstract

The researchers have tended to study on methods which will shorten orthodontic treatment periods due to the fact that orthodontic treatments are long-term treatments with increased side-effect potentials depending on the use of orthodontic force. There is a need for shortening orthodontic treatment time besides minimizing the side effects and achieving permanent results. Therefore, local or systemic application of various chemical agents, some physical-mechanic stimulus, and surgery-assisted methods are used. Surgically assisted methods have a longer clinical history with more predictable and consistent results among the acceleration methods of tooth movement. On the other hand, they include some complication risks due to the interventions as they are invasive methods, which is accepted as the disadvantage of these methods. Outstanding with its ease of implementation and repeatability, "micro-osteoperforation," which is less invasive than other surgical methods, is an up-to-date technique. Animal studies show that micro-osteoperforations increase orthodontic tooth movement rate by enhancing the cellular response. These findings are also supported by a limited number of clinical studies. Although micro-osteoperforations were reported to be included in tooth acceleration techniques as a trustable and applicable method in clinical routine, issues such as application techniques, possible side effects, and combining with different mechanics should be evaluated with further clinical studies.

Keywords: micro-osteoperforations, accelerated orthodontics, tooth movement, bone remodeling

1. Introduction

Many orthodontic patients complain about the physical and social discomfort which is associated with prolonged use of fixed appliances [1]. There are also numerous studies which report that dental and periodontal complications such as apical root resorption, subsequent gingivitis, periodontitis, enamel demineralization, increased levels of dental caries, and open gingival embrasure spaces may occur during orthodontic treatment [2].

However, a major challenge in orthodontics is to shorten treatment time by avoiding undesirable side effects without compromising treatment outcome. The rate of orthodontic tooth movement is primarily determined by the remodeling of tissues surrounding the roots; this in return is under the control of molecular mechanisms regulating cellular behaviors in the alveolar bone and periodontal ligament [3]. Assuming that the clinician optimized mechanics and cooperation for any patient, the main factor controlling the treatment time and rate will be the patient's biological response to the orthodontic forces [4, 5]. Therefore, identifying and controlling the cellular regulators are essential to shorten orthodontic treatment time safely.

The concept of accelerating tooth movement has received increased attention recently [6] with the introduction of various clinical techniques; including local injection of cellular mediators [7], physical or mechanical stimuli [8] and surgically assisted orthodontics [9, 10]. Local or systemic pharmaceutical administration and physical or mechanical stimulation methods might not be applicable to daily clinical practice because of their possible side effects and their outcomes that await validation [11]. Over the past decade, the regional acceleratory phenomenon induced by surgical trauma has received emphasis for accelerating orthodontic tooth movement and reducing the treatment time [11]. However, many techniques which are surgically assisted involve considerably high surgical trauma limiting application of the technique currently.

A new method which uses micro-osteoperforations (MOPs) to stimulate alveolar bone remodeling without the disadvantages of surgery such as the requirement of corticotomies, cuts in cortical bone, raising split-thickness flap, and decorticating the bone has recently been identified [5, 12]. Animal studies revealed that micro-osteoperforations significantly stimulate expression of inflammatory markers and increase the number of osteoclasts and bone resorption. The increase in bone remodeling contributes to the rise in both rate and magnitude of tooth movement [4]. In addition to the requirement of additional studies, similar results are reported in clinical trials [4, 5].

In this chapter, we focused on the biologic basis of orthodontic tooth movement, accelerated tooth movement techniques and application methods, advantages, disadvantages, effects, and possible side effects of micro-osteoperforations as a new, reliable, repeatable and minimally invasive method for accelerating orthodontic tooth movement.

2. Biologic basis of orthodontic tooth movement

Application of mechanical forces to teeth causes orthodontic tooth movement as a result of the biological responses of the periodontal tissues. Alveolar bone remodeling includes selective resorption in some areas and apposition in others. The biologic response to orthodontic therapy includes not only the response of the periodontal ligament and alveolar bone but also the response of growing areas which are distant from the dentition. However, it can be stated that tooth movement is primarily a periodontal ligament phenomenon because the alveolar bone response is also mediated by the periodontal ligament [13].

The first step of the biological response to orthodontic force is "tension and compression in the periodontal ligament" which constricts and deforms blood vessels damaging cells in the periodontal tissues. The initial aseptic acute inflammatory response is realized by releasing chemokines and cytokines from localized cells such as osteoblast, fibroblast, and endothelial cells. Most of these cytokines are pro-inflammatory providing the continuity of the inflammatory response by activating osteoclast precursors of periodontal ligament in extravascular range and inflammatory cells. Infiltration of inflammatory cells causes the increase of chemokine and cytokine levels. This enables differentiation of osteoclast precursors to multinucleated giant cells which will realize alveolar bone resorption that is required for tooth movement. The continuity of the existence of anti-inflammatory chemokines and cytokines is essential in order to suppress destructive pro-inflammatory and osteolytic processes [4]. Therefore; the pro- and anti-inflammatory responses of alveolar bone, periodontal ligament, and inflammatory cells to orthodontic force are required to be known in order to develop safe methods to shorten orthodontic treatment period.

3. Accelerated tooth movement

The methods which accelerate tooth movement can be classified in three groups:

1. Chemical applications (local or systemic applications)
2. Mechanical-physical stimulations
3. Surgical-assisted techniques [14]

3.1. Chemical applications

In this method, substances such as prostaglandins, corticosteroids, vitamin D, cytokines, neuropeptides, leukotrienes, nitric oxide, diazepam, and vasoactive medications, which are considered as physiological agents that transform mechanical forces into cellular response, are used to decrease the resistance to the strength applied during tooth movement that occurs within the cells and to change the environmental factors [15, 16].

Taking systemic effect rather than being limited to the applied area and affecting other target cells in the body are reported as a common side effect of using these hormones and medications [17]. Therefore, there is no medication treatment which safely accelerates tooth movement [18].

3.2. Mechanical-physical stimulations

It was reported that stimulating periodontal ligament mechanically or physically can increase alveolar bone remodeling and tooth movement accordingly. Physical methods frequently include equipment-assisted treatment methods [6] such as low-dose laser applications, electromagnetic field, direct electrical current, and vibrational applications. These methods take effect by inducing signal molecules such as receptor activator of nuclear factor-kappa

B (RANK), receptor activator of nuclear factor-kappa B ligand (RANKL) pathway, mitogen-activated protein kinase (MAPK), c-fos, and nitric oxide [6, 19].

Low-dosage laser applications are reported to increase osteoblastic and osteoclastic activity by stimulating cellular proliferation and differentiation and accelerate orthodontic tooth movement without creating side effects on periodontal ligament [6, 20].

It is also reported that electromagnetic field applications increased levels of a group of enzyme which is responsible from regulating intracellular metabolism and cellular proliferation accordingly by influencing sodium-calcium change speed in cell membrane [21]. Increase in osteoblastic and osteoclastic activity causes an acceleration in the tooth movement. Darendeliler et al. [22] reported that static magnetic field accelerated tooth movement by shortening unproductive period when no tooth movement is observed but the side effect can be a decrease in serum calcium and slight changes in the chemistry of blood.

Applying direct electric current is also among tooth acceleration techniques, but its clinical use is asserted as not appropriate due to some complications such as application difficulty, ionic reactions that cause damages in tissues, and replacing of bone tissue with connective tissue [23].

Resonance vibration and ultrasonic vibration are also among the methods which are used to accelerate tooth movement. Resonance vibration is reported to increase release of peptide which is called RANKL within periodontal ligament and increase tooth movement rate by providing formation, function, and continuity of osteoclasts. Tooth movement can also be accelerated via ultrasonic vibration with the same mechanism but there is a risk that the heat can cause damage in the dental pulp [19].

3.3. Surgical-assisted techniques

The most clinically used and predictable option with stable results among the techniques which accelerate tooth movement is the surgical-assisted technique; it is evaluated as a costly invasive method [6]. It is based on the idea that rapid tooth movement can be achieved by increasing the biological response which is formed in periodontal ligament and alveolar bone. Creating an injury in the bone is a potential physical mechanism which provides rapid tissue recovery. Higher regional tissue response during this tissue remodeling/regeneration period is called as regional acceleratory phenomenon (RAP) [24]. Regional acceleratory phenomenon is a complex physiological case in which initially osteoclastic activity and secondly bone density is decreased followed by a rapid osteoblastic activity and a remodeling process. Orthodontic tooth movement acceleration is provided via the increase in cytokine activity around the teeth and decrease in cortical bone resistance and formation of hyalinization tissue by activation of this recovery mechanisms [25]. The advantages of the dentoalveolar surgical intervention in orthodontic treatment of adult patients are reported as: (a) less treatment time, (b) avoidance of potential periodontal complications, (c) favorable direction of growth, and (d) extensive envelope of the tooth movement [26].

3.3.1. Corticotomy and osteotomy combinations

They were first used by Heinrich Köle who stated that the basic resistance toward tooth movement was in cortical layer so by applying corticotomies and osteotomies might accelerate tooth movement by breaking the resistance [27]. Köle et al. applied vertical corticotomies between the roots of two adjacent teeth buccally and lingually and horizontal osteotomies subapically as to combine corticotomies buccal-lingually. They theorized that the segments which became "blocks of bone" move as a whole to achieve rapid tooth movement without devitalization in long-term monitoring. Düker et al. also reported that pulpal and periodontal tissues of the teeth which were applied orthodontic force similarly were not damaged in their study on dogs with reference to Köle's corticotomies [28].

Although Köle and Düker proposed the opposite, periodontal and pulpal damages can be formed following invasive horizontal subapical osteotomies [29]. Additionally, osteotomy surgery is an invasive intervention with possible complications such as vascular and nerve damages so it is not a widely accepted method [30]. Nonetheless, Köle's studies pioneered surgery-assisted methods which accelerate tooth movement to be involved in the literature of modern orthodontics.

3.3.2. Corticotomy-assisted treatments

Köle's horizontal subapical osteotomies were changed with horizontal subapical corticotomies by Gantes et al. [31] and Suya [32] and it was stated that treatment of the cases was completed in almost 50% less period when compared to conventional methods. Gantes et al. [31] reported that overall vitality of the tooth was preserved and none of the patients had a periodontal damage that can be clinically recognized despite minimal root resorptions and gingival recession. Suya [32] asserted that corticotomy-assisted orthodontics had less root resorption and relapse risk and pain when compared to traditional treatments. In a recent study, Uzuner et al. [33] reported that corticotomy-assisted orthodontics increased the rate of tooth movement during canine retraction in 20% ratio and also relative bodily movement was achieved with the corticotomy-combined treatment.

3.3.3. Periodontal ligament distraction

The method was introduced to orthodontic literature by Liou and Huang [34]. Initially, a distractor device which consists of canine and molar bands was applied to the patients by the researchers and following extraction of upper first premolar teeth, surgical preparation phase which consists of two vertical channels formed buccally and lingually toward canine teeth through the extraction socket and a horizontal incision on the base of the extraction socket that connects the channels was completed at the same session. Interseptal bone was not cut mesiodistally during the surgical intervention. Activation was carried out without a need for latent period different from traditional distraction method and distalization of canine teeth was completed in a short period of 3 weeks with minimal anchorage loss. None of the patients suffered from pain and minimal resorption was observed in the roots of canine teeth in the radiographies at the end of procedure. Suggesting to be used especially in orthodontic treatments with primary premolar extraction which has anterior crowded teeth, Liou and Huang [34] associate the periodontal ligament distraction with this method to the distraction which is formed in midpalatal suture during rapid maxillary expansion.

3.3.4. Dentoalveolar distraction

The method was introduced by Kişnişci et al. [35] in 2002. The researchers applied a distraction device before teeth extraction as in periodontal ligament distraction method but a more rigid device was used. Initially, the osteotomy curved apically at a distance of 3–5 mm from the apex of the canine at the same session with the primary premolar tooth extraction as a surgical preparation. Cortical bone which remained in the buccal of the socket after the extraction was carefully removed. Direct distraction was applied by skipping latent period similar to periodontal ligament distraction method. Canine distraction was reported to be completed within 8–12 days without anchorage loss. Root resorption or vitality loss was not observed in the posttreatment evaluations.

Although a faster canine distalization is achieved with less teeth tilting in dentoalveolar distraction method when compared to periodontal ligament distraction method, it is clear to be a more invasive method [36].

3.3.5. Periodontally accelerated osteogenic orthodontics

The method which is known as "Wilckodontics" or "periodontally accelerated osteogenic orthodontics" was introduced by Wilcko and Wilcko [9, 37–40]. According to the researchers, achieving optimal tooth movement is possible by forming a bone layer of 1.5 mm or less on the root surface in the direction of movement in corticotomy-assisted orthodontic treatment. When the force is applied, soft tissue matrix and osteoid islets remaining from the demineralized layer move with the root and remineralized when the orthodontic movement is completed. Wilcko brothers explained the acceleration of tooth movement following corticotomy with demineralization-remineralization period that is generated from rapid osteoclastic activity in alveolar bone in the beginning of "regional acceleratory phenomenon" which was introduced by Frost [24]. According to this mechanism, less resorption and rapid orthodontic tooth movement is achieved as a result of the decrease in alveolar bone density and increased metabolic activity in bone tissue. Thus, the term "movement of bone blocks" which was defined by Köle [27] was replaced with the term "bone matrix transplantation."

Wilcko and Wilcko discussed the need for applying a bone graft in order to prevent dehiscences, fenestrations, and relapses which can occur in posttreatment period due to the decrease in alveolar bone density within the cases with buccal move of the roots or thin buccal bones following corticotomy. They proposed to use resorbable bone graft by saturating clindamycin phosphate or platelet-rich plasma and creating circular perforations on the surface of the bone in order to increase blooding of graft material if the cortical bone thickness is sufficient [37]. The applied surgery apart from this procedure is almost the same with Suya procedure [32]. In this technique, bonding and applying forces to teeth is initiated 1 week earlier from the surgical intervention and biweekly orthodontic examinations are recommended.

Treatments are completed in three or four times shorter periods with "periodontally accelerated osteogenic orthodontics" method when compared to traditional orthodontic treatments besides its increased root resorption and relapse risks. Its need for additional surgical intervention with an extra cost, possibility of bone loss in alveolar crest, and gingival recession following the surgery and surgical complications such as pain and edema are among the disadvantages of the procedure.

3.3.6. Corticision

The necessity to remove flaps during corticotomy-assisted orthodontic treatment makes the method invasive, decreasing its acceptability by the patients and clinicians. Therefore, corticision was introduced by Park et al. [41] as an alternative approach for corticotomy procedures. The researchers made the patients rinse their mouth with an antiseptic mouthwash and then placed a stabilized scalpel on the attached gingiva interradicularly as to make an angle of 45–60 with the long axle of root of the teeth and applied cortical incisions via a surgical hammer without removing flaps [42]. Incisions were applied as 2/3 of the roots vertically and in 10 mm depth. Corticision area must be cleaned with physiological saline solution until hemorrhage stops. Park reported that fixed orthodontic treatment of a patient without extraction was completed in a short period of 10 months through this method. Although corticision method is minimally invasive with a short surgical intervention, it is not widely accepted as it is not appropriate to grafting and the surgical technique is disturbing for the patience.

3.3.7. Piezocision

In 2009, Dibart et al. [43] introduced a minimally invasive technique that can be applied by piezosurgical tools, the piezoincision method, which can be carried out without any flap surgery as in corticision method but it allows hard or soft tissue grafting differently. In this method, small piezoelectric incisions are placed in the area from the targeted corticotomy area to periost. Piezoincisions of 3 mm length and depth are applied with the piezosaw without removing mucoperiosteal flap. In this stage, mucoperiosteal flap can be removed as a tunnel and a bone graft in pad form can be replaced if necessary. Sutures are required if grafting is applied, otherwise there is no need for sutures. It was reported that no significant difference was found in terms of tooth movement speed and root resorption in the studies which compare corticotomy-assisted methods with piezoincision method [44].

Piezoincision is a practical, minimally invasive, and effective method. Additionally, ultrasonic vibrations which occur during the procedure in piezoincision method also contribute to accelerate tooth movement [3]. Required precautions must be taken before the procedure with patients in high-risk group due to possibility of temporary bacteremia formation risk following the procedure.

3.3.8. Piezopuncture

"Piezopuncture" method, which is applied by using an ultrasonic piezosurgical tool, "piezotome" without gingival incisions in piezoincision method was developed by Kim et al. [45]. In their study on 10 dogs, the researchers created several cortical punctures both buccally and lingually on the mesial and distal sides of the teeth which will be moved and reported that anabolic activity and tooth movement were accelerated at the end of the procedure. Omidkhoda et al. who carried out piezopuncture technique on human reported that tooth movement was accelerated but they observed distal tilt in the canine teeth crowns in their case reports which consist of two cases [46].

"Piezopuncture" method also takes part in literature as a method with promising positive results but it must be evaluated by further clinical studies.

4. Micro-osteoperforations

Orthodontic tooth movement is a biological response which is created by an external force that will prevent the dentofacial complex to be in physiological balance [13]. Orthodontic force creates an aseptic inflammatory response in periodontal tissues. An increase on vascular permeability and cellular infiltration of leucocytes was reported in the early period of orthodontic tooth movement [47]. Along with native cells such as osteoblasts and fibroblasts, migrated immune cells produce inflammatory cytokines that include chemotactic factors, growth factor, monocyte-derived factor, lymphocyte, and colony-stimulating factors [48, 49]. The gingival crevicular fluid of moving teeth includes tumor necrosis factor-α (TNFα), interleukin-1 (IL-1), IL-2, IL-3, IL-6, IL-8, osteoclast differentiation factor, and interferon-γ (IFNγ) [48, 50].

Orthodontic tooth movement rate is basically found associated with the rate of bone resorption which is controlled by osteoclast activity [51]. Therefore, any factors which effect activities of osteoclast precursor cells and their transformations into osteoclasts can be assumed to have significant effects on orthodontic tooth movement. There are a lot of researches that report the increase in the activity of inflammatory markers such as chemokines and cytokines as a response to orthodontic forces [5, 25]. It is reported that several cytokines which play role in osteoclast formation and activity such as TNFα, IL-1, and IL-6 are found in gingival crevicular fluid during orthodontic tooth movement [25]. Although the roles of chemokines and cytokines during orthodontic treatment are not clearly known, they are valued as essential mediators for orthodontic tooth movement in terms of their significant roles on differentiation and activity of osteoclast cells [52–54]. Significant decrease on orthodontic tooth movement rate within the studies in which the effects of these markers are blocked via different techniques such as anti-inflammatory medication or genetic manipulation can be accepted as a proof that these factors are extremely efficient on orthodontic tooth movement rate [55–57]. Previous studies represent that surgical interventions which cause minor bone traumas increase inflammatory cytokines, bone remodeling, and orthodontic tooth movement acceleration together with regional bone density [24, 58]. Surgery-assisted techniques which are applied in order to accelerate orthodontic tooth movement should be studied under subtitles such as corticotomy and osteotomy techniques, dental distraction technique, perisegmental corticotomy, and piezoincision. Corticotomy-assisted orthodontic treatment increases bone remodeling which accelerates recovery and repair mechanisms and tooth movement rate accordingly by creating a mechanical trauma in cortical bone [59]. Although corticotomy-assisted orthodontic treatment was reported to be an efficient method in accelerating tooth movement, the significance of removing flaps is also stated to cause important postoperative complications [60]. Piezoincision technique, which is a minimally invasive technique that includes piezoelectric incisions without removing flaps, was developed in order to overcome these disadvantages [43]. Piezoincision is known to be an effective method for acceleration of tooth movement but it was reported to have high risks of damaging tooth roots [18]. Surgery-assisted techniques are invasive with disadvantages such as bone loss, postoperative pain, edema and infection, avascular necrosis besides low acceptance rates by the patients [37, 40]. Based on this, the hypothesis that small osteoperforations on cortical bone without removing flaps will increase bone remodeling and tooth movement rate accordingly by stimulating release of inflammatory cytokines minimizing these disadvantages was developed (**Figure 1**). Micro-osteoperforation is an up-to-date procedure which is promoted as an auxiliary dentoalveolar procedure which can accelerate tooth movement via minimum surgical interventions.

In their animal study in 2010, Teixeira et al. [25] classified 48 rats, which were applied experimental orthodontic tooth movement, into four groups as one group with only orthodontic forces, a group via application of soft tissue flaps together with orthodontic force, a group that was applied 3 small perforations on cortical plate with soft tissue flaps together and orthodontic force and a control group. The researchers stated that they formed the microperforations in the cortical bone by using a round bur and handpiece. It was observed that at the end of experimental tooth movement period, release of 37 out of the 92 cytokines increased in all experimental groups and 21 of them were at the maximum level in the group which was applied perforation. In addition to that, light and fluorescent microscopy, microcomputed tomography, and immunohistochemistry examinations, which were carried at the end of the experiment, represented a significant increase in osteoclast number which accompanied by generalized osteoporosis and orthodontic tooth rate besides bone remodeling activity [25]. Similar to previous studies, researchers also demonstrated that the increase in bone remodeling was not limited around the loaded teeth but also involved the periodontal structures of the adjacent teeth. The researchers, who argued that the observed effects of osteoperforations on tooth movement can be related to loss in bone structure rather than release of increased inflammatory cytokine, stated that perforations were applied in the smallest amount and number possible and the remaining cortical bone was healthy in order to minimize this possibility. These findings also represent that the perforations that will be applied in order to accelerate tooth movement rate are not necessarily be adjacent to the moved teeth. Stating that inflammation can cause negative effects on periodontium and tooth structure when it is uncontrolled because it is a double-sided injury, it is also reported that applying micro-osteoperforations instead of some surgical interventions such as corticotomy, which are applied for acceleration of tooth movement, can minimize the side effects.

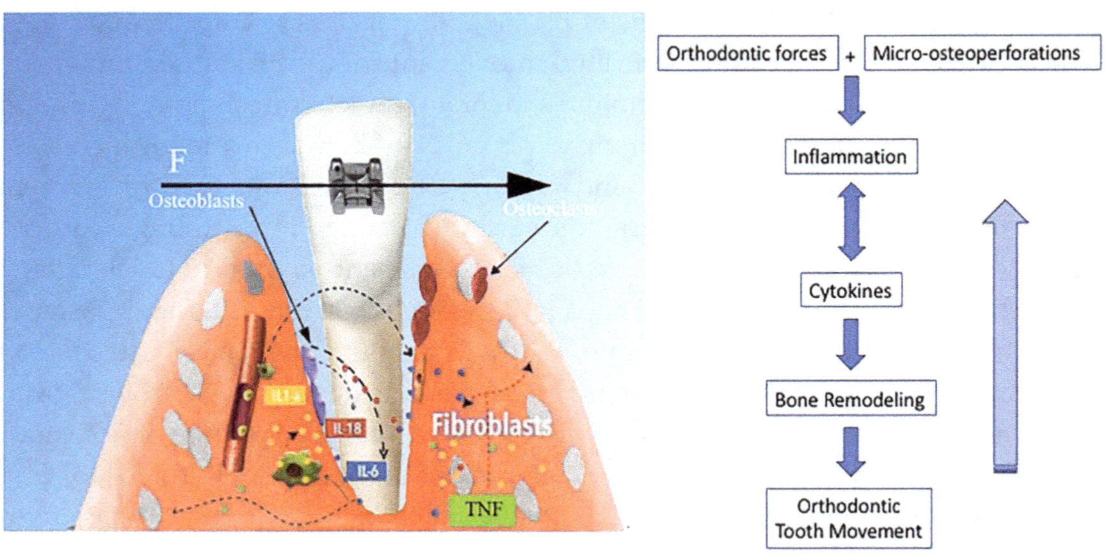

Figure 1. Micro-osteoperforations on cortical bone increase bone remodeling and tooth movement rate by stimulating release of inflammatory cytokines.

Tsai et al. [11] applied both micro-osteoperforations and corticision without removing flaps different from the previous studies and evaluated the differences between the procedures in their animal study which was carried out to evaluate the effects of micro-osteoperforations and corticisions on orthodontic tooth movement rate. It was stated that bone and bone mineral densities were significantly decreased when compared to control group and tooth movement rate was increased in both groups without any significant difference. The rise in tooth movement rate in both groups in this study is smaller than the previous studies. The researchers, who stated that there might be a direct proportion between trauma amount and remodeling rate, reported that the difference was resulted from the smaller amount of the trauma as the flap was not removed.

In 2016, Cheung et al. [12] published a study which evaluated the effectiveness of micro-osteoperforations. Mini-implants were used in order to form micro-osteoperforations different from the previous animal studies and the existence of external apical root resorption was evaluated following the procedure. Similar to previous studies, it was observed that there was a decrease on the density and volume of the bone surrounding moved molar teeth compared with the control side besides the acceleration of orthodontics tooth movement on the side where micro-osteoperforations were applied in the split mouth design study with six rats. Histological examinations also showed that new bone formation increased as well as osteoclast numbers on the side with micro-osteoperforations. This is a proof of the existence of osteoclasts-osteoblast coupling formation with decortication. Despite the fact that resorption and new bone formation were represented together, bone fraction volume and bone mineral density was decreased, which shows that resorption was more than new bone formation during tooth movement period. Contrary to conventional theories which assert osteoclast activity is limited to pressure area, the recent studies show that periodontium was remodeled as a single unit [61]. This study also shows that osteoclast rate in all alveolar bone surrounding the moving teeth is clearly on the pressure areas.

Alikhani et al. [5] designed a clinical trial to evaluate tooth movement with or without micro-osteoperforations in order to investigate whether this phenomenon occurs in human or not. They called the technique of creating micro-osteoperforations in the bone as "alveocentesis." In their study, 20 adults were divided into 2 groups as control and experimental groups. Micro-osteoperforations were applied in the experimental group on one side of the maxilla using a disposable micro-osteoperforation device designed for this purpose by Propel Orthodontics (Ossining NY) and the control group did not receive any micro-osteoperforations. Following 28 days of canine retraction period, amount of the tooth movement was measured and also the activity of inflammatory mediators was determined in gingival crevicular fluid with an antibody-based protein assay. Additionally, the presence of pain or discomfort was evaluated with a numeric rating scale. Results of this first clinical trial about micro-osteoperforations in the literature reported significant increase in the levels of inflammatory markers and also 2.3-times rise in the rate of tooth movement with micro-osteoperforations. However, significant pain or discomfort during or after the procedure was not reported by the patients; also, any other complications were not observed.

It was stated that orthognathic surgery, corticotomies (applying several incisions and perforations with removing flaps), piezoincision (creating injury on the bone with small incisions without removing flaps via a piezoelectric device), and even tooth extractions will increase the release of inflammatory markers and bone remodeling by creating injuries similar to micro-osteoperforations on alveolar bone effecting the rate of tooth movement accordingly [5]. Unfortunately, increase of inflammatory marker release cannot continue for a long period of time and a decrease in cytokine activity is observed regardless of the severity of the trauma after 2–3 months [4] which reveals the necessity for repeating the procedure during orthodontic treatment. Therefore, the extraction is suggested to be applied at the same time with major tooth movement for the patients whose tooth is planned to be extracted. There will not be a need for micro-osteoperforation requirement to accelerate tooth movement process as remodeling will speed up. In other words, it would be appropriate to prefer micro-osteoperforations in the treatments without tooth extraction or when extraction is carried out long after the orthodontic treatment because its effects are similar to tooth extraction. It is considered that as the level of trauma increases, inflammatory response will also rise. The rise on tooth movement rate when micro-osteoperforation number is increased can be shown as a proof. It was stated that regional acceleratory phenomenon (RAP) took effect in 1 or 2 days following the surgical intervention and reached its maximum level in 1 or 2 months [9]. Aboul-Ela et al. [59], Al-Naoum et al. [62], and Leethanakul et al. [63] reported that tooth movement speed was high during 2 months following the creation of traumas in cortical layers but it gradually decreased in this period. Alikhani et al. also stated that cytokine activity decreased after 2 months following micro-osteoperforation so they proposed that the procedure shall be repeated after a month break [4]. Micro-osteoperforations are repeatable which can be considered as an advantage because application time can affect the results in all surgically assisted procedures. On the other hand, there is not a clear information on how frequently micro-osteoperforations can be applied in order to achieve an optimum acceleration in tooth movement rate.

In a recent thesis study in Akdeniz University, Faculty of Dentistry, Department of Orthodontics (Antalya, Turkey), efficiency of micro-osteoperforations on molar distalization rate with cervical headgear was evaluated on 3D digital models [64]. About 17 patients whose molar relations were bilateral class II (minimum teeth to teeth) with class I skeletal anomalies or normal or low vertical growth pattern were included in the study which is regarded as the first study to evaluate the efficiency of micro-osteoperforations on molar distalization. Propel device (Ossining, NY) was used to form three micro-osteoperforations—one mesially and two distally—of 1.5 diameter and 5 mm depth on a random molar teeth, in the session where distalization was initiated with cervical headgears in the split-mouth designed study. Micro-osteoperforations were renewed at least twice during the distalization period every 8 weeks in each sample. The procedure continued until class I relationship was achieved on the side where tooth movement was considered to be slower. Studies were carried out on 3D digital models which were taken just before and after molar distalization in order to compare molar distalization rate and tilt and rotation rate in molar teeth. While no significant difference was observed between tilting and rotation rates, it was concluded that on the micro-osteoperforation side, more tooth movement was seen.

Lee et al. [65], who stated that in the studies which evaluated the efficiency of micro-osteoperforations on orthodontic tooth movement, micro-osteoperforations were generally applied on healthy alveolar bone, planned a study considering that the effects of bone remodeling process that was activated by applying orthodontic tooth movement and micro-osteoperforations on the atrophic ridge could be different. The researchers, who created atrophic alveolar ridge model on eight beagle dogs, evaluated tooth movement rates and atrophic alveolar ridge area on the sides with and without osteoperforations in their study which they planned via split mouth design. Micro-CT based histomorphometry analysis similar to the previous studies suggested that osteoperforations accelerated tooth movement with a decrease in bone density without any differences in atrophic ridge volume. This up-to-date finding can be evaluated as an indicator that the efficiency of micro-osteoperforations on bone remodeling is more related to resorption mechanism and osteoclast activation.

In the literature, there is a limited number of studies which evaluate the effects of micro-osteoperforations on tooth movement in human. Current studies indicate that micro-osteoperforation is a safe method that can accelerate tooth movement but it must be taken into consideration that several factors such as occlusal relations, movement type, applied mechanics, age and gender of the patient, oral hygiene, periodontal illnesses, alveolar bone loss, systemic diseases, and medication use effect tooth movement rate in human. Therefore, the efficiency of micro-osteoperforations must be evaluated with long-term studies in which study groups are standardized as much as possible considering these variable where different tooth movement types (distalization, intrusion, eruption of impacted tooth, etc.) and mechanics are applied containing more sample numbers.

4.1. Micro-osteoperforation application techniques

Micro-osteoperforation is an up-to-date method among the surgery-assisted techniques of accelerating tooth movement. Therefore, in the literature, there are studies in which different methods are used in order to create MOPs on alveolar bones.

We observe that low-speed handpiece and round bur combinations [11, 25] and mini-implants [12] are used within the animal studies which evaluate effects of MOPs on tooth movement and both methods are accepted as effective. Even if in a limited number of clinical trial; micro-osteoperforations are typically applied with a handheld disposable appliance designed by Propel Orthodontics (Ossining, NY). Propel is an appliance which is designed to apply alveocentesis procedure. The foremost part of the device which is like an orthodontic stainless steel screw is patented, allowing perforation of alveolar bone traumatically over keratinized gingiva and moving mucosa. Contrary to other rotatory devices, Propel was reported to have a slight effect on soft issue. It is a device which enables tissue remodeling and micro-osteoperforations between tooth roots over both stable and moving tissue of 1.5 mm diameter and 3, 5, and 7 mm depth without flap surgery in order to accelerate tooth movement. The appliance has an adjustable length and a light signal that turns on when the clinician achieved desired depth [5, 64]. Micro-osteoperforations, which are applied on the defined depth, reach to medullar bone from cortical bone increasing inflammatory mediators. The device was also reported not to cause soft tissue damage while enabling remodeling process [5].

While it is not always possible to create homogenous perforations of same size using micro-osteoperforation methods such as round burs, Propel device which is designed in order to form MOPs has not included in routine clinical use yet. Thus, mini-implants are considered more advantageous than other methods as they are included in clinical routine and frequently used by orthodontists for different purposes and easily tolerated by the patients. On the other hand, in the literature, there are limited studies in which mini-implant-facilitated micro-osteoperforations are carried out with human. Aksakalli et al. [66] applied three micro-osteoperforations distal to the canine teeth with miniscrews just before canine distalization period. In their case report, they reported that MOP method with miniscrews accelerated canine distalization in their 14-year-old male patient with class II malocclusion by almost 1.5-fold and also without harmful effects on root and periodontal structures. On the contrary, Alkebsi et al. [67] could not find any differences of anchorage loss, canine rotation, and tipping between the MOP and control sides in their randomized controlled clinical trial where they investigated the effectiveness of miniscrew-facilitated MOPs on the rate of canine distalization.

All of the methods are applied without a need for additional periodontal surgeries which is considered as a significant advantage but additional clinical studies are required in order to evaluate the efficiency of each technique and their advantages and disadvantages over each other in detail.

4.2. Advantages of micro-osteoperforation over other surgical techniques

When micro-osteoperforations are compared with several surgical techniques, which are proved to accelerate tooth movement, they are considered as more advantageous because they are less invasive with no need for removing flaps eliminating possible side effects of the surgery [4, 5]. Additionally, all techniques which make use of micro-osteoperforation do not include an invasive surgical procedure represent that they are easily applicable in the clinics by the orthodontists and can be added to clinical routine. Patients did not report any pain or discomfort in the clinical studies with micro-osteoperforations which shows that it is easily accepted and tolerated by the patients who are under orthodontic treatment [5, 64]. These advantages also enable the micro-osteoperforations to be periodically repeated until the desired results are achieved [4, 64].

4.3. The relation of micro-osteoperforations with pain and root resorption

There is a limited number of studies that evaluate patients' pain and discomfort levels among the clinical studies in which micro-osteoperforations are applied. Alikhani et al. [5] asked their patients to scale their pain and discomfort levels via a numeric rating scale on the day they replaced the device, the day they began canine distalization, 24 h, 7th and 28th days after canine distalization in their study in which they evaluated the effect of micro-osteoperforations on canine distalization. In this scale, which is reported as having high credibility, "0" presents no pain, while "10" stands for the existence of the worst pain. Data analyses showed that the patients had the most pain in 24 h following canine distalization but no significant difference was observed between experimental and control groups. The patients defined a slight and resistible pain on the micro-osteoperforation side which does not require taking painkillers but no statically significant difference was found. The similar feedbacks were taken in Boz's thesis study in 2018 concluding that micro-osteoperforations did not cause a significant pain or discomfort [64]. In line with these findings, it is possible to state that micro-osteoperforations are easily tolerated by the patients and can be applied to routine clinical use.

Orthodontically induced inflammatory root resorption (OIIRR) is included in negative side effects of orthodontic tooth movement as a frequent research subject. Although its etiology and predictors are not fully understood, it is considered to be resulted from complex interaction of individual sensitivity [68], applied mechanics [69, 70], and specific dental predisposition [71]. Orthodontically induced inflammatory root resorption was stated to be related with periodontal ligament remodeling which is a result of the pressure applied to tooth root during tooth movement and removal of hyalinized necrotic tissues after trauma. Excessive pressure that causes ischemic necrosis [72] of periodontal ligament and root resorption related to orthodontic tooth movement is reported to be frequently observed in the areas in which excessive pressure is applied to periodontal ligament [73]. The underlying biological process of both orthodontic tooth movement and root resorption covers local inflammatory response. Animal studies show that many pro-inflammatory cytokines are common in both pathways. Cytokines such as IL-1, TNFα, and chemokines as IL-8 and MCP-1 are known to have significant roles to initiate and ease root resorption process [74]. These inflammatory mediators have significant roles on activation of tooth movement and osteoclast activity [75]. Inhibition of cytokine activity decreases osteoclast and odontoclast rate as well as tooth movement and root resorption [76]. It is known that accelerated tooth movement techniques increase inflammatory cytokine activation.

In the literature, there are several studies that evaluate the effects of accelerated tooth movement and decortication on root resorption [5]. The cytokines which promote inflammation are also reported to activate cementoclasts which cause root resorption increasing root resorption risk accordingly [77]. On the contrary, there are findings in the literature which state that decortication and demineralization of alveolar bone decrease the pressure toward tooth movement enabling an ease for the movement and decreasing root resorption risk accordingly [12]. It was found out that the effects of tooth movement accelerated via corticotomy on orthodontically induced inflammatory root resorption were similar to conventional orthodontic treatment but it was also reported that periapical radiographies may not be reliable for assessing root resorption in two studies which was carried out by evaluation of periapical radiographies [78, 79]. In an animal study which evaluates the effects of corticotomies on tooth movement, it was found out that there were not any differences between control and experimental groups in terms of root resorption [80].

In the literature, there is a limited number of studies which evaluates the effects of micro-osteoperforations on root resorption. Tsai et al. reported in their study in which they compared the efficiency of micro-osteoperforations and corticisions that root resorption creation risk of minor surgical interventions is lower when compared with conventional orthodontic treatments. The hematoxylin and eosin analysis of the researchers showed that micro-osteoperforation-assisted accelerated tooth movement was resulted in decreased root resorption [11]. Similarly, in the study in which Cheung et al. evaluated effects of micro-osteoperforations on experimental tooth movement in rats, root resorption was observed on the MOP application side on the samples which were colored with hematoxylin eosin reporting that 3D volumetric analysis did not show any volumetric difference in the root of upper molar teeth which was moved [12]. Although all findings support the idea that micro-osteoperforations do not increase root resorption risk showing that mini-implants can be safely used for MOP procedures in terms of root resorption, it is clear that there is a need for further supportive studies with increased sample number.

Cheung et al. [12] included 20 patients whose upper primary premolars are planned to be extracted for orthodontic purposes in their study which is known as the initial clinical study to evaluate the effects of MOPs on OIRR. About 150 g buccal tipping force was applied to premolar tooth which was planned to be extracted and micro-osteoperforations of 5 mm depth were applied to mesial and distal parts of the premolar teeth on the experimental side via Propel device (Propel Orthodontics, San Jose, Calif) evaluating the patient's opposite side as the control group. Following 28 days of tooth movement period, premolar tooth on both sides was extracted and examined by microcomputed tomography, volumes of root resorption craters were calculated and compared. Volumetric root loss average of the premolar tooth on the side which micro-osteoperforations are applied was found to be 42% more than the premolars on the control side. The researchers represented that the side to be applied micro-osteoperforations was not randomly selected (decision was taken in accordance with the availability of the distance between the roots) and evaluation was carried out following a short-term tooth movement as the limitations of the study and suggested further studies with treatments of longer terms and larger sample numbers. Nonetheless, when the findings of the study are considered, it can be stated that special attention shall be paid on planning micro-osteoperforations with patients who are individually prone to root resorption.

As a result, there are studies which report that micro-osteoperforations can cause positive and negative effects on root resorption. Their relations were not clearly explained so there is a need for further studies.

5. Conclusions

- Among several techniques which are defined to accelerate orthodontic tooth movement and treatment periods accordingly, due to numerous studies, surgical techniques that have the most predictable results have been an essential part of modern orthodontics.
- Micro-osteoperforations are outstanding as a minimal invasive, easy-to-use, repeatable, and efficient new method that can eliminate some disadvantages of surgery among the defined invasive techniques.
- Experimental studies have proved that micro-osteoperforations accelerated bone remodeling process and orthodontic tooth movement accordingly together with an increase in osteoclast number and new bone formation and a decrease on bone volume and density. A limited number of clinical studies also support the findings.
- Different techniques are defined to apply micro-osteoperforation in the literature but there is a need for studies that evaluate differences between techniques in order to determine the ideal method.

- Further studies are required for the ideal timing and frequency of the application in order to achieve optimum tooth movement acceleration.
- Although it is reported that side effects such as pain or root resorption are not observed due to micro-osteoperforations, long-term studies with more samples are required.

Author details

Esra Bolat

Address all correspondence to: dtesrabolat@gmail.com

Department of Orthodontics, Faculty of Dentistry, Akdeniz University, Antalya, Turkey

References

[1] Ngan P, Kess B, Wilson S. Perception of discomfort by patients undergoing orthodontic treatment. American Journal of Orthodontics and Dentofacial Orthopedics. 1989;**96**: 47-53. DOI: 10.1016/0889-5406(89)90228-X

[2] Zahrowski J, Jeske A. Apical root resorption is associated with comprehensive orthodontic treatment but not clearly dependent on prior tooth characteristics or orthodontşc techniques. Journal of the American Dental Association. 2011;**142**:66-68. DOI: 10.14219/ jada.archive.2011.0030

[3] Huang H, Williams RC, Kyrkanides S. Accelerated orthodontic tooth movement: Molecular mechanisms. American Journal of Orthodontics and Dentofacial Orthopedics. 2014; **146**:620-632. DOI: 10.1016/j.ajodo.2014.07.007

[4] Alikhani M, Alansari S, Sansuwon C, Alikhani M, Chou MY, Alyami B, et al. Micro-osteoperforations: Minimally invasive accelerated tooth movement. Seminars in Orthodontics. 2015;**21**:162-169. DOI: 10.1053/j.sodo.2015.06.002

[5] Alikhani M, Raptis M, Zoldan B, Sangsuwon C, Lee YB, Alyami B, et al. Effect of micro-osteoperforations on the rate of tooth movement. American Journal of Orthodontics and Dentofacial Orthopedics. 2013;**144**(5):639-648. DOI: 10.1016/j.ajodo.2013.06.017

[6] Nimeri G, Kau CH, Abou-Kheir NS, Corona R. Acceleration of tooth movement during orthodontic treatment—A frontier in orthodontics. Progress in Orthodontics. 2013;**14**: 1-8. DOI: 10.1186/2196-1042-14-42

[7] Yamasaki K, Shibata Y, Imai S, Tani Y, Shibasaki Y, Fukuhara T. Clinical application of prostaglandin E1 (PGE1) upon orthodontic tooth movement. American Journal of Orthodontics. 1984;**85**(6):508-518. DOI: 10.1016/0002-9416(84)90091-5

[8] Fujita S, Yamaguchi M, Utsunomiya T, Yamamoto H, Kasai K. Low-energy laser stimulates tooth movement velocity via expression of RANK and RANKL. Orthodontics & Craniofacial Research. 2008;**11**(3):143-155. DOI: 10.1111/j.1601-6343.2008.00423.x

[9] Wilcko MT, Wilcko WM, Bissada NF. An evidence-based analysis of periodontally accelerated orthodontic and osteogenic techniques: A synthesis of scientific perspectives. Seminars in Orthodontics. 2008;**14**:305-316. DOI: 10.1053/j.sodo.2008.07.007

[10] Aksakalli S, Calik B, Kara B, Ezirganli S. Accelerated tooth movement with piezocision and its periodontal-transversal effects in patients with Class II malocclusion. The Angle Orthodontist. 2016;**86**(1):59-65. DOI: 10.2319/012215-49.1

[11] Tsai CY, Yang TK, Hsieh HY, Yang LY. Comparison of the effects of micro-osteoperforation and corticision on the rate of orthodontic tooth movement in rats. The Angle Orthodontist. 2016;**86**(4):558-564. DOI: 10.2319/052015-343.1

[12] Cheung T, Park J, Lee D, Kim C, Olson J, Javadi S, et al. Ability of mini-implant-facilitated micro-osteoperforations to accelerate tooth movement in rats. American Journal of Orthodontics and Dentofacial Orthopedics. 2016;**150**(6):958-967. DOI: 10.1016/j.ajodo.2016.04.030

[13] Proffit WR, Fields HW, Sarver DM. Contemporary Orthodontics. 5th ed. St. Louis: Elsevier Health Sciences; 2014. 278 p

[14] Ren A, Lv T, Kang N, Zhao B, Chen Y, Bai D. Rapid orthodontic tooth movement aided by alveolar surgery in beagles. American Journal of Orthodontics and Dentofacial Orthopedics. 2007;**131**(2):160.e1-160.10. DOI: 10.1016/j.ajodo.2006.05.029

[15] Bartzela T, Türp JC, Motschall E, Maltha JC. Medication effects on the rate of orthodontic tooth movement: A systematic literature review. American Journal of Orthodontics and Dentofacial Orthopedics. 2009;**135**(1):16-26. DOI: 10.1016/j.ajodo.2008.08.016

[16] Sekhavat AR, Mousavizadeh K, Pakshir HR, Aslani FS. Effect of misoprostol, a prostaglandin E1 analog, on orthodontic tooth movement in rats. American Journal of Orthodontics and Dentofacial Orthopedics. 2002;**122**(5):542-547. DOI: 10.1067/mod.2002.126153

[17] Tunçer Nİ, Yılmaz A. Tooth movement acceleretaion techniques. Türk Ortodonti Dergisi. 2012;**25**:76-91

[18] Shenava S, Nayak K, Bhaskar V, Nayak A. Accelerated orthodontics—A review. International Journal of Scientific Study. 2014;**1**(5):35-39

[19] Nishimura M, Chiba M, Ohashi T, Sato M, Shimizu Y, Igarashi K, et al. Periodontal tissue activation by vibration: Intermittent stimulation by resonance vibration accelerates experimental tooth movement in rats. American Journal of Orthodontics and Dentofacial Orthopedics. 2008;**133**(4):572-583. DOI: 10.1016/j.ajodo.2006.01.046

[20] Ozawa Y, Shimizu N, Kariya G, Abiko Y. Low-energy laser irradiation stimulates bone nodule formation at early stages of cell culture in rat calvarial cells. Bone. 1998;**22**(4): 347-354. DOI: 10.1016/S8756-3282(97)00294-9

[21] Stark TM, Sinclair PM. Effect of pulsed electromagnetic fields on orthodontic tooth movement. American Journal of Orthodontics and Dentofacial Orthopedics. 1987;**91**(2):91-104. DOI: 10.1016/0889-5406(87)90465-3

[22] Darendeliler MA, Sinclair PM, Kusy RP. The effects of samarium-cobalt magnets and pulsed electromagnetic fields on tooth movement. American Journal of Orthodontics and Dentofacial Orthopedics. 1995;**107**(6):578-588. DOI: 10.1001/jama.1982.03320300027017

[23] Basset CA, Mitchell SN, Gaston SR. Pulsing electromagnetic field treatment in ununited fractures and failed arthrodeses. Journal of the American Medical Association. 1982; **247**(5):623-628. DOI: 10.1001/jama.1982.03320300027017

[24] Frost HM. The regional acceleratory phenomenon: A review. Henry Ford Hospital Medical Journal. 1983;**31**(1):3-9

[25] Teixeira CC, Khoo E, Tran J, Chartres I, Liu Y, Thant LM, et al. Cytokine expression and accelerated tooth movement. Journal of Dental Research. 2010;**89**(10):1135-1141. DOI: 10.1177/0022034510373764

[26] Uzuner FD, Darendeliler N. Dentoalveolar surgery techniques combined with orthodontic treatment: A literature review. European Journal of Dentistry. 2013;**7**:257-265. DOI: 10.4103/1305-7456.110201

[27] Köle H. Surgical operations on the alveolar ridge to correct occlusal abnormalities. Oral Surgery, Oral Medicine, and Oral Pathology. 1959;**12**(5):515-529. DOI: 10.1016/0030-4220(59)90153-7

[28] Düker J. Experimental animal research into segmental alveolar movement after corticotomy. Journal of Maxillofacial Surgery. 1975;**3**(2):81-84. DOI: 10.1016/S0301-0503(75)80022-1

[29] Bell WH, Levy BM. Revascularization and bone healing after maxillary corticotomies. Journal of Oral Surgery. 1972;**30**(9):640-648

[30] Hoogeveen EJ, Jansma J, Ren Y. Surgically facilitated orthodontic treatment: A systematic review. American Journal of Orthodontics and Dentofacial Orthopedics. 2014;**145**(4): 51-64. DOI: 10.1016/j.ajodo.2013.11.019

[31] Gantes B, Rathbun E, Anholm M. Effects on the periodontium following corticotomy-facilitated orthodontics. Case reports. Journal of Periodontology. 1990;**61**(4):234-238. DOI: 10.1902/jop.1990.61.4.234

[32] Suya H. Corticotomy in orthodontics. In: Hosl E, Baldauf A, editors. Mechanical and Biological Basis in Orthodontic Therapy. Heidelberg, Germany: Huthig Buch Verlag; 1991. pp. 207-226

[33] Uzuner FD, Yücel E, Göfteci B, Gülşen A. The effect of corticotomy on tooth movements during canine retraction. Journal of Orthodontic Research. 2015;**3**:181-187. DOI: 10.4103/2321-3825.159548

[34] Liou EJ, Huang CS. Rapid canine retraction through distraction of the periodontal ligament. American Journal of Orthodontics and Dentofacial Orthopedics. 1998;**114**(4): 372-382. DOI: 10.1016/S0889-5406(98)70181-7

[35] Kişnişci RS, Işeri H, Tüz HH, Altug AT. Dentoalveolar distraction osteogenesis for rapid orthodontic canine retraction. Journal of Oral and Maxillofacial Surgery. 2002;**60**(4): 389-394. DOI: 10.1053/joms.2002.31226

[36] Kharkar VR, Kotrashetti SM, Kulkarni P. Comparative evaluation of dento-alveolar distraction and periodontal distraction assisted rapidretraction of the maxillary canine: A pilot study. International Journal of Oral and Maxillofacial Surgery. 2010;**39**(11): 1074-1109. DOI: 10.1016/j.ijom.2010.06.012

[37] Wilcko WM, Wilcko T, Bouquot JE, Ferguson DJ. Rapid orthodontics with alveolar reshaping: Two case reports of decrowding. The International Journal of Periodontics & Restorative Dentistry. 2001;**21**(1):9-19

[38] Wilcko MW, Ferguson DJ, Bouquot JE, Wilcko MT. Rapid orthodontic decrowding with alveolar augmentation: Case report. World Journal of Orthodontics. 2003;**4**:197-205

[39] Wilcko MT, Wilcko WM, Pulver JJ, Bissada NF, Bouquot JE. Accelerated osteogenic orthodontics technique: A 1-stage surgically facilitated rapid orthodontic technique with alveolar augmentation. Journal of Oral and Maxillofacial Surgery. 2009;**67**(10):2149-2159. DOI: 10.1016/j.joms.2009.04.095

[40] Murphy KG, Wilcko MT, Wilcko WM, Ferguson DJ. Periodontal accelerated osteogenic orthodontics: A description of the surgical technique. Journal of Oral and Maxillofacial Surgery. 2009;**67**(10):2160-2166. DOI: 10.1016/j.joms.2009.04.124

[41] Park YG, Kang SG, Kim SJ. Accelerated tooth movement by corticision as an osseous orthodontic paradigm. Kinki Tokai Kyosei Shika Gakkai Gakuiyutsu Taikai Sokai. 2006;**48**(6):6-15

[42] Park YG. Corticision: A flapless procedure to accelerate tooth movement. Frontiers of Oral Biology. 2016;**18**:109-117. DOI: 10.1159/000351904

[43] Dibart S, Sebaoun JD, Surmenian J. Piezocision: A minimally invasive, periodontally accelerated orthodontic tooth movement procedure. The Compendium of Continuing Education in Dentistry. 2009;**30**(6):342-344

[44] Abbas NH, Sabet NE, Hassan IT. Evaluation of corticotomy-facilitated orthodontics and piezocision in rapid canine retraction. American Journal of Orthodontics and Dentofacial Orthopedics. 2016;**149**(4):473-480. DOI: 10.1016/j.ajodo.2015.09.029

[45] Kim YS, Kim SJ, Yoon HJ, Lee PJ, Moon W, Park YG. Effect of piezopuncture on tooth movement and bone remodeling in dogs. American Journal of Orthodontics and Dentofacial Orthopedics. 2013;**144**(1):23-31. DOI: 10.1016/j.ajodo.2013.01.022

[46] Omidkhoda M, Radvar M, Azizi M, Hasanzadeh N. Piezopuncture-assisted canine distalization in orthodontic patients: Two case reports. Journal of Dentistry (Shiraz). 2018;**19**(1):74-82

[47] Krishnan V, Davidovitch Z. Cellular, molecular, and tissue-level reactions to orthodontic force. American Journal of Orthodontics and Dentofacial Orthopedics. 2006;**129**(4):469.e1-469.32. DOI: 10.1016/j.ajodo.2005.10.007

[48] Ren Y, Vissink A. Cytokines in crevicular fluid and orthodontic tooth movement. European Journal of Oral Sciences. 2008;**116**(2):89-97. DOI: 10.1111/j.1600-0722.2007.00511.x

[49] Krishnan V, Davidovitch Z. On a path to unfolding the biological mechanisms of orthodontic tooth movement. Journal of Dental Research. 2009;**88**(7):597-608. DOI: 10.1177/0022034509338914

[50] Alhashimi N, Frithiof L, Brudvik P, Bakhiet M. Orthodontic movement induces high numbers of cells expressing IFN-gamma at mRNA and protein levels. Journal of Interferon & Cytokine Research. 2000;**20**(1):7-12. DOI: 10.1089/107999000312685

[51] Henneman S, Von den Hoff JW, Maltha JC. Mechanobiology of tooth movement. European Journal of Orthodontics. 2008;**30**(3):299-306. DOI: 10.1093/ejo/cjn020

[52] Fuller K, Kirstein B, Chambers TJ. Murine osteoclast formation and function: Differential regulation by humoral agents. Endocrinology. 2006;**147**(4):1979-1985. DOI: 10.1210/en.2005-1340

[53] O'Brien CA, Gubrij I, Lin SC, Saylors RL, Manolagas SC. STAT3 activation in stromal/osteoblastic cells is required for induction of the receptor activator of NF-kappaB ligand and stimulation of osteoclastogenesis by gp130-utilizing cytokines or interleukin-1 but not 1,25-dihydroxyvitamin D3 or parathyroid hormone. The Journal of Biological Chemistry. 1999;**274**(27):19301-19308. DOI: 10.1074/jbc.274.27.19301

[54] Jimi E, Ikebe T, Takahashi N, Hirata M, Suda T, Koga T. Interleukin-1 alpha activates an NF-kappaB-like factor in osteoclast-like cells. The Journal of Biological Chemistry. 1996;**271**(9):4605-4608. DOI: 10.1074/jbc.271.9.4605

[55] Taddei SR, Andrade I Jr, Queiroz-Junior CM, Garlet TP, Garlet GP, Cunha Fde Q, et al. Role of CCR2 in orthodontic tooth movement. American Journal of Orthodontics and Dentofacial Orthopedics. 2012;**141**(2):153-160. DOI: 10.1016/j.ajodo.2011.07.019

[56] Iwasaki LR, Haack JE, Nickel JC, Reinhardt RA, Petro TM. Human interleukin-1 beta and interleukin-1 receptor antagonist secretion and velocity of tooth movement. Archives of Oral Biology. 2001;**46**(2):185-189. DOI: 10.1016/S0003-9969(00)00088-1

[57] Knop LA, Shintcovsk RL, Retamoso LB, Ribeiro JS, Tanaka OM. Non-steroidal and steroidal anti-inflammatory use in the context of orthodontic movement. European Journal of Orthodontics. 2012;**34**(5):531-535. DOI: 10.1093/ejo/cjq173

[58] Yaffe A, Fine N, Binderman I. Regional accelerated phenomenon in the mandible following mucoperiosteal flap surgery. Journal of Periodontology. 1994;**65**(1):79-83. DOI: 10.1902/jop.1994.65.1.79

[59] Aboul-Ela SM, El-Beialy AR, El-Sayed KM, Selim EM, El-Mangoury NH, Mostafa YA. Miniscrew implant-supported maxillary canine retraction with and without corticotomy-facilitated orthodontics. American Journal of Orthodontics and Dentofacial Orthopedics. 2011;**139**(2):252-259. DOI: 10.1016/j.ajodo.2009.04.028

[60] Sebaoun JD, Surmenian J, Dibart S. Accelerated orthodontic treatment with piezocision: A mini-invasive alternative to conventional corticotomies. L'Orthodontie Française. 2011;**82**(4):311-319. DOI: 10.1051/orthodfr/2011142

[61] Iglesias-Linares A, Yañez-Vico RM, Moreno-Fernandez AM, Mendoza-Mendoza A, Solano-Reina E. Corticotomy-assisted orthodontic enhancement by bone morphogenetic protein-2 administration. Journal of Oral and Maxillofacial Surgery. 2012;**70**(2):124-132. DOI: 10.1016/j.joms.2011.10.020

[62] Al-Naoum F, Hajeer MY, Al-Jundi A. Does alveolar corticotomy accelerate orthodontic tooth movement when retracting upper canines? A split-mouth design randomized controlled trial. Journal of Oral and Maxillofacial Surgery. 2014;**72**(10):1880-1889. DOI: 10.1016/j.joms.2014.05.003

[63] Leethanakul C, Kanokkulchai S, Pongpanich S, Leepong N, Charoemratrote C. Interseptal bone reduction on the rate of maxillary canine retraction. The Angle Orthodontist. 2014;**84**(5):839-845. DOI: 10.2319/100613-737.1

[64] Boz T. Evaluation the effect of periodontal-accelerated treatment protocols on the rate of tooth movement [thesis]. Antalya: Turkey Akdeniz University; 2018

[65] Lee JW, Cha JY, Park KH, Kang YG, Kim SJ. Effect of flapless osteoperforation-assisted tooth movement on atrophic alveolar ridge: Histomorphometric and gene-enrichment analysis. The Angle Orthodontist. 2018;**88**(1):82-90. DOI: 10.2319/061217-388.1

[66] Aksakalli S, Balaban A, Nazaroglu K, Saglam E. Accelerated tooth movement with orthodontic mini-screws. Case Reports in Dentistry. 2017;**2017**:2327591. DOI: 10.1155/2017/2327591

[67] Alkebsi A, Al-Maaitah E, Al-Shorman H, Abu Alhaija E. Three-dimensional assessment of the effect of micro-osteoperforations on the rate of tooth movement during canine retraction in adults with Class II malocclusion: A randomized controlled clinical trial. American Journal of Orthodontics and Dentofacial Orthopedics. 2018;**153**(6):771-785. DOI: 10.1016/j.ajodo.2017.11.026

[68] Harris EF, Kineret SE, Tolley EA. A heritable component for external apical root resorption in patients treated orthodontically. American Journal of Orthodontics and Dentofacial Orthopedics. 1997;**111**(3):301-309. DOI: 10.1016/S0889-5406(97)70189-6

[69] Roscoe MG, Meira JB, Cattaneo PM. Association of orthodontic force system and root resorption: A systematic review. American Journal of Orthodontics and Dentofacial Orthopedics. 2015;**147**(5):610-626. DOI: 10.1016/j.ajodo.2014.12.026

[70] Weltman B, Vig KW, Fields HW, Shanker S, Kaizar EE. Root resorption associated with orthodontic tooth movement: A systematic review. American Journal of Orthodontics

and Dentofacial Orthopedics. 2010;**137**(4):462-476. Discussion 12A. DOI: 10.1016/j.ajodo.2009.06.021

[71] Sameshima GT, Asgarifar KO. Assessment of root resorption and root shape: Periapical vs panoramic films. The Angle Orthodontist. 2001;**71**(3):185-189

[72] Brezniak N, Wasserstein A. Orthodontically induced inflammatory root resorption. Part I: The basic science aspects. The Angle Orthodontist. 2002;**72**(2):175-179. DOI: 10.1043/0003-3219(2002)072<0175:OIIRRP>2.0.CO;2

[73] Brudvik P, Rygh P. Root resorption after local injection of prostaglandin E2 during experimental tooth movement. European Journal of Orthodontics. 1991;**13**(4):255-263

[74] Asano M, Yamaguchi M, Nakajima R, Fujita S, Utsunomiya T, Yamamoto H, et al. IL-8 and MCP-1 induced by excessive orthodontic force mediates odontoclastogenesis in periodontal tissues. Oral Diseases. 2011;**17**(5):489-498. DOI: 10.1111/j.1601-0825.2010.01780.x

[75] Garlet TP, Coelho U, Repeke CE, Silva JS, Cunha Fde Q, Garlet GP. Differential expression of osteoblast and osteoclast chemmoatractants in compression and tension sides during orthodontic movement. Cytokine. 2008;**42**(3):330-335. DOI: 10.1016/j.cyto.2008.03.003

[76] Jäger A, Zhang D, Kawarizadeh A, Tolba R, Braumann B, Lossdörfer S, et al. Soluble cytokine receptor treatment in experimental orthodontic tooth movement in the rat. European Journal of Orthodontics. 2005;**27**(1):1-11. DOI: 10.1093/ejo/cjh089

[77] Bartok RI, Văideanu T, Dimitriu B, Vârlan CM, Suciu I, Podoleanu D. External radicular resorption: Selected cases and review of the literature. Journal of Medicine and Life. 2012;**5**(2):145-148

[78] Shoreibah EA, Ibrahim SA, Attia MS, Diab MM. Clinical and radiographic evaluation of bone grafting in corticotomy-facilitated orthodontics in adults. Journal of the International Academy of Periodontology. 2012;**14**(4):105-113

[79] Shoreibah EA, Salama AE, Attia MS, Abu-Seida SM. Corticotomy-facilitated orthodontics in adults using a further modified technique. Journal of the International Academy of Periodontology. 2012;**14**(4):97-104

[80] Lee W, Karapetyan G, Moats R, Yamashita DD, Moon HB, Ferguson DJ, et al. Corticotomy-/osteotomy-assisted tooth movement microCTs differ. Journal of Dental Research. 2008;**87**(9):861-867. DOI: 10.1177/154405910808700904

9

Current Approaches in Orthognathic Surgery

Mustafa Sancar Atac

Abstract

The orthognathic surgical procedures are performed for the correction of abnormalities of the facial skeleton that are present from the birth or arise during growth or acquired secondarily during lifetime. Due to the cover of this book as orthodontics, I would prefer to summarize some commonly used techniques to correct the dentofacial deformities. Even we have published all these techniques at their popular time with our orthodontist colleagues; skeletal anchor systems, some basic interdental osteotomies, or complex mechanics that are applying orthopedic corrective forces are currently being used by the orthodontists rather than surgeons. Le Fort I osteotomy in maxilla and sagittal split ramus osteotomies (SSRO) in mandible are commonly used techniques to solve the deformity problems of the facial skeleton; therefore, the scope of this chapter is going to be including my personal experience and some technical details with Le Fort I and SSRO.

Keywords: orthognathic, surgery, dentofacial deformity, Le Fort I osteotomy, sagittal split ramus osteotomy, maxillary osteotomy, mandibular osteotomy, airway, facial esthetics, genioplasty, facial harmony, piezoelectric surgery, piezosurgery

1. Introduction

The orthognathic surgical procedures are performed for the correction of abnormalities of the facial skeleton that are present from the birth or arise during growth or acquired secondarily during lifetime. The variety of the underlying reasons of the facial deformities would require different types of surgical strategies, but mainly orthognathic surgical techniques are preferred for the rehabilitation of the deformities. Due to the cover of this book as orthodontics, I would prefer to summarize some commonly used techniques to correct the dentofacial deformities.

Skeletal anchor systems, some basic interdental osteotomies, or complex mechanics that are applying orthopedic corrective forces are currently being used by the orthodontics rather than surgeons. Even we have published all these techniques at their popular time period with our orthodontist colleagues. Therefore in this chapter, I will focus on the most commonly used surgical applications to solve the skeletal discrepancies mainly called as Le Fort I osteotomy and BSSRO. These techniques can be applied as a single-jaw surgery or double-jaw surgery depending on the magnitude of discrepancy of the jaws to each other. Besides these basic techniques can also be preferred in association with distraction osteogenesis or orthodontic elastic traction forces for gradual and slow motions of the segments as well, but I think it is better to discuss the indication not in this chapter. Therefore the scope of this chapter is going to be including my personal experience and some technical details with Le Fort I and SSRO.

2. Bilateral sagittal split ramus osteotomy (BSSRO)

The history of orthognathic surgical techniques goes back to the mid-1800s. Both in Europe and the USA, the corrective jaw surgeries at their first steps begun to be heard by the population. Schuchardt was the author who first described the sagittal split in 1942 in German literature [1]. In English literature, Trauner and Obwegeser were the pioneers in 1957 who described and discussed the technique in detail [2]. Dal Pont [3], Hunsuck [4], and Epker [5] all added modifications to the technique such as to maintain more surface contact between bony segments at outer cortex, obtaining a minimal horizontal cut in the medial surface of ramus just beneath the lingula and minimal muscle detachment to avoid postoperative blood loss and hematoma.

2.1. Indications

BSSRO is a perfect option for surgical treatment of dentofacial deformities including the mandibular deformities. The mandible can be repositioned in three dimensions of the space such sagittal direction (as advancement, setback), transversal direction (asymmetries and shifting from one side to the other or transversal rotation), and axial plane (clockwise or counterclockwise rotation). For each movement a patient-specific osteotomy and muscle dissection should be kept in mind to avoid postoperative relapse and skeletal disfigurement. On the other hand, while planning such osteotomies, the facial harmony, speech, tongue size, esthetics, and most importantly the airway should be precisely evaluated. As an example huge magnitude of setback of the mandible would result as decreased airway volume and in advance as OSAS. The preoperative evaluation should include a 3D airway evaluation. If such compromise occurs, other osteotomy techniques should be analyzed such as mandibular ostectomy, IVRO. Also in macroglossia patients, tongue reduction surgery should be kept in mind before or during operation in setback surgeries to avoid dentoskeletal relapse. The incision would be placed on the ascending ramus in proximal segment and be carried inferiorly on the distal segment over the external oblique linea, while a mouth gag or a position stabilizator is placed on the opposite side with maximum mouth opening. Care must be taken to avoid dislocation of any condyle during this point (**Figure 1**). An electrocautery knife or a 15 blade would be preferable depending on the surgeon. My choice is the Colorado Needle which may help us for delicate incision without necrosis of the soft tissue with a good bloodless vision. The trick with the electrocautery is to perform repetitive coagulations on the same soft tissue plane to avoid tissue necrosis. A layer-by-layer dissection of mucosa muscles and periosteum is necessary. Adequate amount of soft tissue should be remained on the attached gingival side for wound closure. The mucoperiosteal full thickness flap is raised on the external oblique linea. If the temporal muscle tendons are identified, they can also be reflected. An Obwegeser ramus retractor or a curved hemostat is positioned on the tip of coronoid process. The anterior inferior border of the mandible which is close to the external oblique linea can also be reflected, and during bone osteotomies an Obwegeser channel retractor should be placed on the inferior mandibular border. The lingula and the mandibular foramina should be identified on the medial surface of the mandibular ramus and a Williger or Obwegeser raspatorium is used to protect the neurovascular bundle above its insertion to foramen mandibularis. This maneuver will guide to horizontal medial bone osteotomy just above the foramina. There is no need to perform posterior dissection to the posterior border of the mandible. It is better to create a soft tissue tunnel subperiosteally and keep it just to the posterior of the foramina. This will also reduce the possible intraoperative excessive bleeding arising posteriorly and medially from the adjacent muscle and vessel structures (**Figure 2**). Once all the bony aspects of the desired osteotomy lines have been approached, depending on the surgeon's preference, a cutting instrument like saws, rotary handpiece, or piezoelectric surgery handpiece can be used. If the patient has no cardiac disease like arrhythmias or is not a pacemaker user, my first choice is piezoelectric ultrasonic surgery. The piezoelectric ultrasonic surgery is a well-defined system, the first steps of which were discovered by Pierre and Jacques Curie Brothers in 1880. Piezoelectricity is the electric charge that accumulates in certain solid materials (such as crystals certain ceramics, and biological matter such as bone, DNA and various proteins) in response to applied mechanical stress. The first ultrasonic alveolar bone cut was performed by Horton on the dog alveolus in 1975 [6]. In piezoelectric surgery, the cavitation phenomenon

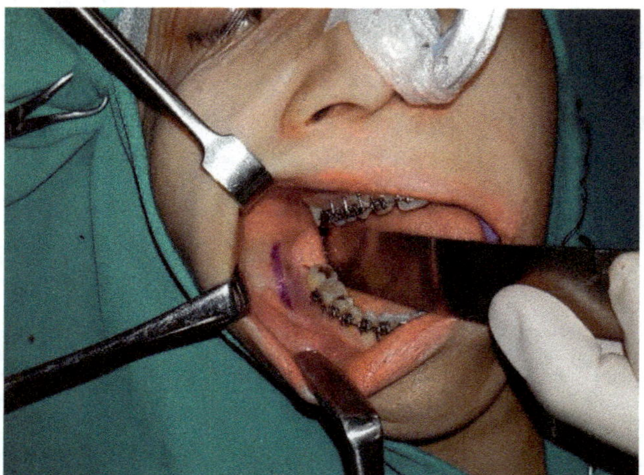

Figure 1. The incision line placed over the external oblique line and ascending ramus. Carrying it to high and medially will cause herniation of temporoparietal fat pad (Bichat's fat pad).

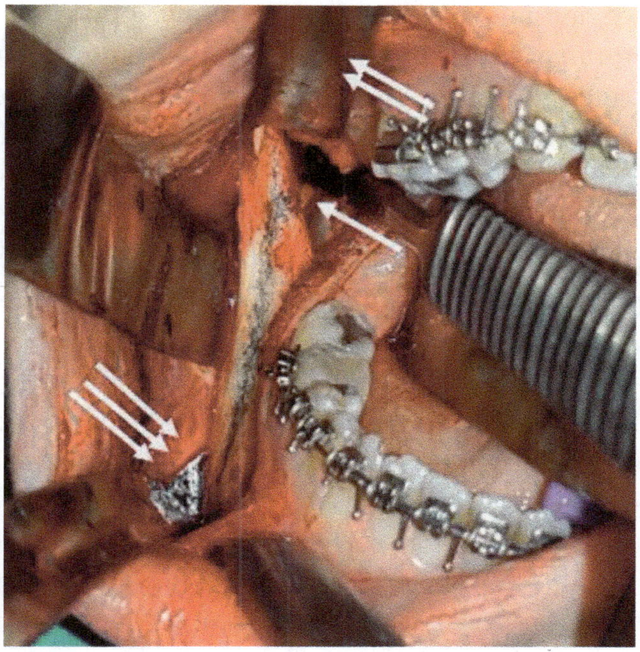

Figure 2. Ramus single white arrow: alveolaris inferior neurovascular bundle; double white arrow: Obwegeser ramus retractor; and three white arrows: Obwegeser ramus channel retractor. Please note that the Obwegeser periosteal raspatorium is placed above the foramina and protecting the neurovascular bundle. Also a sub periosteal dissection has been performed creating a tunnel to avoid haemorrhagia. Also pay attention to pencil drawing along the ascending ramus declining on the external oblique linea finalizing at the anterior most inferior edge of the linea. This cut will create a separation between distal and proximal segments.

describes the process of vaporization, bubble generation, and subsequent implosion (growth and collapse of bubbles) into many minute fractions of its original size (microscopic gas bubbles) that will occur in a flowing liquid because of the decrease and increase in pressure that is caused by the ultrasonic vibrations. In ultrasonic osteotomy, the cavitation phenomenon helps to maintain good visibility in the operative field by dispersing a coolant fluid as an aerosol that causes the blood to essentially be washed away. Furthermore, the cavitation effect will bring about hemostasis, which results in a bloodless surgery. Walmsley et al. have suggested that the cavitation effect fragments the cell walls of bacteria and therefore has an antibacterial efficiency [7]. Also, piezoelectric device has a selective cutting effect and has a sound alert warning system when the tip has reached to a nonresisting part such as neurovascular bundle or sinus membrane that avoids trauma to soft tissues. Therefore, hemorrhagic and neurosensory deficits are rare in piezoelectric surgery. Afterward Vercellotti published his experience with piezoelectric surgery [8]. In orthognathic surgery Landes et al. shared their experience with piezo-osteotomy feasibility as a substitute for the conventional saw in orthognathic surgery that was evaluated regarding operative technique, blood loss, time requirement, and nerve and vessel integrity. Fifty patients who had orthognathic surgery procedures using piezo surgical osteotomy showed that piezoelectric osteotomy reduced blood loss and inferior alveolar nerve injury at no extra time investment, compared with 86 patients who received conventional saw and chisel osteotomies [9]. We have also evaluated piezosurgery in PhD thesis and compared the conventional rotary instruments with piezosurgery. The aim of this study is to comparatively evaluate primary postoperative patient complaints such as edema, paresthesia, and pain and patient satisfaction and operation times of orthognathic surgical operations performed with conventional drills and piezoelectric surgery. A total of 200 patients with completed skeletal growth and malocclusion due to mastication dysfunctions were retrospectively evaluated. These patients were divided into two main groups named control group and piezo group. Each group was divided into three subgroups about the type of surgical procedure performed, which are, Le Fort 1 subgroup, bilateral sagittal split ramus osteotomy (BSSRO) subgroup, and bimaxillary subgroup. The evaluation between the groups is made at postoperative 1 day, 1 week, and 1, 3, and 6 months. To evaluate each subgroup, the data acquired from a specific subgroup was compared to the subgroup with the same name in the other main group. After piezoelectric surgery edema, neurosensory dysfunction and pain levels were found to be lesser than conventional techniques. Patient satisfaction was found to be higher in piezoelectric surgery patients. When operation times were compared, piezoelectric surgery was discovered to take longer to finish the osteotomy because of its lower cutting efficiency. This study shows that the selective cutting ability of the piezoelectric surgery device provides an extremely safe osteotomy for patients by performing a selective osteotomy, thus preserving critical adjacent soft tissues [10]. The piezosurgery begins with the medial aspect of the ramus just over the mandibular foramina, and the cutting tip of the handpiece will be directed 45° angle at posterior start point with around a depth of 2 mm and comes anteriorly. On the ascending ramus, the tip is applied without angulation as deep as possible through the cortex to reach the medullary bone and declines inferiorly on the external oblique linea. If the procedure is a mandibular setback surgery, it is better to extend the osteotomy till the anterior border of the external oblique linea which would help the removal of bony segment for desired positioning of the distal segment similar to Hunsuck-Epker modification. In my experience if a rotational or laterognatic corrective sagittal split osteotomy is going to be performed, the anterior vertical osteotomy on the lateral cortex would be like Obwegeser technique that goes posteriorly to the angulus of the mandible. Besides if the rotation amount is excessive, care must be taken not to dislocate the proximal segment laterally. If such situation occurs, a greenstick fracture must be performed on the posterior part of the distal segment distal to the last molar. In thin and small volumetric mandibles generally, piezoelectric ultrasound surgery is enough to complete the whole osteotomy running from the superior cortex border to the inferior bony cortex border through a fashion without chisel and hammer or separators. Also, this would avoid unfavorable fracture of the segments during rotation split maneuver of the osteotomes that are placed between proximal and distal segments. To avoid undesired inferior border, splitting piezoelectric surgical instruments tips can be directed to the inferior border to maintain a bone cut at the inferior border initiating from the end of the anterior vertical osteotomy back to the posterior end just inferior to orthogonal projection of the lingula. The osteotomy and separation of the proximal and distal segments will simultaneously be completed via this technique without chiseling and hammering. I personally call this technique as Piezotomy Technique®. If the osteotomes are needed to complete the osteotomy, thin osteotomes would be helpful to complete cortex osteotomies keeping them away from the neurovascular bundles. While osteotomizing the inferior border of the mandible, the Obwegeser channel retractor is essential to guard the underlying soft tissues and vital structures. It is better to use a thin osteotome to start separation of the segments seen in **Figure 3**. Completing the osteotomies bilaterally and

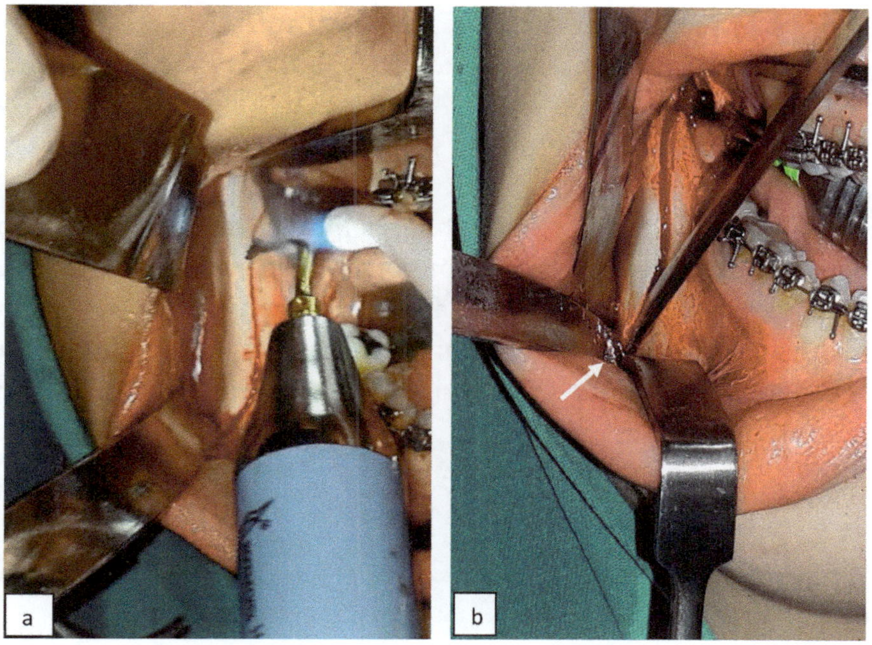

Figure 3. (a) Osteotomy line starting from medial surface of ramus down to ascending ramus to he external oblique linea inferiorly with ultrasonic surgery; (b) thin osteotome is placed for separation of outer cortex of the inferior border.

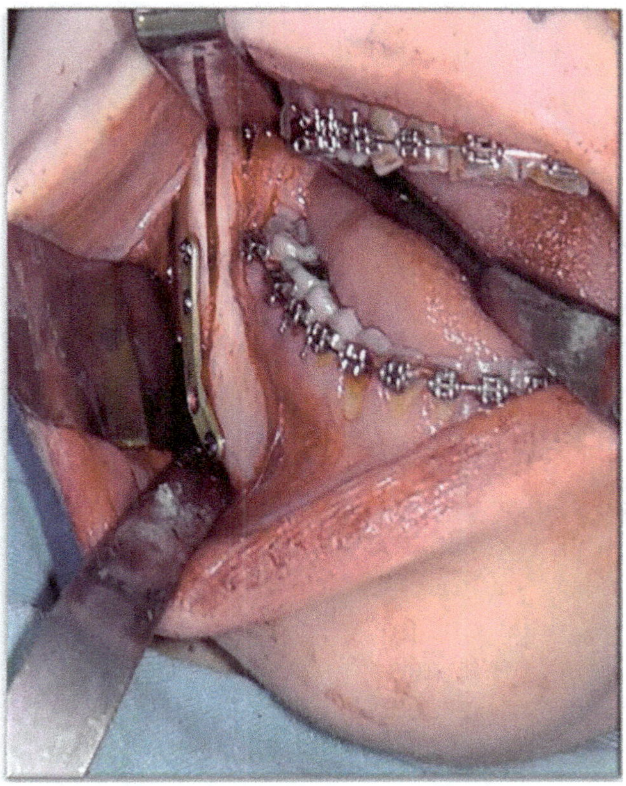

Figure 4. The sagittal mini plate has been bended and passively adopted to proximal and distal segments with monocortical mini self-drive screws and let mandible for early functioning.

detaching the muscle attachments that are resisting for mobilization of distal segment, the surgical splint is placed, and an exact intermaxillary fixation is secured. In this period if it is a setback surgery, the excess bone is removed. At this point, for rigid fixation, the surgeon can prefer lag screws or miniplates with screws to stabilize the segments. My personal choice is to use sagittal plates with self-drive mono cortical screws for rigid fixation. This is essential to avoid condylar sag and distortion of proximal segments as well, especially in the laterognatic and asymmetric cases that require shifting or rotation of the mandible. Also bending the plates geometrically to create a step would stabilize the segments in passive but stable position avoiding the relapse phenomenon. The proximal and distal segments are rigidly fixated (**Figure 4**). After bleeding control the wound edges will be sutured with 3.0 resorbable sutures. Suctioning drains are placed if required.

3. Le Fort I osteotomy

The maxillary discrepancies and the midface abnormalities can easily be corrected by Le Fort I level osteotomy with variable surgical modifications. In 1927, Wassmund performed the first Le Fort I osteotomy for an open-bite deformity [11]. The advancement of maxilla was performed by Axhausen [12], and Bell was the first to show the vascular supply and safety of the procedure at this osteotomy level [13]. The quadrangular Le Fort I was first described by Obwegeser in 1969 [14].

3.1. Technique

The patient is intubated via nasotracheal preformed intubation tube (RAE tube) to avoid nasal deformation during the surgery. Prior the incision a circular infiltrative local anesthesia is administrated with vasoconstrictor agent. A mucosal incision at the vestibular fornix region from one premolar to another is initiated with Colorado Needle electrocautery (**Figure 5a**). To avoid repetitive coagulation, layer-by-layer single application is essential for deeper soft tissue structures down to the periosteum. A mucoperiosteal flap is raised both on sagittal and vertical plans. Laceration of the periosteum would result in discomfortable bleeding and herniation of Bichat fad pad. Depending of the level of the osteotomy, the reflection of the flap may extend up to the infraorbital region. A curved periosteal elevator would be essential for the elevation of the nasal mucosa on the medial sinus wall and midpalatal suture for each side (**Figure 5b**). If a collective fashion of haemorrhagia occurs, a fine rat tail tamponade with tranexamic acid solution will control it. Using piezoelectric ultrasonic surgery device, osteotomy will be initiated at the apertura priformis back to the crista zygomaticus and through the tuberosity of the posterior maxilla. Also via the piezosurgery tip, the medial antral wall osteotomy may be completed. Thanks to its selective cutting effect with cavitation phenomenon, also the palatine bone can be cut via piezosurgery. Even in some cases, from anterior nasal spine to posterior nasal spine, septal separation from midpalatal suture can be performed via piezoelectric surgery (**Figure 5c**). For each maneuver special piezo cutting tips can be preferred even for the pterygomaxillary junction region (**Figure 5d**). When all the

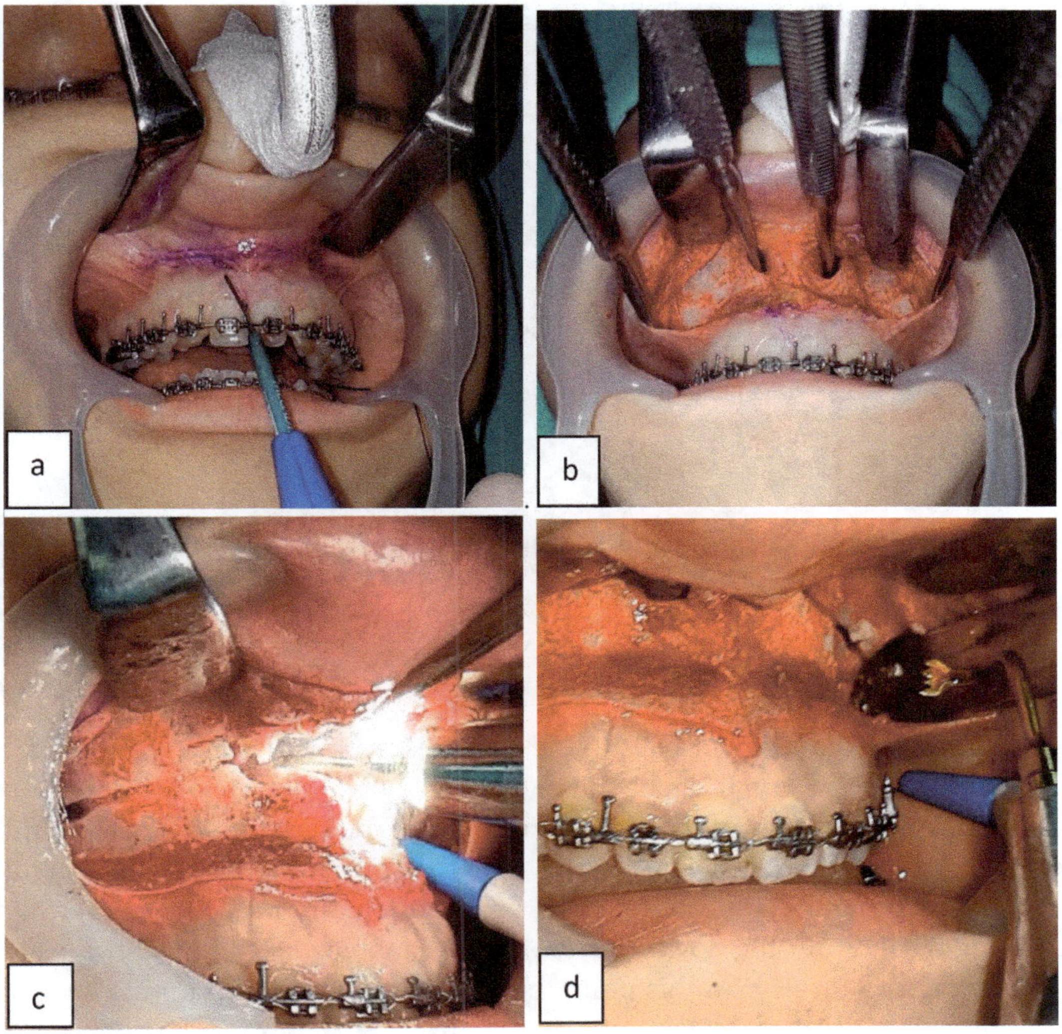

Figure 5. (a) Nasotracheal intubation via RAE tube, Colorado Needle for soft tissue incision, and the at very deepest sulcus, the incision is initiated between premolar regions; (b) soft tissue flaps created by subperiosteal tunneling; (c) anterior nasal spine to posterior nasal spine and also septal separation from mid palatal suture can be performed via piezo electric surgery; and (d) piezo cutting tips can be preferred even for the pterygomaxillary junction region.

osteotomies are performed via piezoelectric surgery, a bi-digital mild pressure on the anterior incisors is applied by the surgeon in vertical and sagittal directions for down fracture of the maxilla. In cases that osteotomies are performed by rotary handpieces or saws, the osteotomy lines are quite similar to piezosurgery, but care must be taken while malleating curved pterygoid osteotome to separate the pterygomaxillary junction. The surgeons' eye should follow the upper occlusion, and the osteotome should be parallel to this line to avoid directing it cranially. One should place the point finger of the assisting hand to the pterygoid hamulus intraorally to feel the tip of the pterygoid osteotome (**Figure 6**). If such malpositioning occurs, there is the risk of laceration of maxillary artery close to the posterior region. Also during medial antral wall osteotomy, care must be taken not to go so far posteriorly due to laceration risk for descending palatinal artery. Because around 3.5 cm posteriorly, the sound will change and a resistance will occur during chiseling. This means that one has reached to the perpendicular lamina of the palatine bone that descending palatine artery is

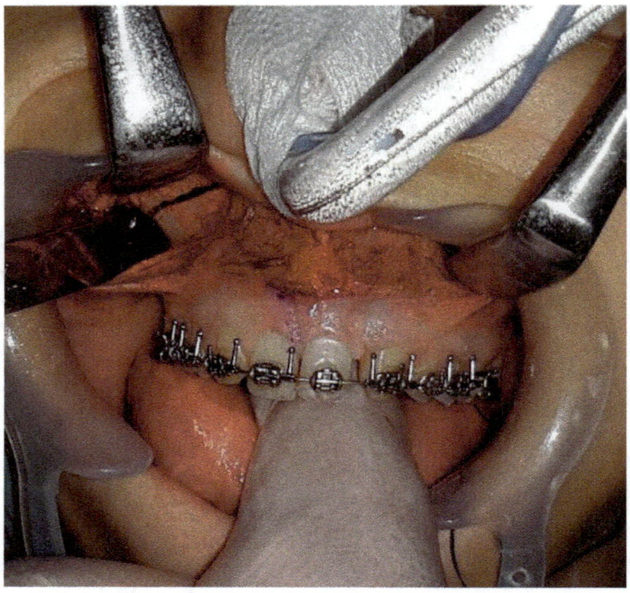

Figure 6. Pterygoid osteotome placed at the pterygomaxillary junction, and the assisting point finger is positioned on the hamulus pterygoideus to feel the disjunction and the tip.

running inside of it. If the surgeon is inexperienced, it is so easy to face an aggressive hemorrhage from the palatine artery. It can be controlled easily by direct packing with a immediate down fracture procedure to isolate the bleeding source. The septal cartilage and midpalatal bone would be separated using nasal septal osteotome. The assisting hand's point finger should be placed posterior-to-posterior nasal spine to feel the tip of the septal osteotome at the end (**Figure 7**). After the down fracture, Tessier mobilizers or Rowe forceps are used to mobilize the maxilla freely. At this point the lacerations on the nasal mucosa is sutured, and posterior reflection of the soft tissues was completed (**Figure 8a**, **b**). If the maxilla is going to be impacted, the septal cartilage would be trimmed as required to avoid deviation of the septum. If the anterior nasal spine is problematic for columella or nasal shape, it can also be removed till the desired level. If the magnitude of the advancement, impaction, or rotation is quite much, surgeon will face resistance; then decompression of the palatal artery and removal of the palatal bone around are necessary. These risky maneuvers can easily be done via piezoelectric surgery without bleeding. As an alternative, a round diamond rotatary burr can be preferred. Surgical saws may lead to hemorrhage. The maxilla will be repositioned with a surgical prefabricated splint followed by intermaxillary fixation. The bone edges are controlled, and interference of excessive bones is removed. When maxilla and mandible act as one unit due to intermaxillary fixation, rotation is completed by gentle force application on both sides of the mandibular premasseteric notches, and rigid fixation is performed (**Figure 9**). If regular micro- or miniplates are going to be used for rigid fixation; I suggest to use two plates on each side in inferior repositioning and advancement surgeries. If the maxilla is impacted, one four-hole L-shaped plate is adequate on each side. For the first time in the literature in 2008, I have published stress distribution both on plates (single- or double-plate fixation on each side) and facial skeleton after rigid fixation in Le Fort I osteotomies for all scenarios, and since 10 years, I clinically follow the guidelines of my publications to choose the number of the plates for each case [15–17].Also as an alternative, I

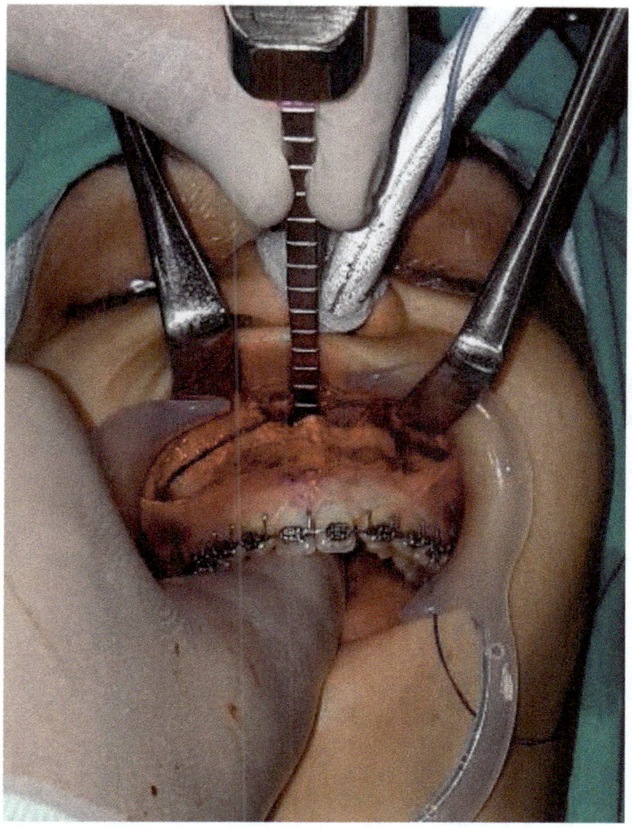

Figure 7. Nasal osteotome is placed on the midline just below the septum to separate the septal cartilage and the mid-palatal bone junction. Assisting point finger placed on to the posterior nasal spine.

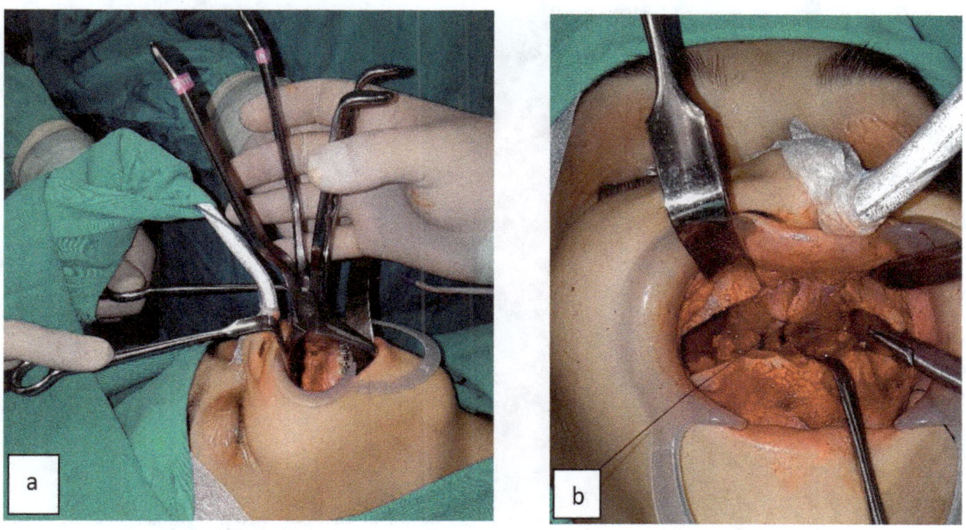

Figure 8. (a) Rowe forceps placed bilaterally on the down fractured maxilla to complete the disjunction, (b) suturing the nasal mucosa ruptures.

suggest to use preformed Le Fort microplates that are currently available on the market with different shoulder sizes (**Figure 10**). Another current advancement in rigid fixation materials is the patient-specific titanium miniplates that are manufactured via 3D printers. The use

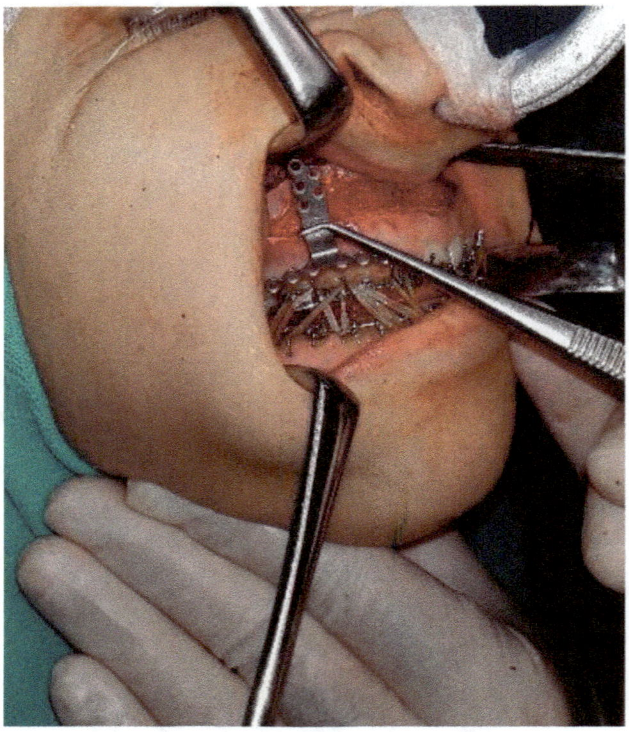

Figure 9. Intermaxillary fixation with a surgical splint, and superior repositioning of the complex with gentle pressure that has been applied bilaterally on both premasseteric notches.

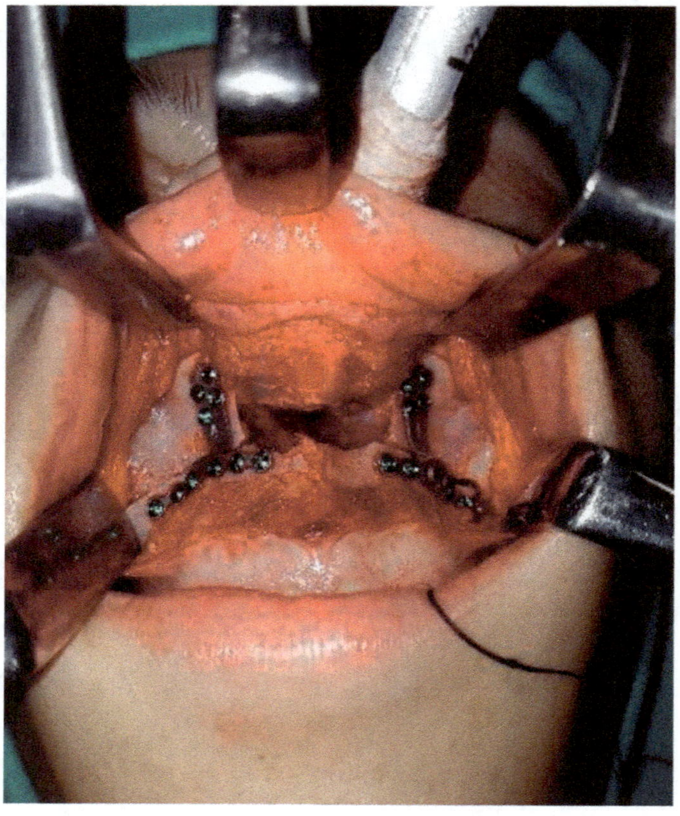

Figure 10. Preformed Le Fort miniplates and self-drive screws used for rigid [18] fixation. This special form supplies enough rigidity with just one plate and there is no need to place posterior plates around zygomatic buttress.

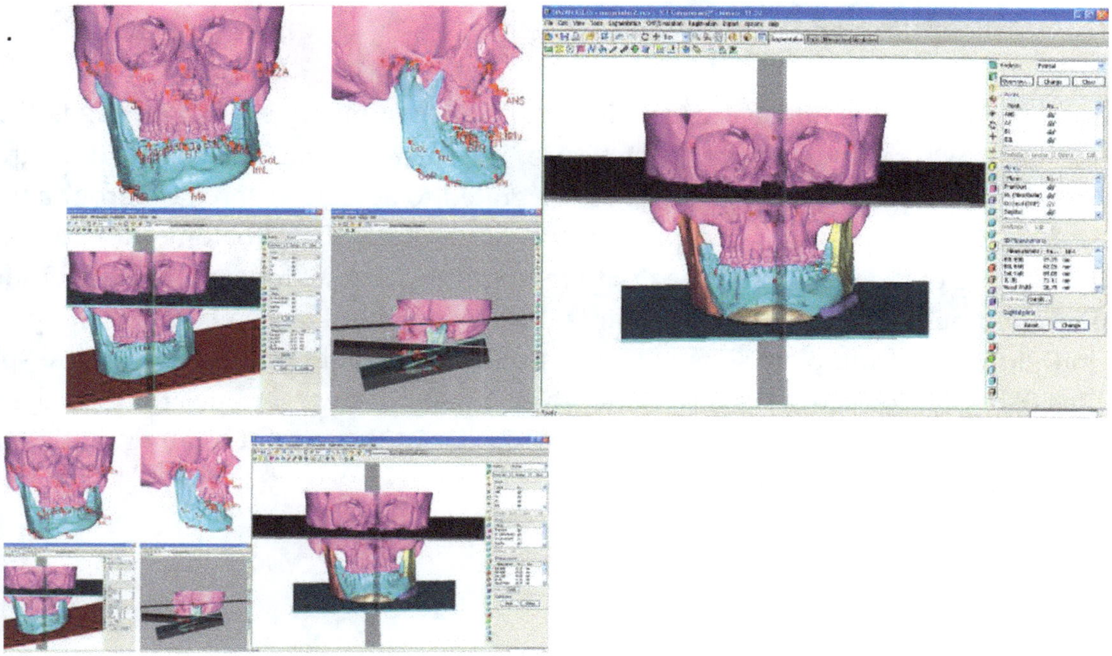

Figure 11. 3D evaluation and planning of a hemimandibular hyperplasia case using DICOM data with a surgical software, published in Journal of Cranio-Maxillofacial Surgery in 2009.

of 3D surgical planning in orthognathic surgery cases is on the market more than 10 years. Meanwhile we also published a paper with 3D tomographic DICOM data transferred to software and completed the operation virtually in 2009 (**Figure 11**) [18]. Depending on surgeons and orthodontist's choice, currently there are many alternatives to each other starting from conventional cast model articulating and model set up on casts, to 3D analyze and 3D printing of surgical splints and titanium fixation plates. On the other hand, higher technology for planning and manufacturing with 3D printers increases the financial expenses. After rigid fixation of the maxilla, the alar wings, nasal tip, and nostril symmetry and projection of the upper lips and the gums should all be evaluated. If the maxilla has been impacted, the nostrils and the nasal soft base will be wider, and alar chinch suture is essential to control the width. Also, a V–Y closure will help to improve the philtrum projection.

4. Bimaxillary surgery

The sequence of these surgeries may vary from surgeon to surgeon. My traditional way to do double jaw is to start with the maxilla first then complete the mandible. But in one indication, one should always start with mandible first which is the double-jaw counterclockwise surgery. Especially Class II with maxillary excess with gummy smile cases associated with OSAS or airway limitations, there is indication for counterclockwise double surgery. The surgical strategy should be mandibular advancement surgery with posterior inferior repositioning and anterior superior rotation. The space created at posterior occlusion is then filled with inferior rotation of the posterior maxilla with anterior maxillary impaction with Le Fort I osteotomy. The pivot point to perform this maneuver is premolar and zygomatic buttress region.

5. Conclusion and the future

As I have briefly explained the basic techniques that are commonly used in orthognathic surgery, for 5 years we are already beyond the future. The current advancements are tomographic evaluation including 3D reformatted frames integrated to advanced software programs with facial scanning to analyze the facial proportions rather than 2D cephalometric radiographs and 3D scanning of the teeth integrated with tomography that let to us perform operation in virtual environment and print out 3D splints. Besides other advancements are; 3D printing of the individual titanium plate screw fixation systems will avoid producing surgical splints, as well as using piezoelectric surgery rather than burs and saws supplies for bloodless and neuro-sensorial deficit-free operations, finally last but not the least, a totally robotic guided surgery will take place within a couple of years.

Author details

Mustafa Sancar Atac

Address all correspondence to: msatac@gmail.com

Faculty of Dentistry, Gazi University, Department of Oral and Maxillofacial Surgery, Ankara, Turkey

References

[1] Schuchardt G. BeitragzurchirurgischenKieferorthopadieunterBerucksichtigungihrer fur tdieBehandlungangeborener und erworbener Kiefer deformitatenbeiSoltaten. Dtsch Zahn MundKieferheilkunde. 1942;**9**:73

[2] Trauner R, Obwegeser H. The surgical correction of mandibular prognathism and retrognathia with consideration of genioplasty. I. Surgical procedures to correct mandibular prognathism and reshaping of the chin. Oral Surgery, Oral Medicine, Oral Pathology, Oral Radiology. 1957;**10**:677-689

[3] Dal PG. Retromolar osteotomy for the correction of prognathism. Journal of Oral Surgery, Anesthesia, and Hospital Dental Service. 1961;**19**:42-47

[4] Hunsuck EE. A modified intraoral sagittal splitting technic for correction of mandibular prognathism. Journal of Oral Surgery. 1968;**26**:250-253

[5] Epker BN. Modifications in the sagittal osteotomy of the mandible. Journal of Oral Surgery. 1977;**35**:157-159

[6] Horton JE, Tarpley TM Jr, Wood LD. The healing of surgical defects in alveolar bone produced with ultrasonic instrumentation, chisel, and rotary bur. Oral Surgery, Oral Medicine, and Oral Pathology. 1975;**39**:536-546

[7] Walmsley AD, Laird WR, Williams AR. Dental plaque removal by cavitation activity during ultrasonic scaling. Journal of Clinical Periodontology. 1988;**15**:539-543

[8] Vercellotti T. Piezoelectric surgery in implantology: A case report–A new piezoelectric ridge expansion technique. The International Journal of Periodontics & Restorative Dentistry. 2000;**20**:358-365

[9] Landes CA, Stübinger S, Rieger J, Williger B, Ha TK, Sader R. Critical evaluation of piezoelectric osteotomy in orthognathic surgery: Operative technique, blood loss, time requirement, nerve and vessel integrity. Journal of Oral and Maxillofacial Surgery. 2008; **66**:657-674. DOI:10.1016/j.joms.2007.06.633

[10] Rzayev S. Retrospective Evaluation of Comparison of Conventional and Piezoelectric Surgery Osteotomies in Orthognathic Surgery Patients [Thesis]. Ankara: Gazi University; 2017

[11] Wassmund M. Lehrbuch der praktischenChirurgie des Mundes und der Kiefer. 1st Bd. Leipzig. Meuser; 1935

[12] Axhausen G. zurbehandlung,veralteterdisloziertgehelteroberkieferbrucke. Deutsche Zahn MundKieferheilkunde. 1934;**1**:334

[13] Bell WH, Fonseca RJ, Kenneky JW, Levy BM. Bone healing and revascularization after total maxillary osteotomy. Journal of Oral Surgery. 1975;**33**:253-260

[14] Obwegeser HL. Surgical correction of small or retrodisplaced maxillae. The "dish-face" deformity. Plastic and Reconstructive Surgery. 1969;**43**:351-365

[15] Ataç MS, Erkmen E, Yücel E, Kurt A. Comparison of biomechanical behaviour of maxilla following Le Fort I osteotomy with 2-versus 4-plate fixation using 3D-FEA. Part 1: Advancement surgery. International Journal of Oral and Maxillofacial Surgery. 2008; **37**:1117-1124. DOI: 10.1016/j.ijom.2008.10.004

[16] Ataç MS, Erkmen E, Yücel E, Kurt A. Comparison of biomechanical behaviour of maxilla following Le fort I osteotomy with 2- versus 4-plate fixation using 3D-FEA part 2: Impaction surgery. International Journal of Oral and Maxillofacial Surgery. 2009;**38**: 58-63. DOI: 10.1016/j.ijom.2008.10.005

[17] Erkmen E, Ataç MS, Yücel E, Kurt A. Comparison of biomechanical behaviour of maxilla following Le Fort I osteotomy with 2- versus 4-plate fixation using 3D-FEA: Part 3: Inferior and anterior repositioning surgery. International Journal of Oral and Maxillofacial Surgery. 2009;**38**:173-179. DOI: 10.1016/j.ijom.2008.10.006

[18] Tuncer BB, Ataç MS, Yüksel S. A case report comparing 3-D evaluation in the diagnosis and treatment planning of hemimandibular hyperplasia with conventional radiography. Journal of Cranio-Maxillo-Facial Surgery. 2009;**37**:312-319. DOI: 10.1016/j.jcms.2009.01.004

10

Cone Beam Computed Tomography in Orthodontics

Emine Kaygısız and Tuba Tortop

Abstract

Cone beam computed tomography (CBCT) is an important source of three-dimensional volumetric data in clinical orthodontics. Due to the progress in the technology of CBCT, for orthodontic clinical diagnosis, treatment and follow-up, CBCT supply much more reliable information compared to conventional radiography. The most justified indications for the use of CBCT in orthodontics are the existence of impacted and transposed teeth. For the management of the impacted teeth, CBCT enhances the ability to localize these teeth accurately and to assess root resorption of adjacent teeth. Patients with craniofacial anomalies like cleft palate cases, the abnormalities of the temporomandibular joint contributing malocclusion, evaluation of airway morphology in obstructive sleep apnea cases, patients needing maxillary expansion or planning orthognathic surgery in severe skeletal discrepancies are also listed among the indications of using CBCT in orthodontics. CBCT is useful in identifying optimal site location for temporary skeletal anchorage device. The use of CBCT for the assessment of treatment outcomes and evaluation of cervical vertebral maturation are still controversial issues. It should be kept in mind that before using CBCT, justification and evaluation of risks and benefits are needed. In order to minimize the radiation dose, the exam should include only the areas of interest.

Keywords: cone beam computed tomography, orthodontics, impacted canine, orthodontic treatment planning, root resorption

1. Introduction

The key of a successful orthodontic treatment is an accurate diagnosis, growth evaluation and treatment planning. Diagnostic records for an orthodontic treatment planning generally begin with history and intraoral and extraoral examination of the patient. Dental casts, intraoral and extraoral photographs are also routine diagnostic materials. Imaging is a necessary diagnostic tool in the practice of orthodontics. For radiographic evaluation, panoramic radiograph, periapical views, upper occlusal radiograph and lateral cephalometric radiograph are obtained if indicated. Imaging should answer the questions that cannot be solved clinically. By using radiographic examination, it is possible to confirm or rule out clinical findings [1].

In recent years, orthodontists have begun to use three-dimensional (3D) cone beam computed tomography (CBCT) images to overcome the inadequateness of two-dimensional (2D) radiographic records. When computed tomography was first introduced into the dental field, because of the high radiation dose, it is not preferred for orthodontic diagnosis. The technology has been evolving ever since, resulting in a reduction in radiation dose and relatively low cost of CBCT systems, so they become popular to visualize the craniofacial complex in three dimensions.

In some studies, it has been suggested that different options for orthodontic treatment plans in some specific cases may change due to use of CBCT [2–4]. Orthodontists should know how to use the radiographic records and what they offer, before deciding which tool they will use [1].

2. Advantages and disadvantages of using CBCT in orthodontics

Although there has been considerable interest in using CBCT as a part of routine orthodontic management, diverse results about the advantages, disadvantages and indications were noted in the literature.

The review of recent literature reveals some advantages [1, 5–15] and disadvantages [16–20] as following:

2.1. Advantages

- Accuracy of image geometry is increased, and real size 3D image is obtained by CBCT. Unlike lateral cephalometric radiographs, CBCT image is more similar to the patient, more accurate and distortion-free.
- It eliminates the magnification, overlapping and distortion of structures.
- It is possible to assess the image from the three planes.
- CBCT images allow to make localized and specific transversal cuts to assess areas of clinical interest.
- For a proper diagnosis and treatment planning, sometimes temporomandibular, postero-anterior cephalograms, periapical, occlusal and bite-wing radiographs are also required besides the routine panoramic and lateral cephalometric examination. But, by using CBCT technology, it is possible to produce several types of radiographic images and to construct study casts from a single scan.
- The reorientation of the images, on the contrary to the lateral cephalometric radiograph, is possible.

- The ease of landmark identification and high precision of superimposed images have been reported.
- By the use of CBCT, less variability and more reproducibility of transverse measurements were demonstrated compared to conventional 2D. CBCT images were reported to be more reliable than posteroanterior cephalograms and offer an unobstructed view for diagnosis of maxillary transverse discrepancies.
- The unerupted tooth sizes, bone dimensions and even soft tissue anthropometric measurements can be assessed precisely by CBCT.
- The fine adjustment of the head position is not essential for CBCT.
- The use of CBCT in orthodontics greatly enhances evaluation of impacted canines and offers comprehensive information.
- The detection of root resorption is reported to be highly accurate with CBCT scanners.
- An occlusal view of the maxilla from CBCT can be used for the customized transpalatal arch design. This might prevent interfering of the wire to the path of eruption of impacted tooth.

2.2. Disadvantages

- The amount of generated radiation is the biggest controversy about the use of CBCT in dental imaging. Although the radiation dose of the CBCT is lower than the medical spiral CT, it is still higher than that of a 2D cephalogram.
- Difficulty in differentiating various soft tissues in the image due to the poor low-contrast resolution compared to medical CT is one of the disadvantages.
- An adequate method to digitize and analyze 3D radiographic images is not still improved.
- The lack of 3D standard population norms has also restricted CBCT from routine orthodontic use.
- Landmark identification on coronal, sagittal and axial views of CBCT is more time consuming to carefully select the best slice.
- The diagnostic accuracy for caries detection with CBCT is less than with conventional periapical radiographs.

3. The usage of CBCT in orthodontics

Many orthodontists interested in using CBCT during their routine diagnosis and treatment planning because of the additional diagnostic information. This brings the risk of unnecessary ionizing radiation. So, it is mandatory to determine exact indications for the use of CBCT in orthodontics.

3.1. Impacted and transposed teeth

Tooth impaction is a commonly observed dental anomaly which needs orthodontic treatment. The most frequent impacted teeth were mandibular wisdom teeth, which were followed by maxillary and mandibular canines [21]. Radiographic examinations play a more critical role than clinical examination especially in the initial diagnosis and treatment planning of impacted teeth. For several years, radiographic evaluation of these teeth was done by using panoramic, periapical, occlusal or lateral cephalograms. These conventional two dimensional radiographs are inadequate in accurately visualizing the location, angulation, spatial position and relationships of the impacted tooth in three dimensions. So, the most justified indications for the use of CBCT in orthodontics are the existence of impacted and transposed teeth (**Figure 1a–c**).

For the management of the impacted teeth, CBCT enhances the ability to localize these teeth accurately, evaluate their proximity to other teeth and structures, determine the alveolar width and follicle size, the presence of pathology and assess root resorption of adjacent teeth, assist in planning surgical access and bond placement, besides determining optimal direction for the extrusion of these teeth into the oral cavity [22–25]. In particular, for impacted teeth, if exposure or forced eruption is planned, it would be possible to determine not only the position of tooth and dilacerated root but also the alveolar boundary conditions. Additionally, it would be much easier to prepare the space needed for the impacted tooth as it is possible to obtain a more accurate size from CBCT images.

Haney et al. [26] reported an approximate 20% lack of agreement among clinicians on the location (palatal versus labial) of the tooth tip between the routine 2D radiographs and 3D CBCT images. Also large differences in treatment approaches were demonstrated when the two imaging methods were compared [27]. On the other hand, in another study, it was reported that the determination of canine position was not significantly different when using panoramic and CBCT systems [3].

Using CBCT improves the clinician confidence in diagnosis and treatment plan as it is helpful in defining the surgical access site, bond position and in designing mechanics [25, 26]. The orthodontists have a different perception of localization and can determine the shortest way for the impacted tooth in three planes of space while avoiding damage to neighboring teeth.

In some studies, it was suggested that orthodontic treatment planning for impacted tooth showed no differences when using 2D- or 3D-based information. On the contrary, findings of some other studies showed that orthodontists changed their treatment planning derived from conventional radiographs for 25% of the impacted teeth when they viewed CBCT images [26, 28]. Alqerban et al. [4, 29] concluded that CBCT allows clinicians to obtain 3D images with visualization of craniofacial structures and significantly increases the orthodontists' confidence level, with more information on canine localization and detection of possible root resorption on adjacent incisors [30].

When the impacted tooth did not move, CBCT is indicated. Becker et al. [31] reported that invasive cervical root resorption is a rare insidious and aggressive form of external

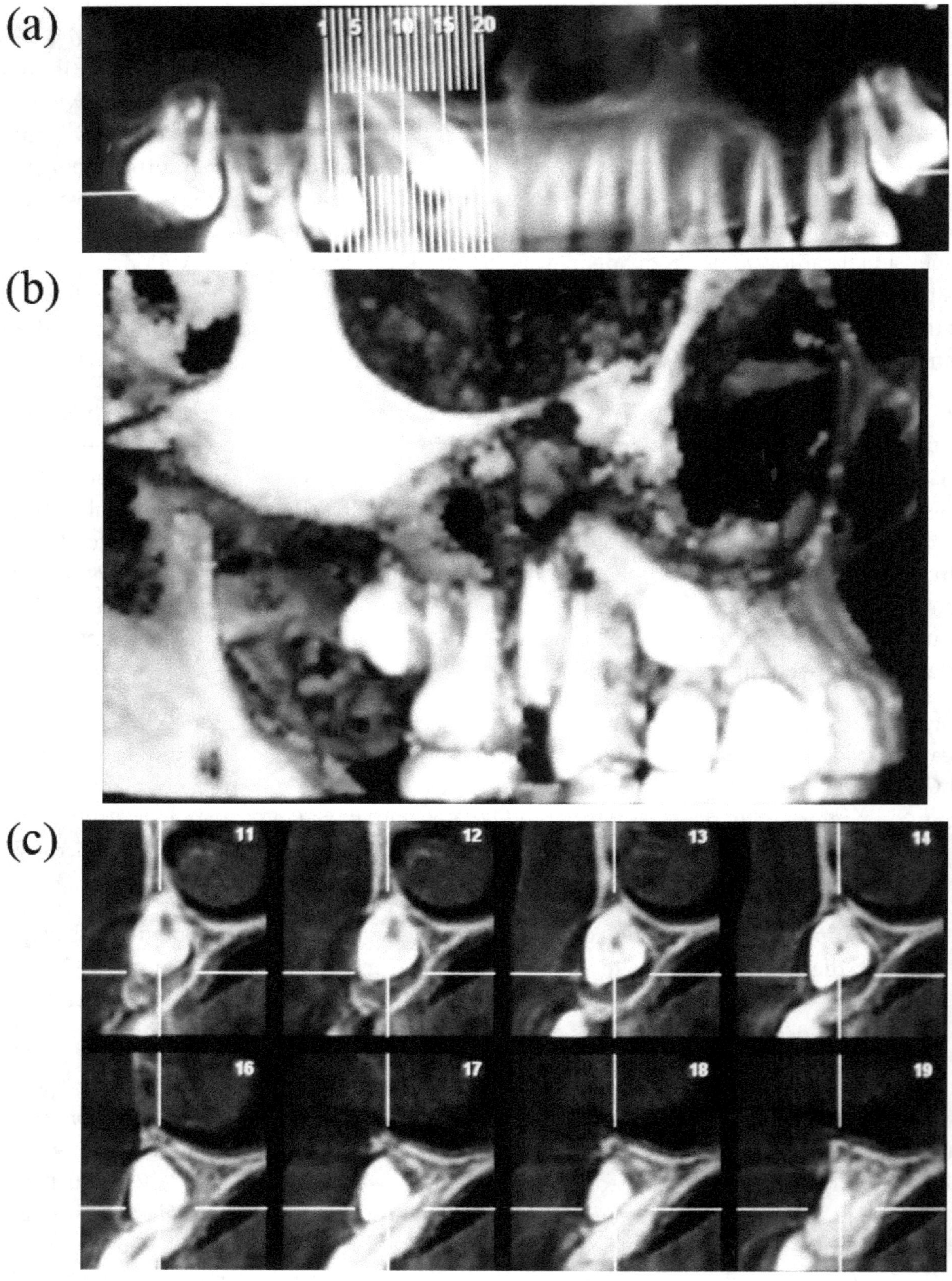

Figure 1. (a) Panoramic view of a maxillary impacted canine. Note that in this case, FOV was restricted only to maxilla. (b) Determination of vestibular location of a maxillary impacted canine. (c) Evaluation of proximity between impacted canine and root of lateral incisor by CBCT.

root resorption and an overlooked cause of failure of orthodontic resolution of impacted canines.

CBCT minimizes superimposition artifacts and provides superior visualization of roots [24, 32]. In extraction cases with an impacted tooth, it is a much more important to decide which tooth to extract, a tooth with a resorbed root or a healthy premolar? Using CBCT images will contribute to a logical clinical outcome, as it provides superior information on root resorption.

Overall, it could be considered to increase efficiency and enhance success rates for the treatment of impacted teeth when the treatment and biomechanics are customized by using CBCT [33].

Field of view (FOV) must be determined according to the needs of the case. If the only problem is an impacted tooth, it would be logical to localize the FOV as the impacted tooth, adjacent teeth and surrounding alveolar structure. In fact, in a recent study, Wriedt et al. [30] recommended small volume FOV CBCT for impacted maxillary canines if the canine inclination on a conventional 2D panoramic radiograph exceeds 30° relative to a perpendicular midline, when adjacent root resorption is suspected, and/or when canine root dilaceration is suspected on conventional panoramic radiographs. But if an orthognathic surgical treatment plan is predicted, cephalometric and panoramic radiograph need must be considered while determining FOV. It is advisable to refer the patient to an oral and maxillofacial radiologist with a note including clinically significant findings and request a report on the region of interest [27].

Maxillary lateral incisor root resorption is most commonly associated with canine impaction. It often remains asymptomatic, limiting early diagnosis. However, early diagnosis is important, because the presence or absence of root resorption will determine the treatment strategy. Furthermore, advanced root resorption can make treatment impossible [34]. Improvement in diagnostic measures for early detection and prevention is therefore essential for ensuring correct treatment, and it might also reduce treatment time, complexity, complications and costs. It has been suggested that by using 3D images, overlapping of structures can be avoided.

Dental transposition represents a multifactorial condition. In the etiology of transposition, both genetic and environmental factors play an important role [35]. For the diagnosis and treatment planning of transposed teeth, several significant variables can be derived from CBCT imaging, especially, critical when deciding whether patient requires extraction or not. So, it would be much easier to evaluate adequately the quality and shape of teeth, location of roots and limitations of the alveolar boundary conditions around the transposed teeth by using CBCT. Kapila et al. [28] recommended to be selective about which cases may benefit from CBCT scans for assessing boundary conditions. Cases with compromised periodontal or gingival conditions, patients with narrow alveolar bone in which it would be critical to manage buccolingual displacements or angulations of teeth, and cases who need shifting position of the teeth are listed as cases that will benefit from CBCT scans.

3.2. Supernumerary teeth

A supernumerary tooth may closely resemble the teeth of the group to which it belongs [36]. In supernumerary cases, radiographic examination aims to determine the localization and the morphology of the supernumerary teeth. As it is critical to decide which teeth to be extracted and which teeth to be retained, CBCT helps to precisely evaluate the position and morphology of these teeth. It is also possible to detect any contact between the supernumerary teeth and adjacent teeth and to evaluate their relation with other anatomical structures. The information obtained from CBCT images also facilitates the determination of the optimal surgical access to these teeth in order to minimize harm to adjacent teeth and to surrounding tissue [37] (**Figure 2**).

3.3. Root resorption

Root resorption is a condition occurs in response to a variety of stimuli resulting in a loss of dentin, cementum or bone [36]. Panoramic radiographs have a week diagnostic efficacy in determining external root resorption. So, root resorption has traditionally been evaluated by periapical radiographs. Nevertheless, in recent years, it is suggested that CBCT can detect precise images of small root defects with a greater sensitivity and specificity compared to 2D radiographs [3, 24]. In a meta-analysis, Yi et al. [38] reported that CBCT is superior to periapical radiographs in the accuracy of diagnosing external root resorption. They emphasized that periapical radiographs provide limited information of external root resorption in the buccal and lingual root surface.

External root resorption of maxillary lateral incisor is a common finding that associates with canine impaction. Early diagnosis is difficult as it is asymptomatic and advanced root resorption makes the treatment planning more complex. In a study evaluating efficacy of CBCT for the diagnosis of root resorption associated with impacted canines, improved detection rates of root resorption (63%) were reported [39]. By using CBCT, it is possible to visualize of root resorptions on buccal and lingual surfaces. This might be critical for the extraction decision during treatment planning. In another study, it was suggested that the combination of thin slices and high resolution caused overestimation of the cavities for moderate root resorption cases [3].

The main problem is to decide how and when a clinician justify taking CBCT scan when a patient has undergone root resorption. Yi et al. [38] suggested that patients with clinically suspected root resorption be first evaluated by periapical radiographs. If positive results are obtained, for further examination, CBCT should be considered.

Alqerban et al. [10] reported that all CBCT systems used in their study showed high accuracy in the detection of root resorption, and there was no significant difference among CBCT systems in the detection of the severity of root resorption. Limitations of using CBCT for external root

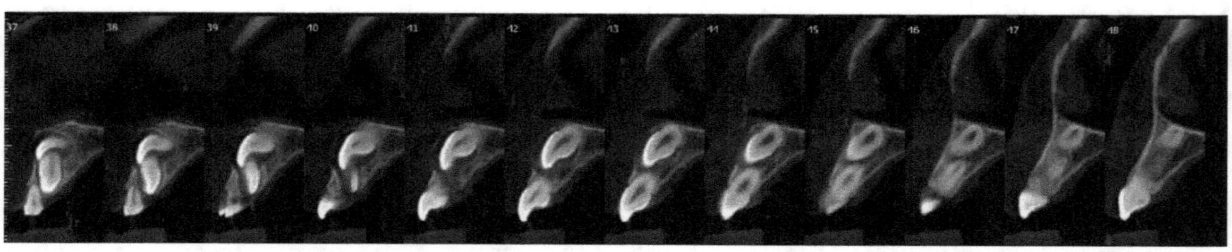

Figure 2. Evaluation of position of a supernumerary tooth and impacted incisor and their relation with neighboring structures.

resorption are the detection of small resorptions in the apical third and the high dose of radiation required [3].

3.4. Evaluation of root angulation and length

CBCT imaging becomes a preferred method for diagnosis by orthodontists because of its three dimensional rendering capability. Root position and morphology are critical issues for an orthodontist as it may affect the final occlusion. Root anatomy, such as short or dilacerated, is a determinant factor for the amount and direction of a tooth movement. Furthermore, because of the concerns about external root resorption, orthodontists need to get precise measurements of root angulation and length before treatment. Using CBCT images also provide detailed information about dysmorphic roots. Root positioning and morphology might be indicators of a disease. Of course, all root anomalies are not identical, but when supported with genetic testing, CBCT imaging will be helpful in interpreting anomalous root morphology in syndromic cases [40].

3.5. Tooth-bone relationship

In bimaxillary protrusion cases, Class 3 patients with an initial symphysis bone width, cases with preexisting periodontal disease, after maxillary expansion treatment, CBCT provides valuable information about tooth-bone relationships, and it might reduce the risk factor for dehiscence. While assessing deficiencies of buccolingual thickness in the alveolar ridge of patients subjected to critical tooth movement, high resolution and a limited FOV is recommended [41].

3.6. Cleft lip and palate (CLP) cases

Patients with CLP are treated by interdisciplinary teams from infancy until adulthood. Several types of surgical procedures are used to reconstruct the anatomy of the alveolar ridge, dentofacial region, lips and nose. The SEDENTEXCT Consortium stated, in regard to the radiation dose, that "the application of CBCT in cleft lip and palate patients was found to be the simplest to support" in dentistry [42]. However, in a recent systematic review, it was suggested that further investigation is necessary to determine the influence of this new 3D facial imaging modality on treatment planning, treatment outcome and treatment evaluation.

The preoperative CBCT may provide reliable estimates on how much expansion and graft material will be needed, aid in appropriate selection of an autogenous graft donor site before surgery and enable the visualization of the three-dimensional morphology of the bone bridge, the relationship between the bone bridge and roots of the neighboring teeth. For alveolar bone graft success, determination of the buccal-palatal width of the bone in CLP cases, the use of CBCT is recommended [43] (**Figure 3**). Pharyngeal space, the results of bone grafting, and the effect of nasoalveolar molding can be evaluated with a post-treatment CBCT.

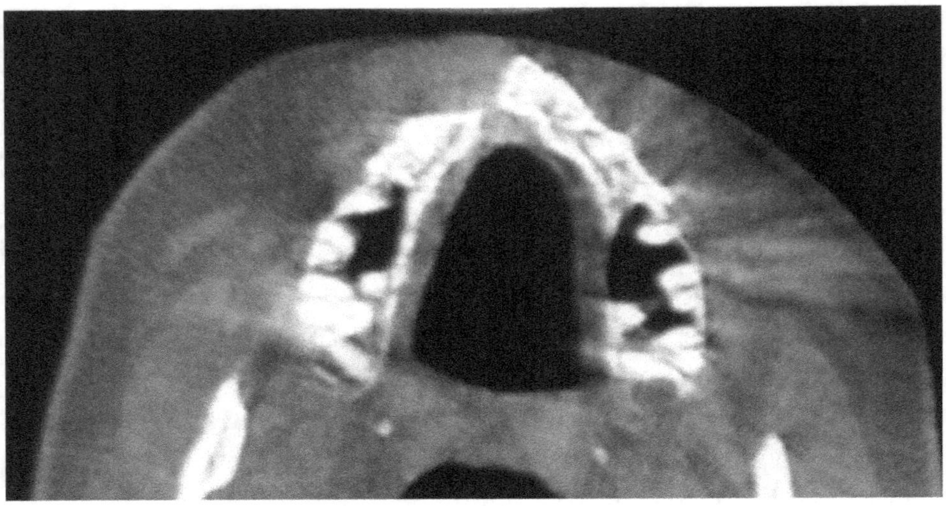

Figure 3. Preoperative CBCT view of a CLP case showing the graft site.

3.7. Temporomandibular joint (TMJ) morphology and pathology contributing to malocclusion

The changes in the size, form and special and functional relationships of the TMJ components might cause pathological TMJ conditions. TMJ disorders which occurred during active growth period might alter jaw, tooth positions and occlusion. Even though signs and symptoms of disturbances in the masticatory system are common, understanding the cause can be very complex. A proper diagnosis is possible, if only a through history and examination were achieved. Various types of imaging techniques can be used to gain additional information regarding the health and function of TMJs. CBCT is indicated for orthodontic cases that require analysis of TMJ bone components accompanied by signs and symptoms [44, 45]. One of the greatest advantages of CT scan is evaluating the condyle-disk relationship [46]. In comparison with panoramic radiograph and linear tomography, CBCT proves more accurate in diagnosing erosion of the condyle [47]. Soft tissue imaging is possible, but bony tissues are best imaged with CT scans [48]. As magnetic resonance imaging enables visualizing the non-mineralized soft tissues, it is preferable for the diagnosis of internal derangements of TMJ. However, it is not possible to observe dynamic joint movements.

Besides the evaluation of TMJ disorders, CBCT has been used to evaluate the condylar changes after orthodontic treatment. It allows volumetric evaluation of TMJ and provides better landmark identification on curved surfaces like condyle. Literature review showed that CBCT evaluation was preferred to determine respond of TMJ to mandibular advancement [49] or extraction treatment [50] and effects of the distraction splint therapy in mandibular asymmetry cases.

3.8. Airway morphology and obstructive sleep apnea (OSA)

Sleep-disordered breathing is a spectrum of conditions with abnormal respiratory pattern, and OSA is the severe end of that spectrum. Orthodontics takes place in the management of OSA by using mandibular advancement appliances and by planning orthognathic surgery in these cases. It is also crucial to evaluate the dimensional changes in the nasopharyngeal area and airway obstruction in CLP [51]. Until recent years, lateral cephalometric radiography was used for the evaluation of the upper airway. But, changes which occur in the transverse dimension cannot be visualized. Three-dimensional analysis and evaluation of airway have got a significant attention in the literature. CBCT allows orthodontists to measure cross-sectional area, minimum cross section and total volume of the patient's airway accurately. Also, it has been used to investigate the effects of orthodontic treatments and orthognathic surgery on airway dimensions.

Studies of the upper airway based on CBCT scans are considered to be reliable in providing important information about the morphology of the pharyngeal airway; however, they have limitation in distinguishing different types of soft tissues [52]. Variations in airway dimensions and morphology due to patient's swallowing movement and head posture are also among the limitations of this technique [53].

3.9. Maxillary transverse dimension and maxillary expansion

In the treatment of transverse maxillary deficiencies, it is important to assess transverse dimension as early as possible and accurately diagnose the need for transverse maxillary expansion using proper diagnostic tools. Before CBCT, post-treatment skeletal changes on patients treated with RME were measured on dental casts, lateral and posterior-anterior cephalometric and occlusal radiographs. Researches to date on rapid maxillary expansion have focused on determining treatment outcomes like dental tipping, alveolar bone bending, skeletal expansion and soft tissue changes, rather than the benefits of CBCT in diagnosis and treatment planning. Nowadays, it is claimed that CBCT images appear to be more reliable than posteroanterior cephalograms, offer an unobstructed view for the assessment of transversal intermaxillary discrepancies and provide much greater resolution and minimal image distortion [15]. However, the radiation dosage and its effect on growing patients must be taken into account.

The mid-palatal suture becomes more fused after the completion of the adolescent growth spurt [54], as prediction of mid-palatal suture maturation is possible by using CBCT [55]. It is a reliable diagnostic tool, while planning surgically assisted rapid maxillary expansion (SARME) in skeletally mature patients or using bone-borne devices, which have recently gained popularity. It is possible to determine treatment outcomes of SARME and also permits the detection of the complications, such as tooth tilting of the anchoring teeth and bone fenestration due to periodontal stress [56].

3.10. Temporary anchorage device (TAD) placement

In recent years, TADs are considered as a prerequisite for the resistance of unwanted tooth movements during the treatment of various orthodontic problems without patient compliance. The most common indications for treatment with TADs are molar protraction followed by indirect skeletal anchorage for space closure, intrusion of supraerupted teeth, intrusion of anterior to manage anterior open bite, anterior en-masse retraction, molar uprighting, intrusion of maxillary cant, molar distalization, traction on impacted canine, and attachment for protraction facemask. CBCT images can be helpful to anchor the miniscrew and miniplate securely in the surrounding bone and to visualize neighboring structures for avoiding damage or complications during TAD placement and be useful in identifying optimal site location (**Figure 4**).

CBCT technology enables us to evaluate the interradicular distance and thickness, transverse bone thickness, bone density and thickness, cortical bone dimensions and quality. Even though anterior palate offers the greatest bone thickness, Holm et al. [57] recommended a CBCT evaluation for maximum screw length, as there is considerable variation of bone thickness between individuals. Before placing a miniscrew by using CBCT, it is also possible to define even cranial and caudal boundaries, besides alveolar boundary conditions, and eliminate the risk of bone and root perforations. Surgical guides fabricated using CBCT images will help to avoid possible root and maxillary sinuses damage. Finite element analysis constructed using CBCT will also guide the evaluation of mechanical advantages or disadvantages of the orthodontic appliances with TADs by simulating stress distribution.

There are several factors that affect the stability and success rate of TADs. If cortical bone thickness is less than 1 mm, primary stability may not be achieved, and the TAD may loosen during orthodontic treatment [58]. Evaluation of cortical bone quantity and quality is also critical for long-term stability. With finite element analysis, it has been shown that root contact is also one of the factors that can cause loss of miniscrew stability [59]. The information gathered from CBCT will be determinant for some of these factors, such as the dimension and insertion

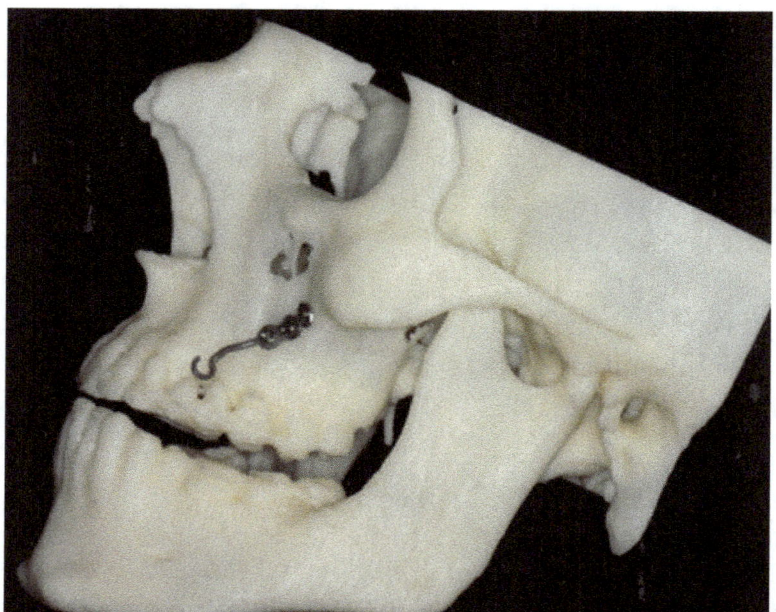

Figure 4. Planning and preparation of TAD (zygomatic skeletal anchorage) on a 3D model obtained from CBCT before surgery.

angle of the miniscrew, the insertion procedure, the depth of the screw insertion and insertion torque [38, 57, 60].

In some cases, routine panoramic, lateral and frontal cephalometric radiographs may not provide all information needed to optimize the location of a miniscrew placement. However, it should be kept in mind that in regions with a high bone quality, such as paramedian palate and palatal region, lateral cephalometric radiographs are usable to determine the location of TADs. Therefore, it is not necessary to take a CBCT in all cases [61].

It is recommended to use the smallest possible FOV unless the CBCT is needed for the diagnosis of another condition in which case a large FOV may be preferred [60].

3.11. Dentofacial deformities and craniofacial anomalies

Evaluation of changes in the craniofacial region during growth and with treatment using lateral cephalograms makes a great contribution to the science of orthodontics. However, in recent years, researches discussed the validity of evaluating a 3D craniofacial structure in a 2D plane. CBCT imaging can provide valuable information about dentofacial deformities and craniofacial anomalies, like facial asymmetry which affects three dimensions of the face, and it can be used to simulate virtual treatment plans for orthopedic corrections, orthognathic surgeries and distraction osteogenesis. By capturing images and analyzing the craniofacial hard and soft tissues and by generating virtual patient models, CBCT imaging permits the clinicians to reposition and reconstruct craniofacial structures (**Figure 5a**, **b**).

Several studies were conducted to determine reference planes, to develop cephalometric analysis, to evaluate the accuracy of these measurements, to establish the mean normality values and to assess the differences of gender and ethnic groups for 3D evaluations [62]. Besides morphological analysis, these images are used to evaluate the spatial relationship of the neighboring structures. CBCT technology enables carrying out the model surgery. So, computer assisted orthognathic surgery permits the design and fabrication of the occlusal surgical splints. By using virtual models, constructing anatomically grafts and correct replacement can be achieved (**Figure 6**). The data obtained from CBCT provide a better prediction of soft tissue response to the changes in the hard tissue after orthognathic surgery [63]. In the literature, CBCT is recommended for the assessment of preoperative orthodontic decompensation of maxillary and mandibular incisors [64]. This is an additional information from CBCT that is taken for orthognathic surgery planning, and it could not be one of the main purpose of using CBCT. Furthermore, CBCT proves a good method to assess TMJ after orthognathic surgery, particularly when there is considerable potential for resorption of the condyle [14].

3.12. Treatment outcomes

Taking CBCT at the end of orthodontic treatment is a controversial issue. However, it must be taken into consideration that studies on response to treatment can help elucidate clinical questions on variability of outcomes of treatment. There are studies assessing treatment

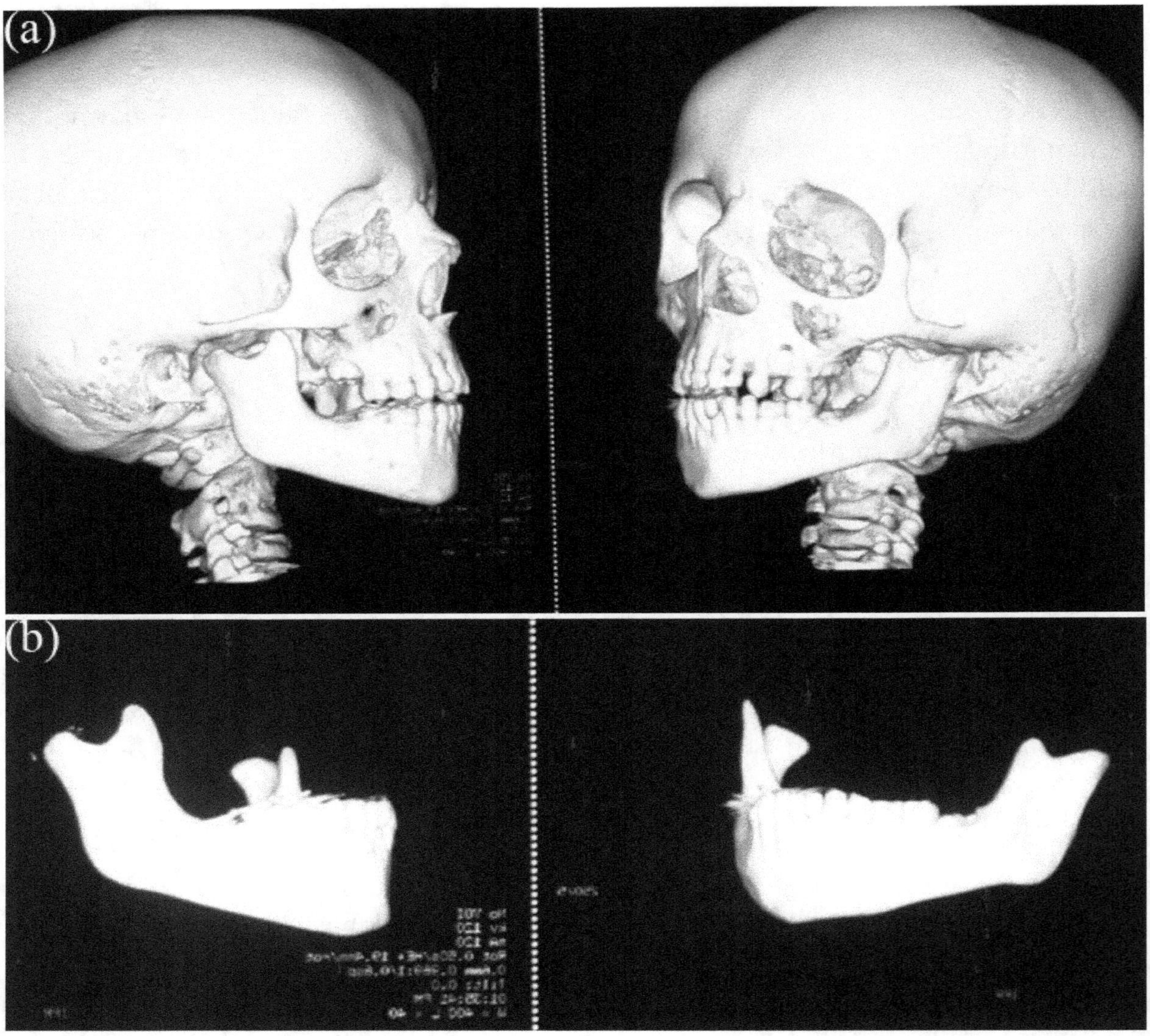

Figure 5. (a) 3D view of a case with Golden Haar syndrome. Note the asymmetric growth of left and right condyles. (b) 3D evaluation of mandible and condyles in this case.

outcomes of orthognathic surgery, maxillary expansion, bone grafting and several orthopedic appliances. A review of literature showed that jaw and teeth relationships, soft tissue, hyoid bone position, pharyngeal airway dimensions and morphology were evaluated after orthodontic and surgical treatments. To facilitate the evaluation of treatment outcomes, superimposition methods for CBCT images were also offered [28].

3.13. Evaluation of cervical vertebral maturation (CVM)

Skeletal maturation of patients is an important factor while planning orthodontic treatment. Hand-wrist and CVM methods were used for assessing the adolescent growth peak. It is suggested that the CBCT images may be useful for estimates of skeletal maturation, although they should not be used solely for that purpose [65]. Shim et al. [66] claimed that the esti-

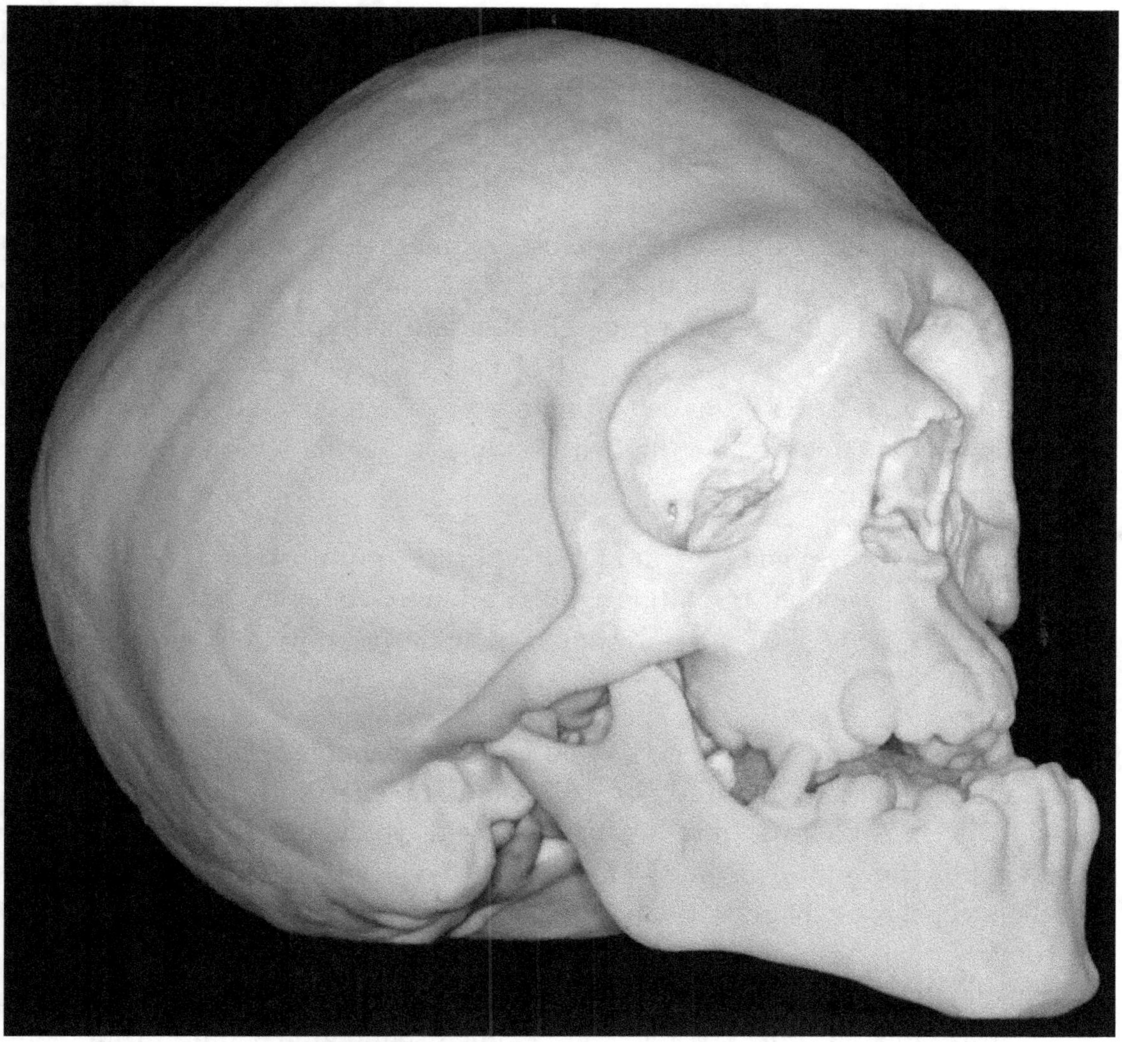

Figure 6. Presurgical 3D model of a case with Crouzon syndrome obtained from CBCT.

mate of maturation stages of the cervical vertebrae on CBCT provided a reliable evaluation of pubertal growth support and strongly positive correlations with lateral cephalograms and hand-wrist radiographs.

4. Radiation dose

Radiation dose depends on the CBCT scanner's specifications, milliampere setting, peak kilovoltage (kVp), voxel size, sensor sensitivity and number of images obtained, the time of scanning, and FOV. It is recommended to apply the 3D evaluation when the use of CBCT can be justified. Clinicians should always keep in mind that the radiation exposure to a human being should be kept "As Low As Reasonably Achievable" (ALARA) principle.

SEDENTEXCT project guidelines include a variety of topics, like justification, referral criteria, optimization, training, quality assurance and staff protection aspects [67]. Justification of using CBCT in dentistry can be considered if only a patient history and clinical information are available, if additional new information is expected, and if 2D radiographs are inadequate for diagnosis. The orthodontist should weigh the potential benefits of a CBCT against the chance of causing cancer for each patient. The chance may be small, but it is never negligible.

To reduce the patient dose, the smallest available volume size should be preferred. kVp and mAs of CBCT used in dental and maxillofacial region vary in a wide range and patients' doses varies considerably. It is recommended to standardize exposure parameters in dental and maxillofacial CBCT for each imaging task [68]. Gamache et al. [7] suggested that the total radiation exposure from CBCT scans can be reduced by while maintaining adequate image quality using low kV and moderate-to-high mA settings rather than the manufacturer-recommended settings.

Voxel size should be determined according to the purpose of the exam. When voxel dimension decreases, a better spatial resolution will be achieved, but the radiation dose will be increased [70]. Voxel sizes of 0.3–0.4 mm should be preferred if there is no need for a high level of detail [41].

Using child dose is offered because effective doses are higher compared with adults if exposure factors are not adapted. In a study on estimation of pediatric organ and effective doses from dental CBCT in 2012, it was reported that the average effective doses to the 10-year-old and adolescent phantoms were 116 and 79 mSv, respectively, which are similar to adult doses. So, the authors concluded that dental CBCT examinations on children should be fully justified over conventional X-ray imaging due to the higher radiosensitivity of children and that dose optimization by FOV collimation is particularly important in young children [69]. FOV should be restricted as much as possible [42]. So, the examination should include only the areas of interest in order to minimize radiation dose and ALARA principle must be followed. Repeated CBCT examinations should be avoided. The patient must be informed, and consent of the patient or parents must be obtained.

Technical properties of CBCT units were given inadequately in several studies. To make a comparison based on effective dose between studies, these properties must be reported and more evidence base studies on effective dose and image quality relation are still needed [70].

5. Future of CBCT in orthodontics

Further research-based technological developments are needed to achieve CBCT imaging, which is cost-effective, more precise on landmark identification and providing more accurate image quality with reduced radiation dose. By technological evolution and innovation of this technique, indications and the usage of CBCT in orthodontics will advance in the future. Future investigations are needed to investigate the dose levels for pediatric imaging protocols and to assess the use of a thyroid collar as a dose reduction technique.

6. Conclusions

In recent years, the use of CBCT in orthodontics has gained popularity and preferred as an imaging method by many clinicians for diagnosis and treatment planning. In this chapter, the indications and usage of CBCT in orthodontics are summarized. Clinicians should have comprehensive knowledge about advantages, disadvantages, limitations and potential risks due to increased radiation dose before deciding to use CBCT. Evidence-based studies are still needed whether using CBCT has any effect on clinical decision and lead to an improvement in treatment outcome.

Acknowledgements

We like to thank for their valuable contributions Dr. Sema Yuksel, Dr. Neslihan Ucuncu, Dr. Nilufer Darendeliler, Dr. Erdal Bozkaya, Dr.Secil Acar, Dr. Gülce Tosun who shared 3D views of their cases.

Author details

Emine Kaygısız* and Tuba Tortop

*Address all correspondence to: dt.emineulug@mynet.com

Faculty of Dentistry, Department of Orthodontics, Gazi University, Ankara, Turkey

References

[1] Palomo JM, Valiathan M, Hans MG. Orthodontic Diagnosis and Treatment Planning. Available from: http://pocketdentistry.com/11-3d-orthodontic-diagnosis-and-treatment-planning/3D

[2] Edwards R, Alsufyani N, Heo G, Flores-Mir C. Agreement among orthodontists experienced with cone-beam computed tomography on the need for follow-up and the clinical impact of craniofacial findings from multiplanar and 3-dimensional reconstructed views. American Journal of Orthodontics and Dentofacial Orthopedics. 2015;**148**(2):264-273

[3] Alqerban A, Jacobs R, Souza PC, Willems G. In-vitro comparison of 2 cone-beam computed tomography systems and panoramic imaging for detecting simulated canine impaction-induced external root resorption in maxillary lateral incisors. American Journal of Orthodontics and Dentofacial Orthopedics. 2009;**136**(6):764.e1-e11; discussion 764-5

[4] Alqerban A, Willems G, Bernaerts C, Vangastel J, Politis C, Jacobs R. Orthodontic treatment planning for impacted maxillary canines using conventional records versus 3D CBCT. European Journal of Orthodontics. 2014;**36**(6):698-707

[5] Ludlow JB, Gubler M, Cevidanes L, Mol A. Precision of cephalometric landmark identification: Cone-beam computed tomography vs conventional cephalometric views. American Journal of Orthodontics and Dentofacial Orthopedics. 2009;**136**(3):312.e1-e10

[6] Ludlow JB, Laster WS, See M, Bailey LJ, Hershey HG. Accuracy of measurements of mandibular anatomy in cone beam computed tomography images. Oral Surgery, Oral Medicine, Oral Pathology, Oral Radiology, and Endodontology. 2007;**103**(4):534-542

[7] Gamache C, English JD, Salas-Lopez AM, Rong J, Akyalcin S. Assessment of image quality in maxillofacial cone-beam computed tomography imaging. Seminars in Orthodontics. 2015;**21**(4):248-253

[8] Seet KY, Barghi A, Yartsev S, Van Dyk J. The effects of field-of-view and patient size on CT numbers from cone-beam computed tomography. Physics in Medicine and Biology. 2009;**54**(20):6251-6262

[9] Varghese S, Kailasam V, Padmanabhan S, Vikraman B, Chithranjan A. Evaluation of the accuracy of linear measurements on spiral computed tomography-derived three-dimensional images and its comparison with digital cephalometric radiography. Dentomaxillofacial Radiology. 2010;**39**:216-223

[10] Alqerban A, Jacobs R, Fieuws S, Nackaerts O, SEDENTEXCT Project Consortium, Willems G. Comparison of 6 cone-beam computed tomography systems for image quality and detection of simulated canine impaction-induced external root resorption in maxillary lateral incisors. American Journal of Orthodontics and Dentofacial Orthopedics. 2011;**140(3)**:129-139

[11] Larson BE. Cone-beam computed tomography is the imaging technique of choice for comprehensive orthodontic assessment. American Journal of Orthodontics and Dentofacial Orthopedics. 2012;**141**(4):402, 404, 406 passim

[12] Kusnoto B, Kaur P, Salem A, Zhang Z, Galang-Boquiren MT, Viana G, Evans CA, Robert Manasse, Monahan R, BeGole E, Abood A, Han X, Sidky E, Pan X. Implementation of ultra-low-dose CBCT for routine 2D orthodontic diagnostic radiographs: Cephalometric landmark identification and image quality assessment. Seminars in Orthodontics. 2015;**21**(4):233-247

[13] Cevidanes LH, Bailey LJ, Tucker GR Jr, Styner MA, Mol A, Phillips CL, Proffit WR, Turvey T. Superimposition of 3D cone-beam CT models of orthognathic surgery patients. Dentomaxillofacial Radiology. 2005;**34**(6):369-375

[14] Cevidanes LH, Bailey LJ, Tucker SF, Styner MA, Mol A, Phillips CL, Proffit WR, Turvey T. Three-dimensional cone-beam computed tomography for assessment of mandibular changes after orthognathic surgery. American Journal of Orthodontics and Dentofacial Orthopedics. 2007;**131**(1):44-50

[15] Sawchuk D, Currie K, Vich ML, Palomo JM, Flores-Mir C. Diagnostic methods for assessing maxillary skeletal and dental transverse deficiencies: A systematic review. The Korean Journal of Orthodontics. 2016;**46**(5):331-342

[16] Baumrind S. The road to three-dimensional imaging in orthodontics. Seminars in Orthodontics. 2011;**17**(1):2-12

[17] Scholz R. The radiology decision. Seminars in Orthodontics. 2011;**17**:15-19

[18] Bayome M, Park JH, Kim Y, Kook Y. 3D analysis and clinical applications of CBCT images. Seminars in Orthodontics. 2015; 21: 254-262

[19] Valizadeh S, Tavakkoli MA, Karimi Vasigh H, Azizi Z, Zarrabian T. Evaluation of cone beam computed tomography (CBCT) system: Comparison with intraoral periapical radiography in proximal caries detection. Journal of Dental Research, Dental Clinics, Dental Prospects. 2012;**6**(1):1-5

[20] Chang ZC, Hu FC, Lai E, Yao CC, Chen MH, Chen YJ. Landmark identification errors on cone-beam computed tomography-derived cephalograms and conventional digital cephalograms. American Journal of Orthodontics and Dentofacial Orthopedics. 2011;**140**(6):e289-e297

[21] Alling CC, Helfrick JF, Alling RD. Impacted Teeth. Philadelphia, Pa: W.B. Saunders; 1993

[22] Oberoi S, Knueppel S. Three-dimensional assessment of impacted canines and root resorption using cone beam computed tomography. Oral Surgery, Oral Medicine, Oral Pathology, Oral Radiology. 2012;**113**(2):260-267

[23] Scarfe WC, Farman AG, Sukovic P. Clinical applications of cone beam computed tomography in dental practice. Journal - Canadian Dental Association. 2006;**72**(1):75-80

[24] Alqerban A, Jacobs R, Lambrechts P, Loozen G, Willems G. Root resorption of the maxillary lateral incisor caused by impacted canine: A literature review. Clinical Oral Investigations. 2009;**13**(3):247-255

[25] Walker L, Enciso R, Mah J. Three-dimensional localization of maxillary canines with cone-beam computed tomography. American Journal of Orthodontics and Dentofacial Orthopedics 2005;**128**(4):418-423

[26] Haney E, Gansky SA, Lee JS, Johnson E, Maki K, Miller AJ, Huang JC. Comparative analysis of traditional radiographs and cone-beam computed tomography volumetric images in the diagnosis and treatment planning of maxillary impacted canines. American Journal of Orthodontics and Dentofacial Orthopedics. 2010;**137**(5):590-597

[27] Kapila S, Nervina JM. 3D image-aided diagnosis and treatment of impacted and transposed teeth. In: Kapila S, editor. Cone Beam Computed Tomography in Orthodontics. John Wiley & Sons; 2014. pp. 349-382

[28] Kapila S, Conley RS, Harrell WE Jr. The current status of cone beam computed tomography imaging in orthodontics. Dentomaxillofacial Radiology. 2011;**40**(1):24-34

[29] Alqerban A, Hedesiu M, Baciut M, Nackaerts O, Jacobs R, Fieuws S; SedentexCT Consortium., Willems G. Pre-surgical treatment planning of maxillary canine impactions using panoramic vs cone beam CT imaging. Dentomaxillofacial Radiology. 2013;**42**(9):20130157

[30] Wriedt S, Jaklin J, Al-Nawas B, Wehrbein H. Impacted upper canines: Examination and treatment proposal based on 3D versus 2D diagnosis. Journal of Orofacial Orthopedics. 2012;**73**(1):28-40

[31] Becker A, Abramovitz I, Chaushu S. Failure of treatment of impacted canines associated with invasive cervical root resorption. The Angle Orthodontist. 2013;**83**(5):870-876

[32] Alqerban A, Jacobs R, Fieuws S, Willems G. Comparison of two cone beam computed tomographic systems versus panoramic imaging for localization of impacted maxillary canines and detection of root resorption. European Journal of Orthodontics. 2011;**33**:93-102

[33] Kapila SD, Nervina JM. CBCT in orthodontics: Assessment of treatment outcomes and indications for its use. Dentomaxillofacial Radiology. 2015;**44**(1):20140282

[34] Westphalen VP, Gomes de Moraes I, Westphalen FH, Martins WD, Souza PH. Conventional and digital radiographic methods in the detection of simulated external root resorptions: A comparative study. Dentomaxillofacial Radiology. 2004;**33**(4):233-235

[35] Ely NJ, Sherriff M, Cobourne MT. Dental transposition as a disorder of genetic origin. European Journal of Orthodontics. 2006;**28**(2):145-151

[36] Shafer WG, Hine MK, Levy BM. A Textbook of Oral Pathology. Philadelphia: WB Saunders Co; 1985

[37] Toureno L, Park JH, Cederberg RA, Hwang EH, Shin JW. Identification of supernumerary teeth in 2D and 3D: review of literature and a proposal. Journal of Dental Education. 2013;**77**(1):43-50

[38] Yi J, Sun Y, Li Y, Li C, Li X, Zhao Z. Cone-beam computed tomography versus periapical radiograph for diagnosing external root resorption: A systematic review and meta-analysis. The Angle Orthodontist. 2017;**87**(2):328-337

[39] Jawad Z, Carmichael F, Houghton N, Bates C. A review of cone beam computed tomography for the diagnosis of root resorption associated with impacted canines, introducing an innovative root resorption scale. Oral Surgery, Oral Medicine, Oral Pathology, Oral Radiology, and Endodontology. 2016;**122**(6):765-771

[40] Nervina JM, Kapila SD. Assessment of root position and morphology by Cone Beam Computed Tomography. In: Kapila S, editor. Cone Beam Computed Tomography in Orthodontics. John Wiley & Sons; 2014. pp. 319-348.

[41] Garib DG, Calil LR, Leal CR, Janson G. Is there a consensus for CBCT use in Orthodontics? Dental Press Journal of Orthodontics. 2014;**19**(5):136-149

[42] European Commission. Radiation protection no 172. Cone beam CT for dental and maxillofacial radiology (evidence based guidelines). 2012. Available: http://www.sedentexct.eu/files/radiation_protection_172.pdf. [Accessed 2014 Mar 16]

[43] Hamada Y, Kondoh T, Noguchi K, Iino M, Isono H, Ishii H, et al. Application of limited cone beam computed tomography to clinical assessment of alveolar bone grafting: a preliminary report. The Cleft Palate-Craniofacial Journal. 2005;**42**(2):128-137

[44] American Academy of Oral and Maxillofacial Radiology. Clinical recommendations regarding use of cone beam computed tomography in Orthodontics. Position statement by the American Academy of Oral and Maxillofacial Radiology. Oral Surgery, Oral Medicine, Oral Pathology, Oral Radiology, and Endodontology. 2013;**116**(2):238-257

[45] Scarfe WC, Farman AG. What is cone-beam CT and how does it work? Dental Clinics of North America. 2008;**52**(4):707-730

[46] Okeson JP. Management of Temporomandibular Disorders and Occlusion. Mosby Co.; 1998. pp. 281-303

[47] Honey OB, Scarfe WC, Hilgers MJ, Klueber K, Silveira AM, Haskell BS, et al. Accuracy of cone-beam computed tomography imaging of the temporomandibular joint: comparisons with panoramic radiology and linear tomography. American Journal of Orthodontics and Dentofacial Orthopedics. 2007;**132**(4):429-438

[48] Tuncer BB, Ataç MS, Yüksel S. A case report comparing 3-D evaluation in the diagnosis and treatment planning of hemimandibular hyperplasia with conventional radiography. Journal of Cranio-Maxillo-Facial Surgery. 2009;**37**(6):312-319

[49] Knappe SW, Bakke M, Svanholt P, Petersson A, Sonnesen L. Long-term side effects on the temporomandibular joints and orofacial function in patients with obstructive sleep apnoea treated with a mandibular advancement device. Journal of Oral Rehabilitation. 2017;44(5):354-362

[50] Alhammadi MS, Fayed MS, Labib A. Three-dimensional assessment of condylar position and joint spaces after maxillary first premolar extraction in skeletal Class II malocclusion. Orthodontics & Craniofacial Research. 2017. doi: 10.1111/ocr.12141

[51] Massie JP, Runyan CM, Stern MJ, Alperovich M, Rickert SM, Shetye PR, Staffenberg DA, Flores RL. Nasal septal anatomy in skeletally mature patients with cleft lip and palate. JAMA Facial Plastic Surgery. 2016;**18**(5):347-353

[52] Aboudara CA, Hatcher D, Neilsen IL, Miller A. A three-dimensional evaluation of the upper airway in adolescents. Orthodontics & Craniofacial Research. 2003;**6**(Suppl 1):173-175

[53] Lenza MG, Lenza MM, Dalstra M, Melsen B, Cattaneo PM. An analysis of different approaches to the assessment of upper airway morphology: A CBCT study. Orthodontics & Craniofacial Research. 2010;**13**(2):96-105

[54] Goldenberg DC, Alonso N, Goldenberg FC, Gebrin ES, Amaral TS, Scanavini MA, et al. Using computed tomography to evaluate maxillary changes after surgically assisted rapid palatal expansion. Journal of Craniofacial Surgery 2007;**18**:302-311

[55] Jang HI, Kim SC, Chae JM, Kang KH, Cho JW, Chang NY, Lee KY, Cho JH. Relationship between maturation indices and morphology of the midpalatal suture obtained using cone-beam computed tomography images. The Korean Journal of Orthodontics. 2016;**46**(6):345-355

[56] Koudstaal MJ, Wolvius EB, Schulten AJ, Hop WC, van der Wal KG. Stability, tipping and relapse of bone-borne versus tooth-borne surgically assisted rapid maxillary expansion: A prospective randomized patient trial. International Journal of Oral and Maxillofacial Surgery. 2009;**38**:308-315

[57] Holm M, Jost-Brinkmann PG, Mah J, Bumann A. Bone thickness of the anterior palate for orthodontic miniscrews. The Angle Orthodontist. 2016;**86**(5):826-831

[58] Motoyoshi M, Yoshida T, Ono A, Shimizu N. Effect of cortical bone thickness and implant placement torque on stability of orthodontic mini-implants. The International Journal of Oral & Maxillofacial Implants. 2007;**22**(5):779-784

[59] Motoyoshi M, Ueno S, Okazaki K, Shimizu N. Bone stress for a mini-implant close to the roots of adjacent teeth-3D finite element analysis. International Journal of Oral and Maxillofacial Surgery. 2009;**38**(4):363-368

[60] Baumgaertel S. Planning and placing temporary anchorage devices with the aid of cone beam computed tomography. In: Kapila S, editor. Cone Beam Computed Tomography in Orthodontics. John Wiley & Sons; 2014. pp. 411-426

[61] Baumgaertel S, Hans MG. Buccal cortical bone thickness for mini-implant placement. American Journal of Orthodontics and Dentofacial Orthopedics. 2009;**36**(2):230-235

[62] Porto OC, de Freitas JC, de Alencar AH, Estrela C. The use of three-dimensional cephalometric references in dentoskeletal symmetry diagnosis. Dental Press Journal of Orthodontics. 2014;**19**(6):78-85

[63] Schendel SA, Lane C, Harrell WE Jr. 3D Orthognathic surgery simulation using image fusion. Seminars in Orthodontics. 2009;**15**:48-56

[64] Sun B, Tang J, Xiao P, Ding Y. Presurgical orthodontic decompensation alters alveolar bone condition around mandibular incisors in adults with skeletal Class III malocclusion. International Journal of Clinical and Experimental Medicine. 2015;**8**(8):12866-12873

[65] Bonfim MA, Costa AL, Fuziy A, Ximenez ME, Cotrim-Ferreira FA, Ferreira-Santos RI. Cervical vertebrae maturation index estimates on cone beam CT: 3D reconstructions vs sagittal sections. Dentomaxillofacial Radiology. 2016;**45**(1):20150162

[66] Shim JJ, Heo G, Lagravère MO. Assessment of skeletal maturation based on cervical vertebrae in CBCT. International Orthodontics. 2012;**10**(4):351-362

[67] Menezes CC, Janson G, Cambiaghi L, Massaro C, Garib DG. Reproducibility of bone plate thickness measurements with cone-beam computed tomography using different image acquisition protocols. Dental Press Journal of Orthodontics. 2010;**15**(5):143-149

[68] ICRP. Radiological protection in Cone Beam Computed Tomography. ICRP Publication. 129. Annals of the ICRP. 2015;**44**(1)

[69] Theodorakou C, Walker A, Horner K, Pauwels R, Bogaerts R, Jacobs R. SEDENTEXCT Project Consortium. Estimation of paediatric organ and effective doses from dental cone beam CT using anthropomorphic phantoms. The British Journal of Radiology. 2012;**85**(1010):153-160

[70] Al-Okshi A, Lindh C, Sal'e H, Gunnarsson M, Rohlin M. Effective dose of cone beam CT (CBCT) of the facial skeleton: A systematic review. The British Journal of Radiology. 2015;**88**:20140658

11

Orthodontics in Relation with Alveolar Bone Grafting in CLP Patients

Aslıhan Uzel

Abstract

Alveolar bone grafting is an essential step in the overall management of patients with cleft lip and palate (CLP). The numerous advantages of this procedure have been reported in the literature. Failure to rehabilitate the alveolar cleft may give rise to a variety of problems. Lack of investing alveolar bone often precludes the correction of anterior tooth irregularities and limits orthodontic treatment and/or prosthodontic rehabilitation. The success of the graft is multifactorial. The periodontal health of the surrounding graft tissues, the experience and ability of the surgeon, the timing of surgery, and orthodontic management of the cleft area before and after grafting are shown to be the most important factors in this issue. In this chapter, current orthodontic approaches in relation with alveolar bone grafting (ABG) in cleft patients will be discussed.

Keywords: cleft palate, alveolar bone grafting, orthodontics

1. Introduction

Cleft lip and palate (CLP) are among the most common of all congenital facial deformities which affect approximately 1 in every 600 newborn babies worldwide [1]. Congenital CL/P can arise in isolation or together with other syndromes. Alveolar cleft (osseous defect in the alveolus of upper jaw) affects approximately 75% of cleft lip and palate patients [2, 3].

The rehabilitation of individuals with CL/P requires interdisciplinary care by centralization of treatment [1, 4].

As the facial cleft affects the whole stomatognathic system, orthodontics is a core element of the overall treatment process. The orthodontist should aim to provide a dentition that functions well and is capable of lifetime maintenance by routine oral hygiene and dental care. However, the underlying skeletal deformity that reflects intrinsic variation and the consequences of surgery severely restricts occlusal change [5].

There are two major factors which effect orthodontic treatment in patients with CLP:

1. Facial growth disruption

It is well known that facial growth in patient with CP is disturbed. Besides the intrinsic defect, surgery itself contributes to further disruption [3, 6]. A significant feature of facial growth in repaired CP patients is that the maxilla fails to grow at the same rate as the mandible during the adolescent growth spurt. Progressive midfacial retrusion is usually seen by the mid- to late teens. The results of the facial growth studies revealed the general characteristics of the individuals with UCLP: a short retrusive maxilla and vertical elongation of the anterior face, a retrusive mandible, and a reduction in posterior face height [6–9].

2. Alveolar bone deficiency

Lack of the alveolar bone may give rise to a variety of problems, including oronasal fistula, fluid reflux, speech pathology, impaired tooth eruption, lack of bone support for the anterior teeth, dental crowding, periodontal recession and eventual loss of teeth, and maxillary and facial asymmetry. Alveolar defect also limits orthodontic treatment and/or prosthodontic rehabilitation [10–12].

Thus, orthodontic treatment for children with cleft should aim to achieve an optimal occlusion and dentofacial esthetics within the constraints imposed by the underlying skeletal pattern [5].

The integration of orthodontics into the overall treatment of CLP starts any point between birth and end of the teens and highly related to surgical procedures, including lip repair, alveolar bone grafting, distraction, and orthognathic surgery [5].

This chapter reviews current orthodontic approaches in relation with alveolar bone grafting (ABG) in nonsyndromic cleft patients.

2. Alveolar bone grafting

Alveolar bony defect is the main limiting factor for orthodontic treatment. Elimination of the bony defect is provided by alveolar bone grafting (ABG). Since the introduction of secondary alveolar bone grafting (SABG) in 1972, this technique has become an essential step in the overall management of patients with cleft lip and palate (CLP). Providing bone tissue for cleft has following benefits: [10, 12–21]

1. To permit eruption of the permanent canine in the cleft site into sound bone.
2. To provide bony support for teeth on either side of the cleft site.
3. To permit orthodontic tooth movement.

4. To obviate or minimize the need for prosthetic replacement of teeth in the cleft site.
5. To permit placement of osseointegrated implants into the cleft area when indicated.
6. To stabilize maxillary dental arch.
7. To facilitate fistula closure.
8. To improve the contour of the alar base.

The long-term success of the alveolar graft is crucial for providing and lifetime maintaining optimal occlusion and dentofacial esthetics in patients with CLP.

Postgraft stimulation of maturation through remodeling of the graft is extremely important and is provided primarily by natural tooth eruption. Thus, it is generally agreed that the optimum timing for ABG is in the mixed dentition stage (8–11 years), just before the eruption of the permanent canine in line with the cleft side [10, 13, 16, 19, 22–29]. There is no precise recommended chronological age but, when one-half to two-thirds of the canine root is formed [10]. Canines are mostly the reference teeth because lateral incisors in patient with CLP are frequently absent. However, if lateral incisor is present, earlier bone grafting can be indicated at an age around 7–8 years. It has been found that the success rate is significantly reduced when ABG is performed after eruption of the canine. Resorption of the bone graft is a common situation, and the success of ABG depends on several factors. The periodontal health of the surrounding graft tissues, the experience and ability of the surgeon, and graft material are also shown to be the general factors determining success [13, 19, 20, 23, 30, 31].

The importance of the orthodontist in planning, preparations, and follow-up around ABG procedure is also widely recognized. Successful alveolar bone grafting necessitates a joint orthodontic and surgical involvement pre-, peri-, and postoperatively [10, 32, 33].

Before treatment, orthodontists should be able to explain the predicted outcome of bone grafting to patients and their parents [34].

At that point, diagnostic information is very important for planning pre- and post-orthodontic management.

3. Advantages of CBCT in diagnosing and treatment planning of patients with CLP

A bony bridge with sufficient height and width is important for successful bone grafting in the alveolar cleft and to guide eruption and movement of permanent teeth [15, 35–37]. The outcome of the procedure is considered satisfactory when a sufficient volume of remodeled bone tissue is obtained; otherwise, the surgery has to be repeated. Thus, volumetric measurements of CBCT images have been using to evaluate the success of alveolar graft outcomes in the current literature [38]. CBCT, an alternative approach to conventional CT that provides similar diagnostic information with much less radiation exposure, avoids the problems associated with traditional 2D imaging such as image enlargement and distortion, structure

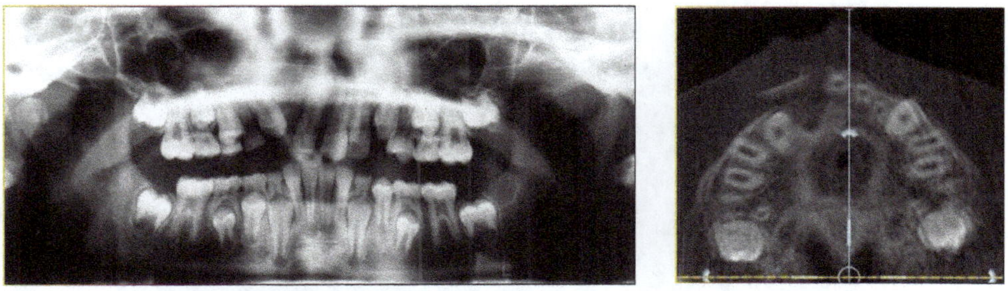

a b

Figure 1. Superimpositions on the 2D imaging might led to misdiagnosis. (a) Grafted area seems to be filled successfully on the pantomograph; (b) axial view of the CBCT image shows that graft is not successful as seen on the panoramic radiograph.

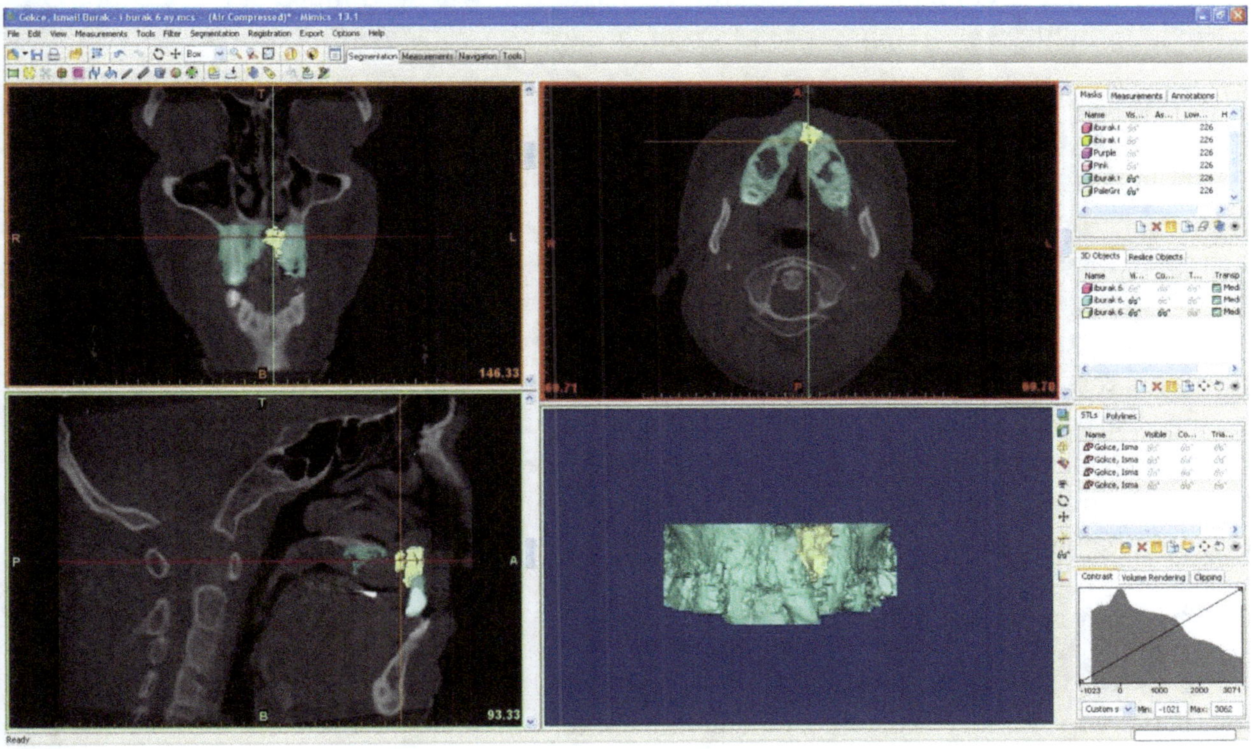

Figure 2. The precise volume and density can be measured by using various software.

overlap, positional problems, and limited number of identifiable landmarks (**Figure 1**). It has been used to quantify the average volume of the graft, location of the bone loss, and periodontal bone support of the cleft-adjacent teeth. CBCT-derived volumetric assessment of alveolar grafts has been reported as a reliable method [24, 29, 37, 39, 40] (**Figure 2**). The success rate of an alveolar graft has been found to be significantly lower with volumetric evaluation than that with conventional radiographic imaging [39, 41, 42].

4. Mixed dentition stage (phase I orthodontic treatment)

Orthodontic treatment of patients with CLP takes much more time (is more extensive) than routine treatment because of the underlying skeletal pattern. There is no need to attempt

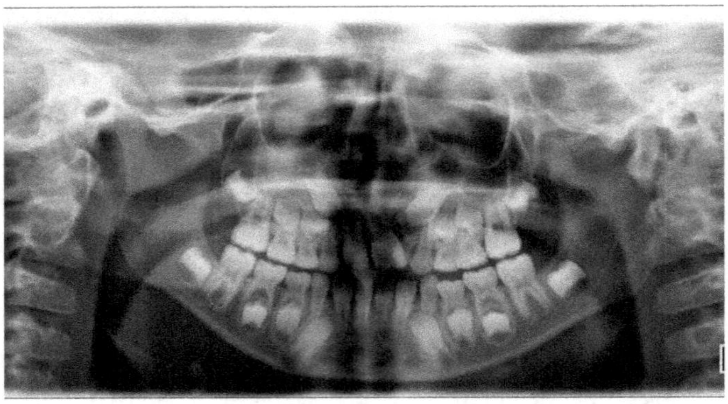

Figure 3. Malpositioned lateral incisor in the cleft area should be extracted 3–4 weeks before ABG.

orthodontic treatment in deciduous dentition stage. This will need much more retention procedures and will impose unnecessary burden of care [5].

Monitoring eruption of the teeth is important by the age 6–7.Radiographic evaluation is needed at the age of 8–9 (after eruption of upper incisors) to detect any possible teeth positioned in the cleft area and to see if lateral incisor is missing or not. If lateral incisor is present, earlier bone grafting can be planned. It is often advisable that any supplemental, deciduous teeth and also malformed and/or malpositioned lateral incisors in the cleft area should be extracted 3–4 weeks before surgery that permits healing of the mucosa (**Figure 3**). Thus, CBCT 6–8 months before ABG is recommended for detailed evaluation of bony support and position of the cleft-related teeth. This time frame will provide enough time to accomplish all necessary pregraft preparations such as tooth extraction and/or orthodontic tooth movement on time and not to delay bone grafting. Sometimes an additional CBCT just before the grafting might be needed to assess the root position of the cleft-related teeth after orthodonticmovement.

4.1. Pre-graft orthodontics

Presurgical orthodontics plays an important role in correcting misaligned incisors or repositioning displaced maxillary alveolar segments. Severe central or canine inclination toward the cleft defect can also interfere with cleft mucoperiosteal dissection. Presurgical orthodontics allows the surgeon better access for placement of the graft and closure of the soft tissue (**Figure 4**). Furthermore, correction of central incisor rotation and inclination prior to SABG enables patients to achieve better oral hygiene and prevents plaque formation. This can therefore prevent chronic, low-grade inflammation activating proteases that degrade grafted bone [5, 32, 33, 38].

One of the presenting problems which occurs early in both unilateral and bilateral clefts is the anteroposterior malpositioning of the incisors. If the anteroposterior malpositioning of the incisors is not corrected, lingual lock of the anterior teeth will further inhibit the development of the maxilla. The proper overjet relationship will allow appropriate growth of the maxilla [19]. By age 7–8, incisor alignment and correction of anterior crossbite can be provided to maximize the forward development of the maxillary dentoalveolar process. However, orthodontic movement of maxillary anterior teeth must be done with great caution because of the closeness of the roots to the bony defect. A very thin bony covering of the central incisor next to the cleft site is a common feature. Often there is just a lamina dura with no cancellous bone.

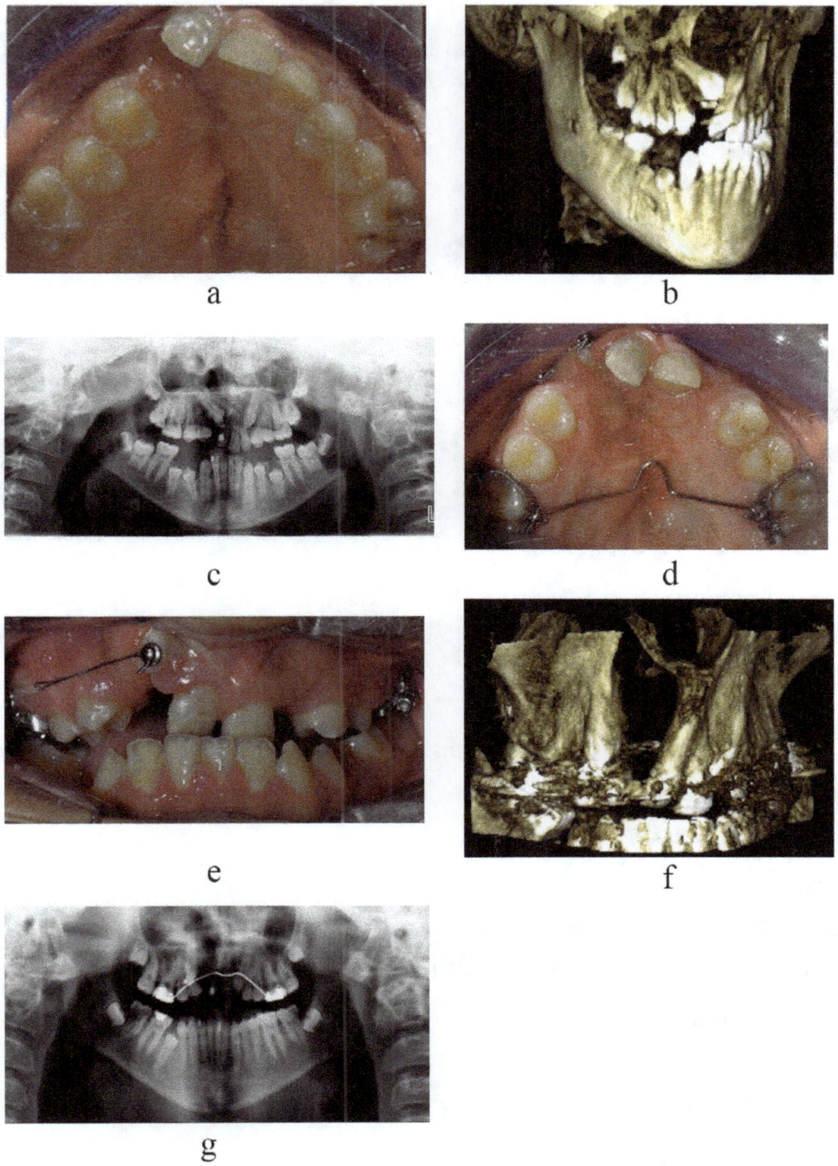

Figure 4. Severe canine inclination toward the cleft defect should be corrected before ABG. (a,b,c) initial views, a. intraoral, b. 3D image c. panoramik radiograph of the patient. (d,e) orthodontic traction of the cleft related canine. (f,g) pregraft 3D image and panoramic radiograph.

The incisor should not be bodily uprighted before successful ABG because of the possibility of bone loss and fenestration of the thin cortical lamina [10, 43].

4.2. Transverse expansion

Constriction of maxillary segments is a very common situation in patients with cleft palate. As the individuals with complete cleft lip and palate do not have midpalatal suture, constriction occurs mostly by the rotation of the lateral segment(s) inward, toward bony defect. Both the absence of the midpalatal bone and the soft tissue traction produced by lip and palate repair promote arch constriction [5, 44, 45].

Significant segmental displacement requires pre-bone graft expansion to rotate the lateral segment(s) outward, facilitate placement of the graft, and provide the surgeon working

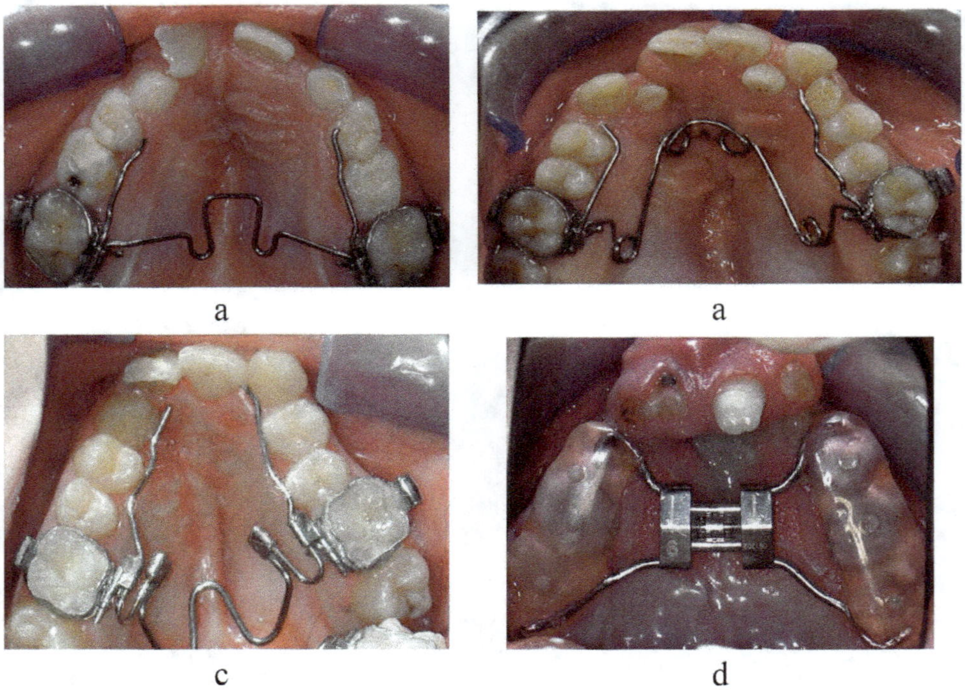

Figure 5. Various types of expanders for maxillary expansion. (a) TPA with lateral expansions, (b) quad helix, (c) NiTi expander, and (d) hyrax.

facility during surgery. If possible, transverse expansion can be combined with the correction of incisor irregularities. In the mixed dentition stage, arch expansion is very important because this process also normalizes the morphology and induces eruption of the canine into the symmetrical maxillary arch [10, 13, 19, 46].

Several types of expanders have been used, and there is no universal protocol for maxillary expansion prior to secondary alveolar bone grafting (**Figure 5**). Both slow maxillary expansion (SME) and rapid maxillary expansion (RME) have been advocated [5, 47, 48].

SME using the quad helix or its variations is frequently used for segmental repositioning as selective expansion anteriorly is required [5]. It has been shown that slow expansion forces are apparently already sufficient to allow a skeletal expansion of the maxilla in complete cleft palate patients [45, 47, 48]. There were *no differences* found between the dentoalveolar effects of SME and RME in patients with BCLP [45, 47].

RME with Haas type or hyrax expanders is also widely used for correcting the maxillary constriction. Asymmetric expansions were found by several authors [46, 48–53]. Isaacson and Murphy reported no correlation between the cleft location and the relative amount of lateral movement of each maxillary segment, emphasizing that RME laterally repositioned the maxillary segments in an unpredictable manner [49]. For greater amount of anterior displacement of the maxilla, fantype or double-hinged RPE expanders have been advocated [54].

According to our clinical experience, there is usually no need for RPE in patients with UCLP. Quad helix or TPA with lateral expansions can solve the problem. However, in some patients with BCLP, significant constriction of the segments necessitates RPE. Thus, patient selection is important in this issue.

5. Postgraft stabilization

The quad helix and/or stabilizing archwire used in BCLP may be removed during the bone grafting procedure for improved surgical access, but these appliances should be replaced before the patient leaves the operating room and left in place for 3 months.

As the bone grafting alone cannot be relied upon to maintain the expansion, a simple palatal arch would be advisable until the permanent dentition has erupted.

Stabilizing a mobile premaxilla with orthodontic arch wire is needed in patients with complete BCLP. Typically the arch wires will be removed during surgery and replaced at the end of the operation to provide retention [5, 10, 19].

6. Postgraft orthodontics

If the graft is done at proper time, before eruption of the cleft-related permanent canine, observation of the permanent dentition is generally all that is necessary. The status of cleft side unerupted teeth does need careful monitoring [5]. Physiologic eruption of the adjacent canine will provide enough stimulation for the alveolar graft. Sometimes orthodontic traction might be needed if the position of the canine is not appropriate for spontaneous eruption. High degrees of canine inclination indicate risk for altered eruption and impaction [5, 32].

If graft is done at age 7–8, correction of incisor irregularities provides also favorable stimulation to the graft.

Orthodontic movement of the cleft-adjacent teeth in the direction of the grafted bone can be instituted at an average of 3 months after the bone grafting, if needed. Combined interceptive bone grafting and orthodontic treatment at an early age avoid more extensive prolonged treatment later in the patient's life [5, 13, 19, 34].

It has been recommended not to delay orthodontic treatment more than 6 months after grafting, in cases in which an a-p crossbite or a residual transverse posterior crossbite exists. One- to two year delay in stimulation of the ABG of the premaxilla (by orthodontic treatment) can lead to serious postoperative problems. Where there is no stimulation of the graft, there tends to be "locking" or lingual collapse of the maxillary central incisors and collapse of the premaxillary arch [19].

6.1. Maxillary space management choice

In patients with CLP, the lateral incisor is missing in about 50% of cases in the permanent dentition. There are two options when maxillary lateral incisors are absent: space closure or space preservation [5].

The success of the bone graft is the determinant factor for this choice. When bone graft is properly done before the eruption of the permanent canine, canine can simultaneously migrate

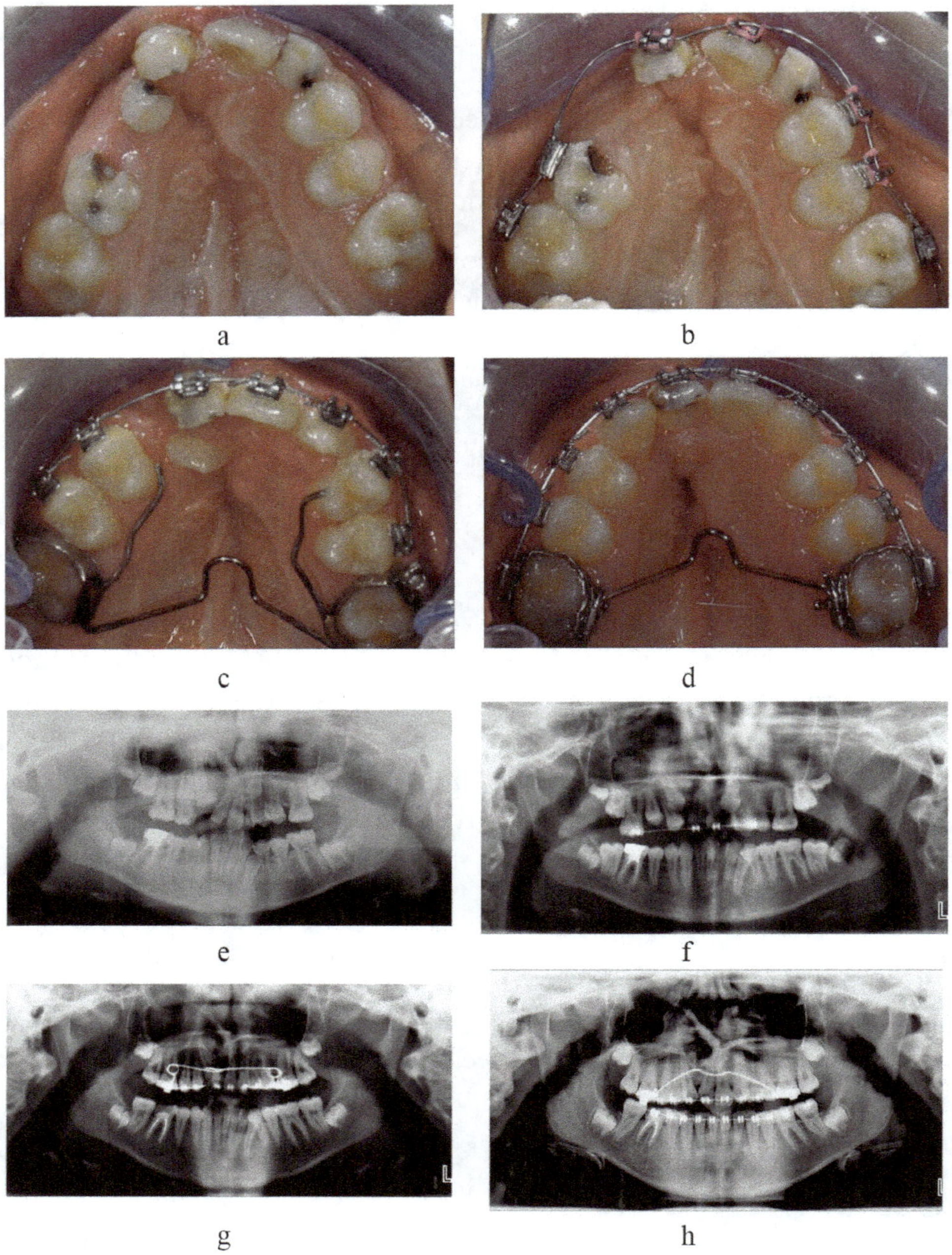

Figure 6. Space closure with canine substitution in patient with successful ABG. (a-d) intraoral occlusal views of the case. a. pre-graft, b. post-graft, c. after eruption of the canine, d. levelling of the upper dentition. (e-h) panoramic radiographs of the case. a. pre-graft, b. post-graft, c. eruption of the canine, h. levelling of the upper arch.

into the newly formed bone and increases its vertical height. Maintaining the alveolar bone height in the cleft area is important to prevent long-term complications, such as gingival retractions and periodontitis [32, 33].

Moreover, the natural dentition has the best prognosis for long-term health of the dentition. Thus, space closure with the canine substitution should be the first treatment choice for patients with CLP [5, 32, 33] (**Figure 6**). The functional stress imposed by orthodontic treatment influences the volume and prevents resorption of the grafted bone. Higher grafting success was found in the case of space closure than in the case of space openings [5, 33].

However, in patients with severely impaired maxillary growth, multiple missing teeth, and/or failure of bone graft, orthodontic space closure may not be feasible, and some form of prosthesis might be needed.

6.2. Extraction choice

Extraction of maxillary teeth may be required in UCLP in non-cleft quadrant, either because of crowding or to allow correction of the dental midline. As the second premolar is frequently malformed, it is the most commonly removed tooth. In some patients removal of the non-cleft lateral incisor allows the rapid restoration of the symmetry. However, this should be considered when compliance with space closure is assured [5].

In the lower arch, the absence of the second premolars is frequent and should be assessed carefully where extractions are necessary to relieve lower incisor crowding.

Extraction of the lower teeth to compensate class III skeletal pattern should be avoided in the early teens.

7. Management of maxillary deficiency in growing cleft patients

Hypoplastic maxilla and progressive midface retrusion are typical characteristics of patients with CLP.

Therefore, maxillary protraction (MP) has been frequently applied in the orthodontic treatment of growing patients with cleft lip and palate to improve the maxillomandibular relationship, occlusion, and facial esthetics. Optimal timing for initiating maxillary protraction for non-cleft children is shown as in the early mixed dentition before age 10. Early mixed dentition is favored over late, because of the closure of the sutures of the nasomaxillary complex [55].

However, SABG is optimally carried out between 9 and 11 years, and there is no consensus on the treatment sequencing of maxillary protraction and SABG in patients with CLP.

Two studies of three-dimensional finite element analysis suggested the advantage of SABG before maxillary protraction [55–57].

In a recent clinical study, short-term results showed that facemask therapy after alveolar bone grafting led to enhance maxillary skeletal advancement and minimize mandibular clockwise rotation more than those in the ungrafted group.

Maeda-lino found that the root lengths of U1 were comparatively short on the cleft side in patients with UCLP treated with MPA before SABG. Thus, they concluded that orthodontic force exerted by the MPA before SABG might result in short dental roots [58].

Moreover, it has been advocated that protraction of severely retruded cleft maxilla, even at an early stage, does not provide lasting skeletal benefit. Its effect in individual cases with CLP is difficult to predict, and many patients require orthognathic surgery after MP treatment [5, 59, 60] (**Figures 7** and **8**). Thus, explanation of the expected effects and associated problems should be given to the patients and parents before MP treatment.

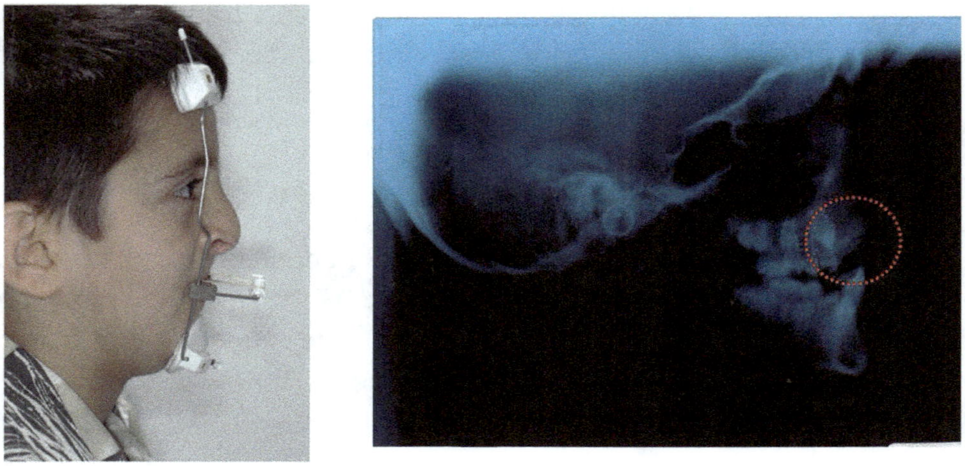

a b

Figure 7. Face mask application using bonded hyrax in patient with BCLP. (a) extraoral view of the patient. (b) initial lateral cephalogram.

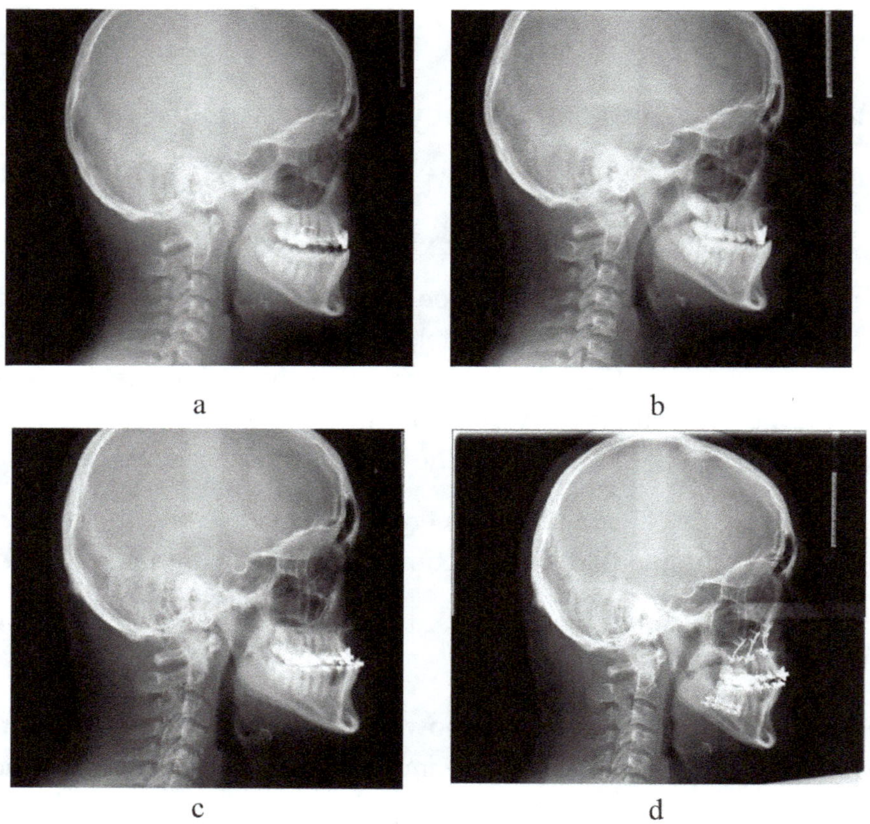

Figure 8. Cephalometric radiographs of the patient after facemask therapy between 10 and 19 years of age and after orthognathic surgery. (a) age 10, after face mask therapy, (b) age 14, follow-up, (c) age 19, ğre-orthogntic surgery, (d) after orthognatic surgery.

7.1. Patients with no to mild skeletal discrepancy

Providing proper overjet relationship at the early mixed dentition by correcting lingual lock of the anterior teeth using either removable or fixed appliances will be sufficient to maximize the forward development of the maxillary dentoalveolar process. Facemask can be a valuable source of anchorage for advancing posterior teeth during space closure after SABG [5, 19].

7.2. Patients with moderate to severe skeletal discrepancy

Early determination of the eventual need for maxillary osteotomy is a very important decision for the orthodontist.

Extracting lower premolar to correct anterior crossbite and trying to camouflage skeletal discrepancy are not appropriate in growing children. In that case, leveling only the upper arch, finishing with crossbite, and monitoring the growth are the best options. Early surgical options can be considered if needed [5].

7.3. Summary of treatment sequencing for mixed dentition stage

Evaluation CBCT–maxillary expansion and/or ortho-tooth movement–fistula closure and alveolar graft–maxillary protraction if needed.

Maxillary protraction protocol: 350–450 gram per side protraction force is adequate 14–15 hours a day for 6–12 months. MP can be started 4–6 weeks after SABG.

Part of this force should be transmitted as intermittent force to the maxillary anterior teeth through oral appliances such as an arch wire and/or lingual arch.

7.4. Unfavorable conditions

If maxillary deficiency accompanies with a wide alveolar cleft and/or fistula, it will be more challenging for both orthodontist and surgeon to treat growing patients [54] (**Figure 9**).

Late bone grafting or prolonged orthodontic treatment prior to bone grafting leads to loss of orthodontic control, marked instability of the premaxilla, and difficulty in maintaining

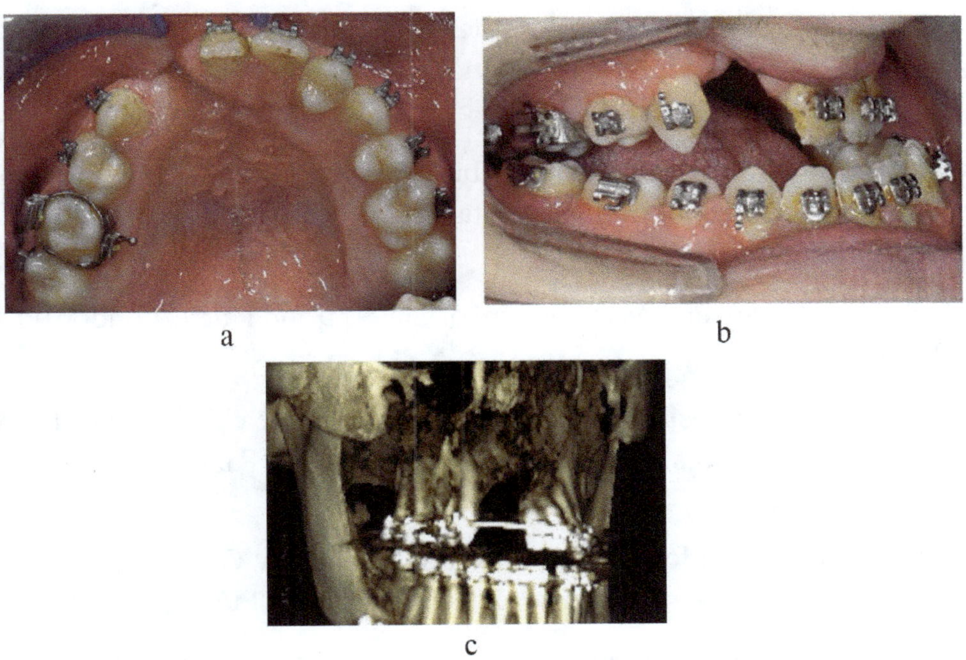

Figure 9. Wide alveolar cleft limits both orthodontic treatment and maxillary osteotomy. (a, b) intraoral views of a wide cleft, (c) 3D image of the case.

anteroposterior growth. In patients with BCLP, the unstable premaxilla with the small amount of maxillary bone attached to the vomer is usually incapable of being maintained with good stability without grafting.

When the premaxilla has been effectively grafted, any need to forward the maxilla at a later date can be accomplished by Le Fort osteotomy with a much diminished possibility of relapse [19].

8. Summary

The success of the orthodontic treatment and SABG is strongly interrelated. Carefully coordinated orthodontic and surgical involvement is critical for the well-being of the patients with CLP.

Author details

Aslıhan Uzel

Address all correspondence to: aslihanuzel@gmail.com

Department of Orthodontics, Faculty of Dentistry, Cukurova University, Adana, Turkey

References

[1] WHO. Global strategies to reduce the health-care burden of craniofacial anomalies. In: Report of WHO Meetings on International Collaborative Research on Craniofacial Anomalies. Geneva, Switzerland: Human genetics programme; 2002

[2] IPDTOC Working Group. Prevalence at birth of cleft lip with or without cleft palate: Data from the international perinatal database of typical oral clefts. The Cleft Palate-Craniofacial Journal. 2011;**48**(1):66-81

[3] ACH W, Sell DA, Grunwel P. Management of Cleft Lip and Palate. London, Philadelphia: Whurr Publishers; 2004

[4] Shaw WC, Semb G. Choosing the best treatment for the child with a cleft. In: ACH W, Sell DA, Grunwel P, editors. Management of Cleft Lip and Palate. London, Philadelphia: Whurr Publishers; 2004. p. 400

[5] Semb G, Shaw WC. Orthodontics. In: Watson ACH, Sell DA, Grunwel P, editors. Management of Cleft Lip and Palate. London, Philadelphia: Whurr Publishers; 2004. p. 299

[6] Kreiborg S, Hermann NV, Darvann TA. Characteristics of facial morphology and growth in infants with clefts. In: Berkowitz S, editor. Cleft Lip and Palate. 2nd ed. Germany: Springer-Verlag Berlin Heidelberg; 2006. pp. 25-235

[7] Semb G. A study of facial growth in patients with unilateral cleft lip and palate treated by the Oslo CLP team. The Cleft Palate Journal. 1991;**28**:1-21

[8] Semb G. A study of facial growth in patients with bilateral cleft lip and palate treated by the Oslo CLP team. The Cleft Palate Journal. 1991;**28**:22-39

[9] Mars M. Facial growth. In: Watson ACH, Sell DA, Grunwel P, editors. Management of Cleft Lip and Palate. London, Philadelphia: Whurr Publishers; 2004. pp. 44-67

[10] Mars M. Alveolar bone grafting. In: Watson ACH, Sell DA, Grunwel P, editors. Management of Cleft Lip and Palate. London, Philadelphia: Whurr Publishers; 2004. pp. 326-337

[11] Semb G. Alveolar bone grafting. Frontiers of Oral Biology. 2012;**16**:124-136

[12] Goudy S, Lott DG, Burton R, Wheeler J, Canady J. Secondary alveolar bone grafting: Outcomes, revisions, and new applications. The Cleft Palate-Craniofacial Journal. 2009; **46**:610-612

[13] Bergland O, Semb G, Abyholm F. Elimination of the residual alveolar cleft by secondary bone grafting and subsequent orthodontic treatment. The Cleft Palate-Craniofacial Journal. 1986;**23**:175-205

[14] Daskalogiannakis J, Ross RB. Effect of alveolar bone grafting in the mixed dentition on maxillary growth in complete unilateral cleft lip and palate patients. The Cleft Palate-Craniofacial Journal. 1997;**34**:455-458

[15] Kindelan JD, Roberts-Harry D. A 5 year post-operative review of secondary alveolar bone grafting in the Yorkshire region. British Journal of Orthodontics. 1999;**26**:211-217

[16] Eppley BL, Sadove AM. Management of alveolar cleft bone grafting-state of art. The Cleft Palate-Craniofacial Journal. 2000;**37**:229-233

[17] Kawakami S, Hura K, Yokozeki M, Takahashi T, Seike T, Nakanishi H, et al. Longitudinal evaluation of secondary bone grafting into the alveolar cleft. The Cleft Palate-Craniofacial Journal. 2003;**40**:569-576

[18] Murthy AS, Lehman JA Jr. Evaluation of alveolar bone grafting: A survey of ACPA teams. The Cleft Palate-Craniofacial Journal. 2005;**42**:99-101

[19] Boyne PJ, Herford AS, Stringer DE. Prevention of relapse following cleftal bone grafting and the future use of BMP cytokines to regenerate osseous clefts without grafting. In: Berkowitz S, editor. Cleft Lip and Palate. 2nd ed. Germany: Springer-Verlag Berlin Heidelberg; 2006. p. 587

[20] Craven C, Cole P, Holier L Jr, Stal S. Ensuring success in alveolar bone grafting: A three-dimensional approach. The Journal of Craniofacial Surgery. 2007;**18**:855-859

[21] Guo J, LI C, Zhang Q, Wu G, Deacon SA, Chen J, et al. Secondary bone grafting for alveolar cleft in children with cleft lip or cleft lip and palate (review). The Cochrane Collaboration issue. 2011;**6**:1-44

[22] Boyne PJ, Sands NR. Secondary bone grafting of residual alveolar and palatal clefts. Journal of Oral Surgery. 1972;**30**:87-92

[23] Boyne PJ, Sands NR. Combined orthodontic-surgical management of residual palato-alveolar cleft defects. American Journal of Orthodontics. 1976;**70**:20-37

[24] Yoshida S, Suga K, Nakano Y, Sakamoto T, Takaki T, Uchiyama T. Postoperative evaluation of grafted bone in alveolar cleft using three-dimensional computed data. The Cleft Palate-Craniofacial Journal. 2013;**50**:671-677

[25] Enemark H, Krantz-Simonsen E, Schramm JE. Secondary bone grafting in unilateral cleft lip palate patients: Indications and treatment procedure. International Journal of Oral Surgery. 1985;**14**:2-10

[26] Feichtinger M, Mossböck R, Karcher H. Assessment of bone resorption after secondary alveolar bone grafting using three-dimensional computed tomography: A three-year study. The Cleft Palate-Craniofacial Journal. 2007;**44**:142-148

[27] Ozawa T, Omura S, Fukuyama E, Matsui Y, Torikai K, Fujita K. Factors influencing secondary alveolar bone grafting in cleft lip and palate patients: Prospective analysis using CT image analyzer. The Cleft Palate-Craniofacial Journal. 2007;**44**:286-291

[28] Sindet-Pedersen S, Enemark H. Comparative study of secondary and late secondary bone-grafting in patients with residual cleft defects. Short-term evaluation. International Journal of Oral Surgery. 1985;**14**:389-398

[29] Tai C-CE, Sutherland IS, McFadden L. Prospective analysis of secondary alveolar bone grafting using computed tomography. Journal of Oral and Maxillofacial Surgery. 2000; **58**:1241-1249

[30] Kalaaji A, Lilja J, Friede H, Elander A. Bone grafting in the mixed and permanent dentition in cleft lip and palate patients: Long-term results and the role of the surgeon's experience. Journal of Cranio-Maxillo-Facial Surgery. 1996;**24**:29-35

[31] Uzel A. Computed tomographic evaluation of secondary alveolar bone grafting in patients with cleft lip and palate. GÜ Diş Hek Fak Derg. 2012;**29**:11-18

[32] Jabbari F, Skoog V, et al. Optimization of dental status improves long-term outcome after alveolar bone grafting in unilateral cleft lip and palate. The Cleft Palate-Craniofacial Journal. 2015;**52**(2):210-218

[33] Liao YF, Huang CS. Presurgical and postsurgical orthodontics are associated with superior secondary alveolar bone grafting outcomes. Journal of Cranio-Maxillo-Facial Surgery. 2015;**43**(5):717-723

[34] Maeda A, Uehara S, Suga M, Nishihara K, Nakamura N, Miyawaki S. Changes in grafted autogenous bone during edgewise treatment in patients with unilateral cleft lip/palate or alveolus. The Cleft Palate-Craniofacial Journal. 2014;**51**(5):525-532

[35] Feichtinger M, Mossböck R, Karcher H. Evaluation of bone volume following bone grafting in patients with unilateral clefts of lip, alveolus and palate using a CT-guided

three-dimensional navigation system. Journal of Cranio-Maxillofacial Surgery. 2006; **34**:144-149

[36] Hamada Y, Kondoh T, Noguchi K, Lino M, Isono H, Ishii H, et al. Application of limited cone beam computed tomography to clinical assessment of alveolar bone grafting: A priliminary report. The Cleft Palate-Craniofacial Journal. 2005;**42**:128-137

[37] Honma K, Kobayashi T, Nakajima T, Hayasi T. Computed tomographic evaluation of bone formation after secondary bone grafting of alveolar clefts. Journal of Oral and Maxillofacial Surgery. 1999;**57**:1209-1213

[38] Chang CS, Wallace CG, Hsiao YC, Chiu YT, et al. Difference in the surgical outcome of unilateral cleft lip and palate patients with and without pre-alveolar bone graft orthodontic treatment. Scientific Reports. 2016;**6**:23597. 1-7

[39] Rosenstein SE, Ross EL Jr, Dado DV, Vinson B, Alder ME. Comparison of 2-D calculations from periapical and occlusal radiographs versus 3-D calculations from CAT scans in determining bone support for cleft-adjacent teeth following early alveolar bone grafts. The Cleft Palate-Craniofacial Journal. 1997;**34**:199-205

[40] Nagashima H, Sakamoto Y, Ogata H, Miyamoto J, Yazawa M, Kishi K. Evaluation of bone volume after secondary bone grafting in unilateral alveolar cleft using computer-aided engineering. The Cleft Palate-Craniofacial Journal. 2014;**51**:665-668

[41] Feichtinger M, Zemanna W, Mossbock R, Kärcher H. Three-dimensional evaluation of secondary alveolar bone grafting using a 3D-navigation system based on computed tomography: A two-year follow-up. The British Journal of Oral & Maxillofacial Surgery. 2008;**46**:278-282

[42] Shirota T, Kurabayashi H, Ogura H, Seki K, Maki K, Shintani S. Analysis of bone volume using computer simulation system for secondary bone graft in alveolar cleft. International Journal of Oral and Maxillofacial Surgery. 2010;**39**:904-908

[43] Long RE Jr, Semb G, Shaw WC, et al. Cleft Palate-Craniofacial Journal. 2000;**37**(6):533-546

[44] Garib DG, Lauris RCMC, Calil LR, Medeiros Alves AC, Janson G, Almeida AM, et al. Dentoskeletal outcomes of a rapid maxillary expander with differential opening in patients with bilateral cleft lip and palate: A prospective clinical trial. American Journal of Orthodontics and Dentofacial Orthopedics. 2016;**150**(4):564-574

[45] de Almeida AM, Ozawa TO, de Medeiros Alves AC, Janson G, Lauris JRP, Ioshida MSY, et al. Slow versus rapid maxillary expansion in bilateral cleft lip and palate: A CBCT randomized clinical trial. Clinical Oral Investigations. 2017;**21**:1789-1799

[46] Ayub PV, Janson G, Gribel BF, Lara TS, Garib DG. Analysis of the maxillary dental arch after rapid maxillary expansion in patients with unilateral complete cleft lip and palate. American Journal of Orthodontics and Dentofacial Orthopedics. 2016;**149**:705-715

[47] de Medeiros Alves AC, Garib DG, Janson G, de Almeida AM. Calil LR analysis of the dentoalveolar effects of slow and rapid maxillary expansion in complete bilateral cleft lip and palate patients: A randomized clinical trial. Clinical Oral Investigations. 2016; **20**:1837-1847

[48] Holberg C, Holberg N, Schwenzer K, Wichelhaus A, Rudzki-Janson I. Biomechanical analysis of maxillary expansion in CLP patients. The Angle Orthodontist. 2007;**77**(2):280-287

[49] Isaacson RJ, Murphy TD. Some effects of rapid maxillary expansion in cleft lip and palate patients. The Angle Orthodontist. 1964;**34**:143-154

[50] Pan X, Qian Y, Yu J, Wang D, Tang Y, Shen G. Biomechanical effects of rapid palatal expansion on the craniofacial skeleton with cleft palate: A three-dimensional finite element analysis. The Cleft Palate-Craniofacial Journal. 2007;**44**:149-154

[51] Wang D, Cheng L, Wang C, Qian Y, Pan X. Biomechanical analysis of rapid maxillary expansion in the UCLP patient. Medical Engineering & Physics. 2009;**31**:409-417

[52] Gautam P, Zhao L, Patel P. Biomechanical response of the maxillofacial skeleton to transpalatal orthopedic force in a unilateral palatal cleft. The Angle Orthodontist. 2011; **81**:503-509

[53] Façanha AJ, Lara TS, Garib DG, da Silva Filho OG. Transverse effect of Haas and hyrax appliances on the upper dental arch in patients with unilateral complete cleft lip and palate: A comparative study. Dental Press Journal of Orthodontics. 2014;**19**:39-45

[54] Liou EJW, Chen PKT. Management of maxillary deformities in growing cleft patients. In: Berkowitz S, editor. Cleft Lip and Palate. 2nd ed. Germany: Springer-Verlag Berlin Heidelberg; 2006. pp. 535-554

[55] Zhang Y, Jia H, Fu Z, Huang Y, Wang Z, Guo R, et al. Dentoskeletal effects of facemask therapy in skeletal class III cleft patients with or without bone graft. American Journal of Orthodontics and Dentofacial Orthopedics. 2018;**153**:542-549

[56] Yang IH, Chang YI, Kim TW, Ahn SJ, Lim WH, Lee NK, et al. Effects of cleft type, facemak anchorage method, and alveolar bone graft on maxillary protraction: A three-dimentional finite element analysis. The Cleft Palate-Craniofacial Journal. 2012;**49**:221-229

[57] Chen Z, Pan X, Shao Q, Chen Z. Biomechanical effects on maxillary protraction of the craniofacial skeleton with cleft lip and palate after alveolar bone graft. The Journal of Craniofacial Surgery. 2013;**24**:446-453

[58] Maeda-Iino A, Marutani K, Furukawa M, Nakagawa S, Kwon S, Kibe T, et al. Evaluation of maxillary central incisors on the noncleft and cleft sides in patients with unilateral cleft lip and palate—Part 1: Relationship between root length and orthodontic tooth movement. The Angle Orthodontist. 2017;**87**:855-862

[59] Kuijpers-Jagtman AM, Long RE Jr. The influence of surgery and orthodontic treatment on maxillofacial growth and maxillary arch development in patients treated for orofacial clefts. The Cleft Palate-Craniofacial Journal. 2000;**37**:1-12

[60] Susami T, Okayasu M, Inokuchi T, Ohkubo K, Uchino N, Uwatoko K, et al. Maxillary protraction in patients with cleft lip and palate in mixed dentition: Cephalometric evaluation after completion of growth. The Cleft Palate-Craniofacial Journal. 2014;**51**(5):514-524

12

Orthosurgical Correction of Severe Vertical Maxillary Excess: Gummy Smile

Fayez Saleh and Wisam Al Hamadi

Abstract

Gummy smile which is commonly described as excessive gingival display in full smile has become a major esthetic concern for patients and healthcare providers in recent years. Because of the complex etiologic factors and severity of this orofacial deformity including skeletal, dentoalveolar, muscular, and gingival, it is essential that a differential diagnosis be established so that a relevant therapy can be selected from a wide range of treatment options. The complex etiologic factors of this dentofacial deformity necessitates coordination between a team of health care providers, especially between orthodontist and maxillofacial surgeon, to improve diagnosis and treatment planning, accurately predict the outcome, and minimize orthosurgical complications. In this chapter, the author will present several clinical cases and briefly review available treatment modalities for excessive gingival display in full smile. Emphasis will be put on orthosurgical treatment of severe vertical maxillary excess as the optimal solution to restore facial balance and harmony, attractive smile, and patients' satisfaction.

Keywords: gummy smile, vertical maxillary excess, dentofacial deformity, orthosurgery, interdisciplinary approach

1. Introduction

Orthosurgical correction of dentofacial deformities aims to obtain more harmonious and esthetically pleasing facial proportions in addition to normal and stable functional occlusion. Facial esthetics cannot be considered apart from an attractive smile and vice versa.

Despite the variety of ethnic, racial, and individual perception of facial attractiveness and a pleasant smile, there are general consensus among health care professionals that harmony and balance of the facial features are equally important as intrinsic dentogingival, lips, and perioral soft tissue components to be considered before designing a beautiful smile [1–3].

Gummy smile caused by vertical maxillary excess and dentofacial disharmony cannot be treated satisfactorily with adjunctive nonsurgical approaches such as botulinum toxin injection or a crown lengthening procedures or temporary anchorage devices (TDAs). An ideal treatment option for vertical maxillary excess (VME) is the reduction of the maxillary vertical excess by LeFort I osteotomy with superior maxillary repositioning [4, 5]. However, when gummy smile is not associated with severe skeletal discrepancy in three dimensions (3Ds), intrusion of anterior teeth using TDAs may be indicated provided that the anterior esthetic occlusal plane and smile arc are well preserved [6, 7].

Many nonsurgical orthodontic treatment modalities proposed to treat gummy smile in adult patients with severe skeletal facial problems were of limited use with no benefit on the skeletal vertical discrepancy [8]. Depending on the magnitude and severity of the gummy smile, combined orthosurgical techniques offer better esthetics and long-term stability [9].

Increased vertical dimension in class III cases is the most important and deciding factor to be considered when formulating a treatment planning and deciding the technique of orthognathic surgery [10].

Computer simulation of orthosurgical outcome which was once of great concern that showing predictions to patients might lead to unrealistic expectations and disappointments. Nowadays, image prediction is becoming more likely satisfying and acceptable as it allows patients to visualize possible soft tissue profile changes and help them to decide whether surgery would be worth in terms of the additional risk and cost [11, 12].

2. Orthosurgical treatment modalities of vertical maxillary excess: gummy smile

Because not all dentofacial deformities are alike, different treatment modalities were developed and advances in surgical orthodontics added a new dimension to the health profession and assured patients' satisfaction. The following case series intended to share experience with colleagues and students.

2.1. Case #1

A healthy patient (39 year 9 month old) presented with a chief complaint of "I am not happy with my smile, arrangement of my teeth, and prominent chin." Cursory examination revealed that the patient has skeletal and dental class III malocclusion with reverse overjet, narrow maxilla, long face, concave profile, and gummy smile. The case was complicated by old extraction of lower left first molar. Thorough clinical examination and diagnostic data collected assured limitation of orthodontic treatment alone to achieve treatment objectives and therefore, combined orthosurgical correction was suggested and the patient agreed after detailed discussion and joint meeting with the clinicians.

2.1.1. *Diagnosis, treatment objectives, and treatment planning*

Figures 1 and **2** explain the extra-oral, intra-oral clinical examination and radiographic assessment of the dentofacial components in 3Ds.

2.1.2. *Treatment objectives*

The objectives were directed to the listed problems to include: achieving esthetic facial features and pleasant smile; in addition to restoring normal occlusion in three dimensions (3Ds) as a prerequisite to ideal lip-teeth relationship. Retaining the treatment outcome is equally important, and all measures were taken to establish effective retention means before appliance removal.

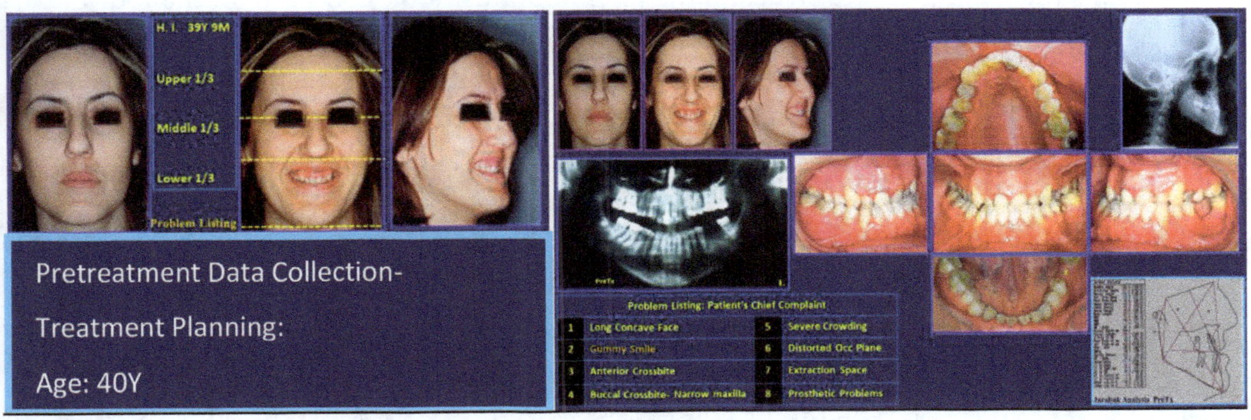

Figure 1. Initial clinical (extra-oral and intra-oral) and radiographic examination that allow to formulate an appropriate treatment planning and setting the treatment objectives.

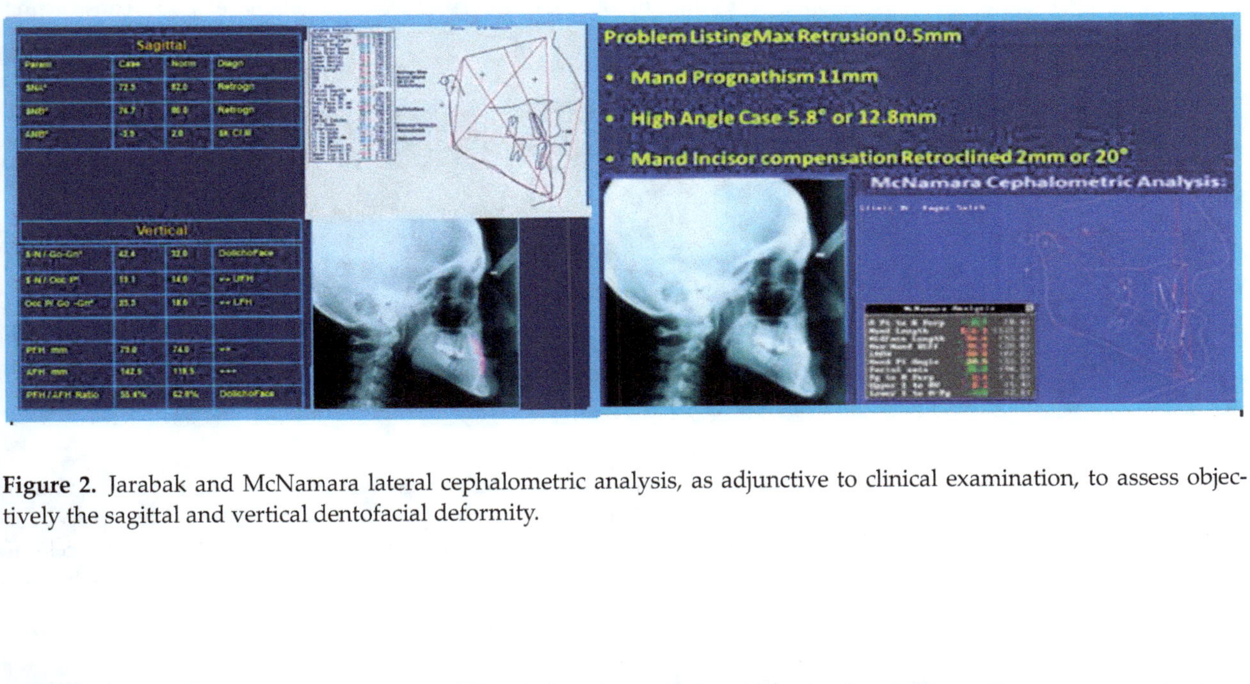

Figure 2. Jarabak and McNamara lateral cephalometric analysis, as adjunctive to clinical examination, to assess objectively the sagittal and vertical dentofacial deformity.

2.1.3. Treatment progress

2.1.3.1. Presurgical phase

Preparing the dentoalveolar arches for orthognathic surgery necessitated leveling and alignment of teeth, decompensating the retroclination of lower incisors, and achieving ideal arch form that allows surgical expansion through median maxillary split. **Figures 3** and **4** depict the sequence of orthodontic work and the simulation of surgical movements in 3Ds.

2.1.3.2. Postsurgical phase

Maintaining normal anterior overjet and overbite, plus ideal incisors, canines, and molar relationship during this phase is crucially important. The healing of bony parts during detailing of occlusion and any minor corrections if they ever exist is the key for success at this stage. Full-time wear of heavy elastics for 2 weeks after surgery to assure full dental interdigitation, arch symmetry, and stable treatment outcome. 4 month later, the appliance was removed, and the necessary retainers were constructed, the prosthodontist took good care of the four maxillary incisors upon the patient's request. Follow up for almost 5 years was planned, and the interdisciplinary approach yielded realistic adequate treatment outcome (**Figures 5–7**).

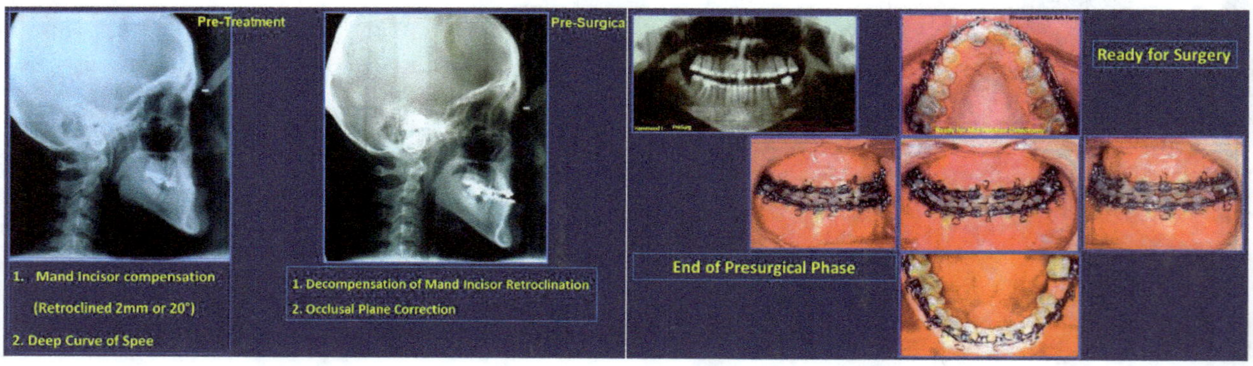

Figure 3. Treatment progress: decompensation of the incisor inclination and uprighting buccal teeth, leveling and alignment of teeth, flattening curve of Spee, restoring normal arch form, preparing model surgery, and constructing surgical hooks prior to surgery.

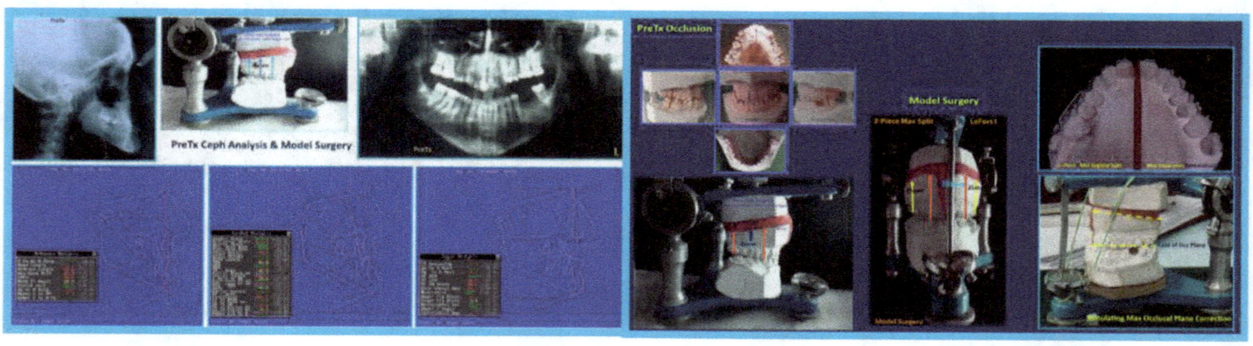

Figure 4. Models of the presurgical arches were constructed and mounted on semi-adjustable articulator, simulation of the surgical act included: superior maxillary repositioning and advancement, splitting the maxilla into two pieces for expansion, displaying final movements of the jaws and cant of the occlusal plane, and monitoring any possible occlusal interference to be resolved.

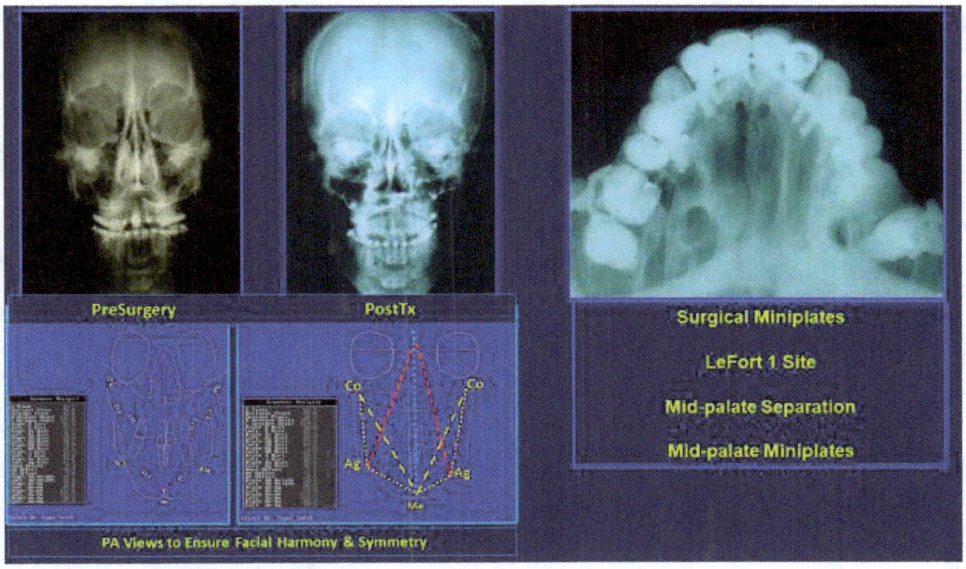

Figure 5. Pre- and postfrontal (PA) cephalometric analysis and occlusal view depicting the transverse surgical expansion of the maxilla with relevant min-plates in situ.

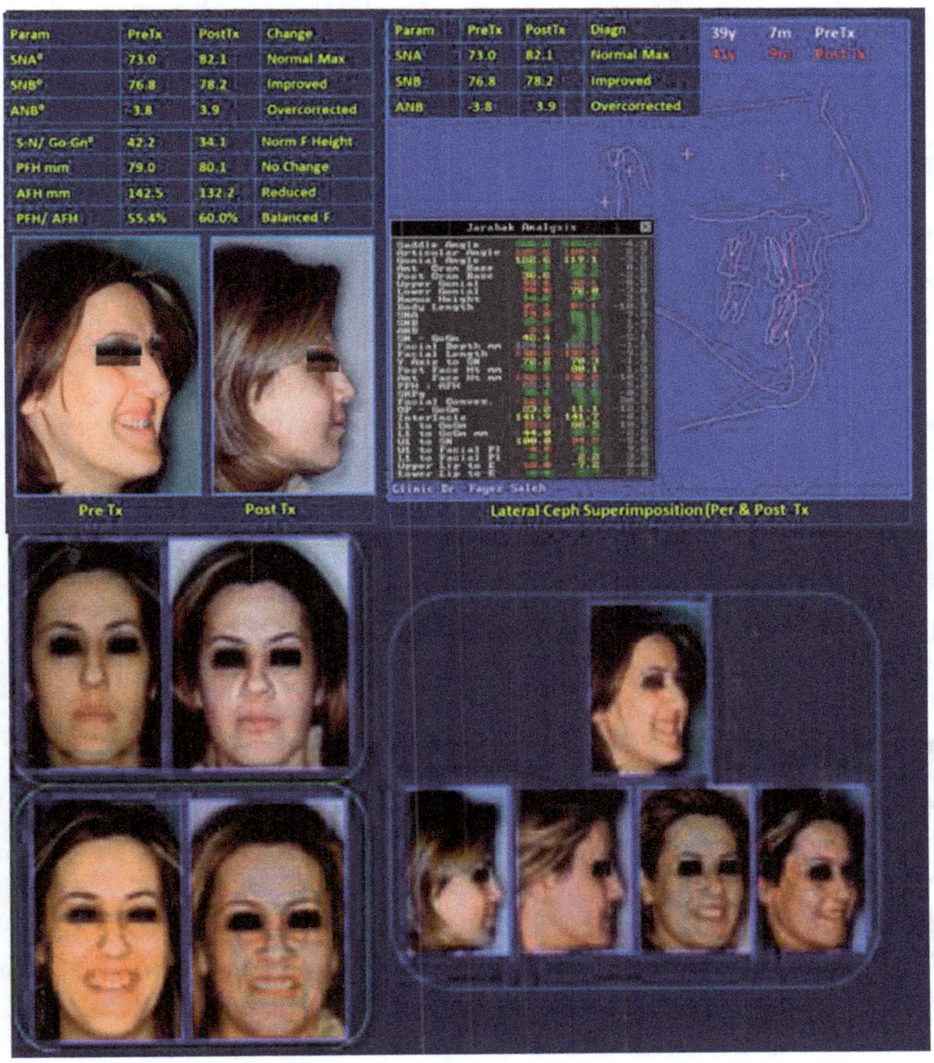

Figure 6. Pre and post photos and Lat Ceph analysis of Jarabak depicting the changes in profile.

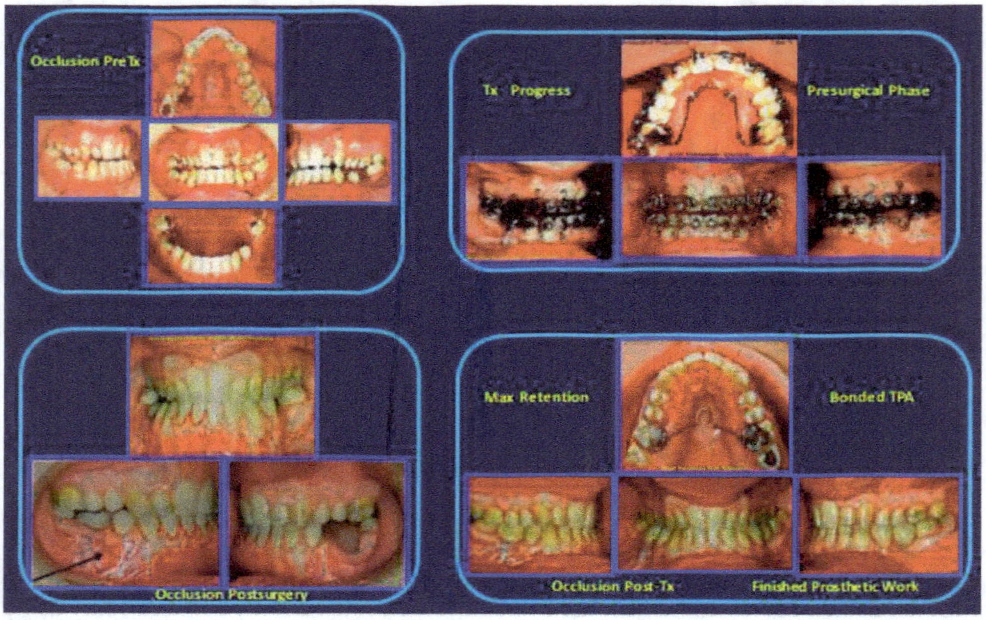

Figure 7. Pretreatment occlusion, presurgical orthodontic preparation, postsurgical occlusion, and final prosthetic reconstruction of occlusion.

2.1.4. Treatment results

The following photos and radiographs reveal the impeccable improvement in the harmony and balance of the facial form in 3Ds, successful surgical expansion, and superior repositioning of the maxilla resulted in ideal functional and static occlusion. Postoperative radiographs have shown a well seated condyle in the glenoid fossa in an appropriate physiologic rest position. Patient's satisfaction was rewarding (**Figures 8–10**).

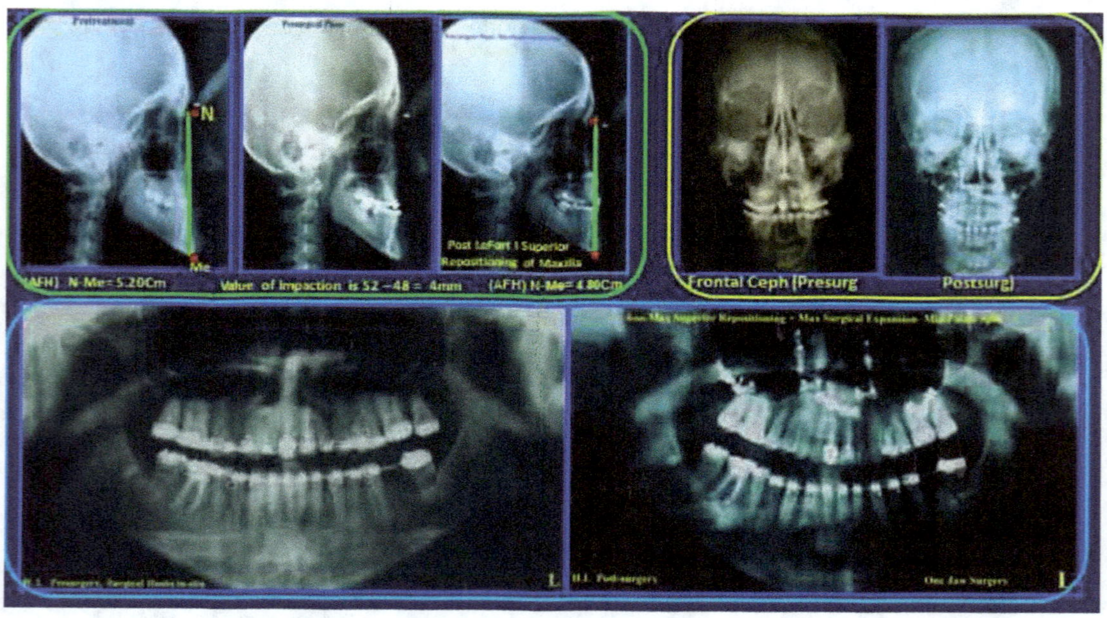

Figure 8. Pretreatment, presurgical preparation phase, postsurgical phase, and postsurgical radiographs.

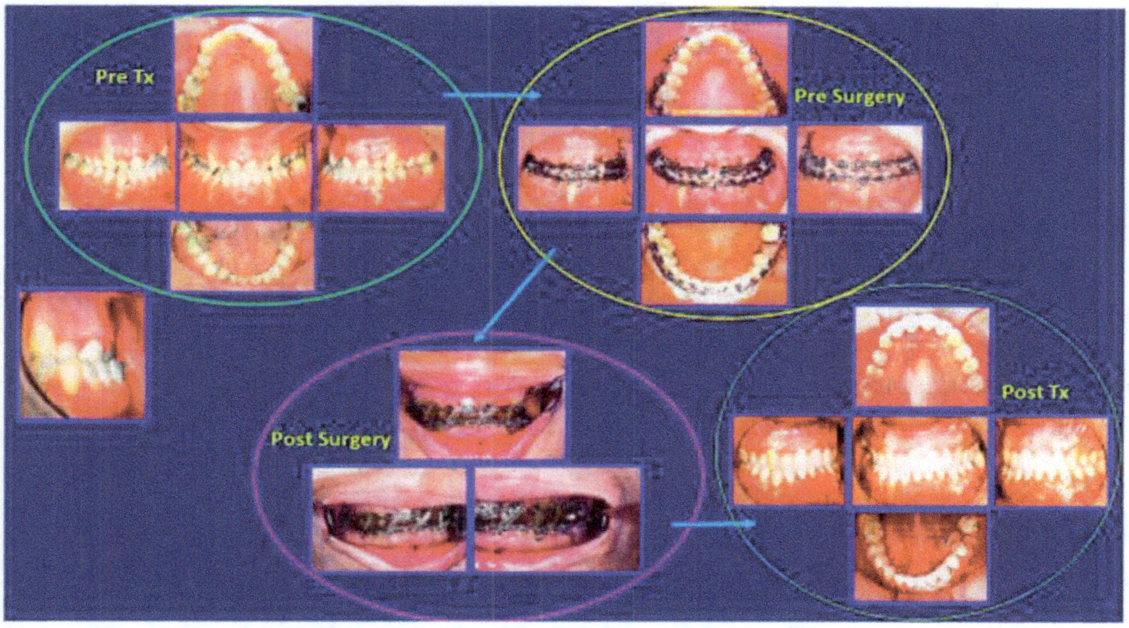

Figure 9. Pretreatment occlusion, presurgical preparation phase, surgical procedures, postsurgical phase to detail the occlusion, and posttreatment occlusion.

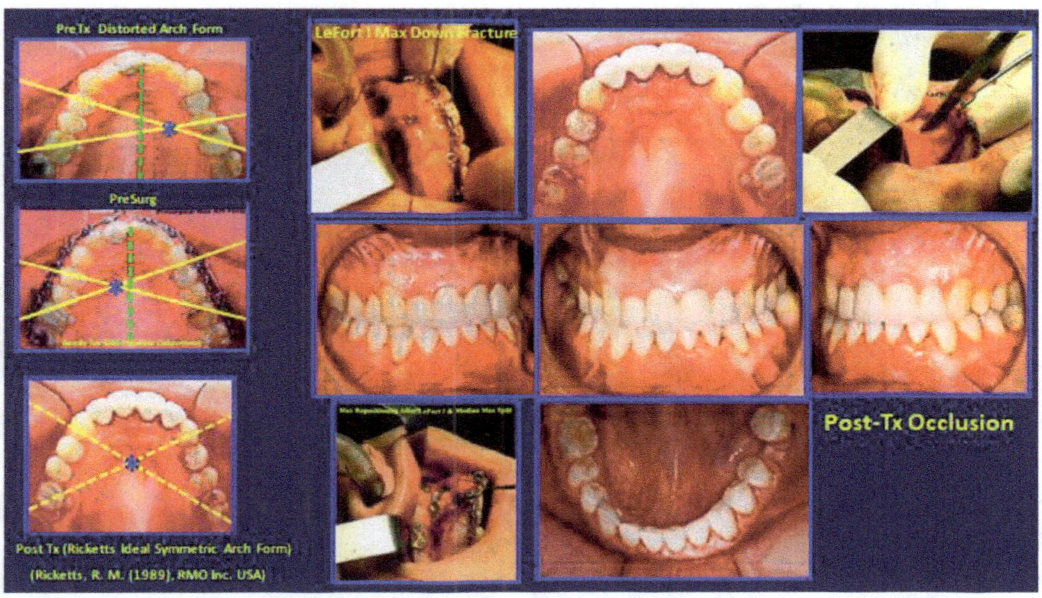

Figure 10. The final occlusion 5 year postretention focusing on the median maxillary surgical split to restore ideal arch form stable occlusion.

2.1.5. Conclusions

Attempt to treat dentofacial deformities without comprehensive data analysis and collaboration with other health care providers will not yield acceptable results and may need retreatment. Medical ethics obligate us to consider the patients' interest and welfare. This case, from the very beginning, was diagnosed as severe skeletal deformity in 3Ds and disproportionate dentoalveolar arches. The dentofacial imbalance and disharmony imposed the orthosurgical treatment approach which was agreed upon by orthodontist and maxillofacial surgeon and readily accepted by the patient.

2.2. Case #2

A healthy female (24 year 5 month old) presented with apparent long face syndrome, convex profile, vertical maxillary excess causing gummy smile, incompetent lips, and deficient chin. Intra-oral examination revealed a class II division 1 malocclusion associated with narrow maxilla, deep palatal vault, micrognathia, moderate crowding mild anterior open bite, and distorted occlusal planes.

2.2.1. Diagnosis

Figures 11–14 exhibit the clinical and diagnostic aids that facilitate the formulation of appropriate treatment planning to achieve optimum treatment outcome.

2.2.2. Treatment planning and treatment objectives

Because of the diagnosed severe skeletal dentofacial deformity, joint consultation and thorough patient's data analysis took place by the orthodontist, and the maxillofacial surgeon, the treatment modality offered to the patient, after detailed discussion and displaying of the possible outcome, was a combined orthosurgical care which was willingly accepted.

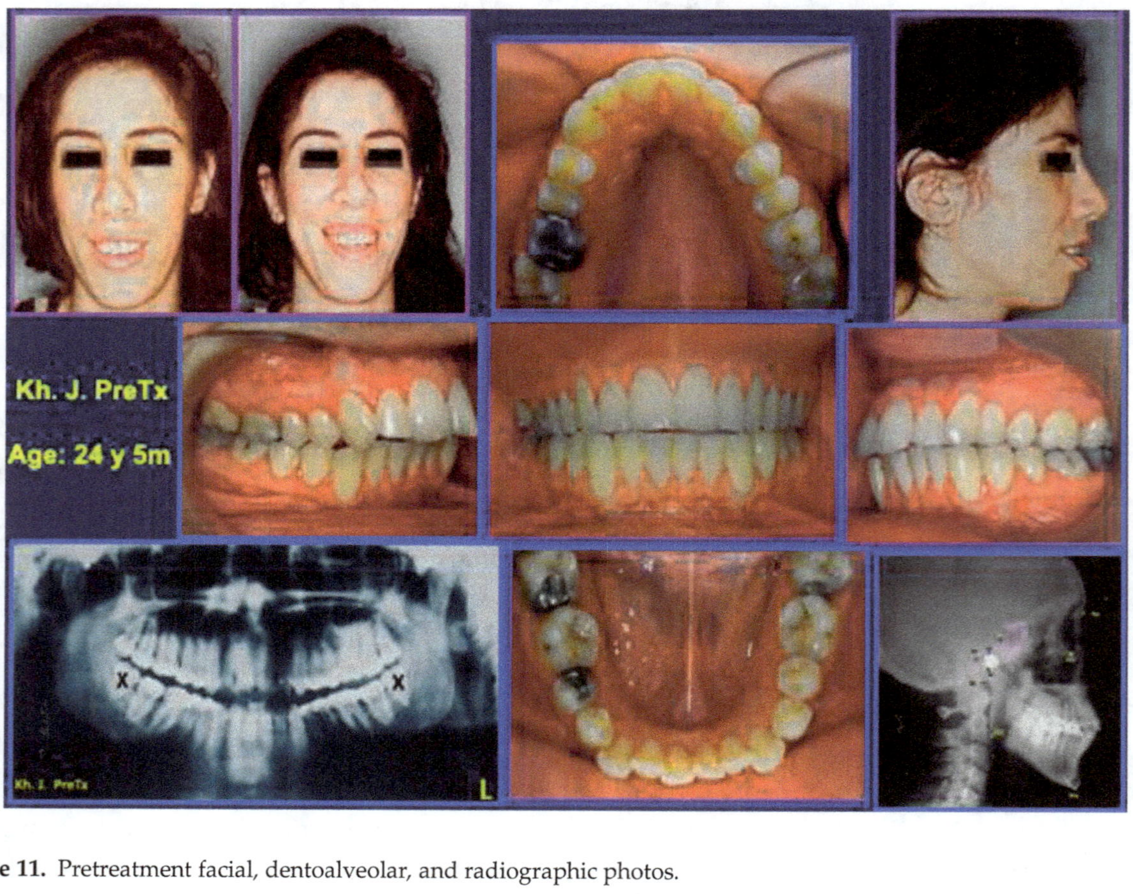

Figure 11. Pretreatment facial, dentoalveolar, and radiographic photos.

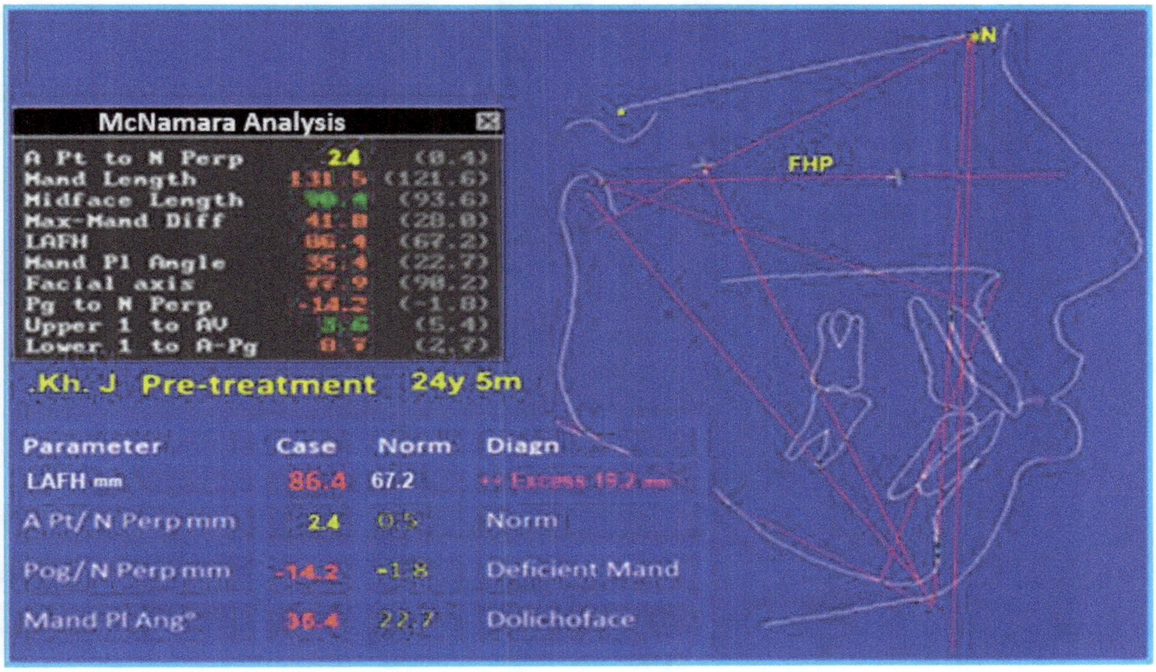

Figure 12. Pretreatment lateral cephalometric analysis of McNamara confirming the long face deformity and retrognathic mandible. Tipped down occlusal plane buccally caused backward rotation of the mandible.

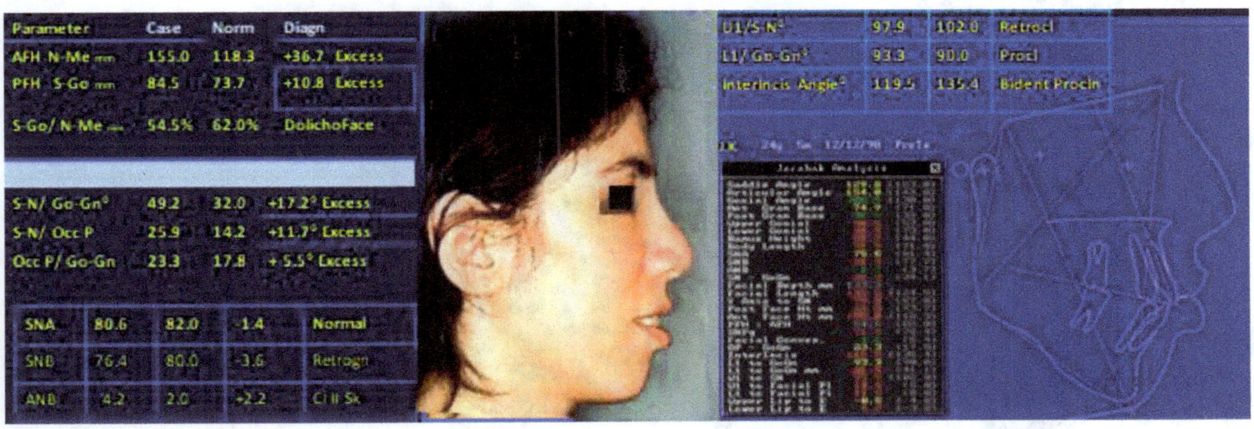

Figure 13. Pretreatment cephalometric analysis of Jarabak (sagittal, vertical, and dentoalveolar findings).

2.2.3. Treatment progress and results

Presurgical orthodontic phase intended to restore ideal arch form and dentoalveolar alignment (teeth decrowding, root parallelism, and occlusal plane leveling). This will facilitate the surgical mobilization of the arches in 3Ds; so that the appropriate canting of the occlusal plane and proper lip-teeth relationship secures satisfying treatment outcome (**Figures 15** and **16**).

2.2.4. Conclusions

When malocclusion is a consequence of facial musculoskeletal imbalance, any attempt to restore facial esthetics and beautiful smile by orthodontic dentofacial orthopedics alone will

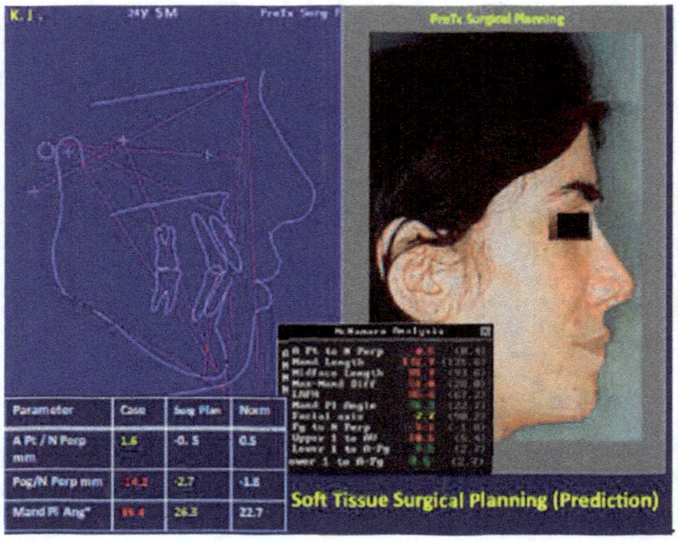

Figure 14. Soft tissue and dentoalveolar surgical planning of the case, surgical mobilization of the maxilla, and chin to restore harmony and balance of the facial profile, in addition to dentoalveolar sagittal and vertical orthodontic movements.

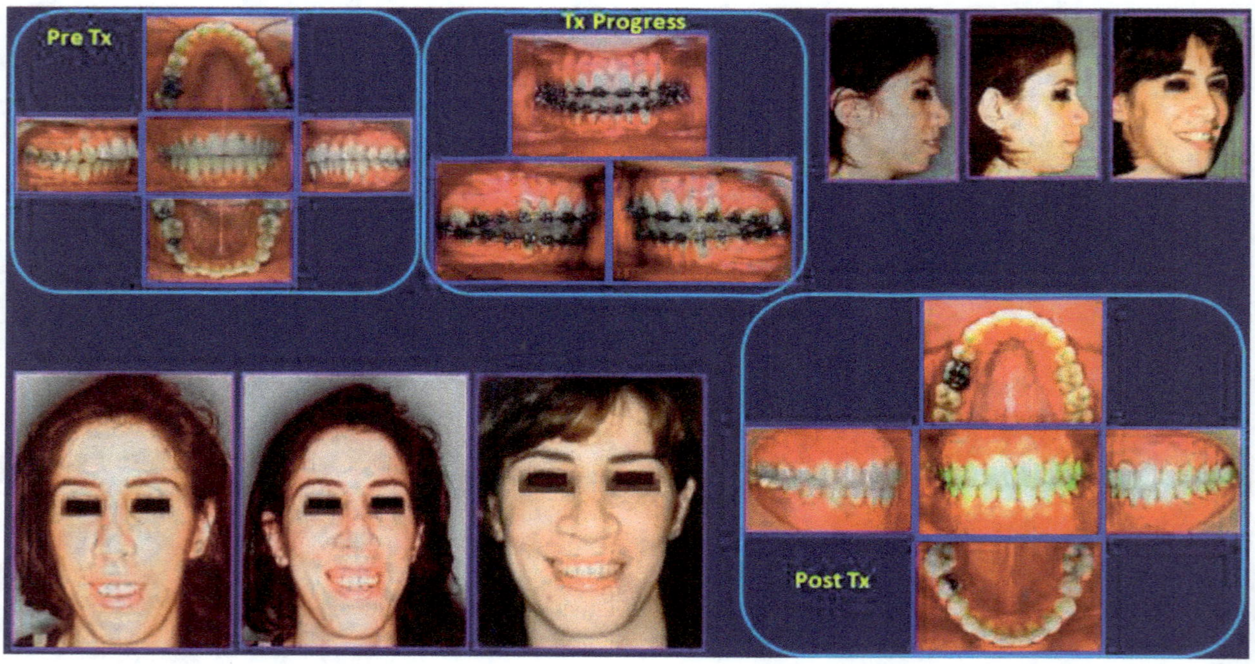

Figure 15. Phases of treatment (facial esthetics, pleasant smile, and ideal occlusion).

relationship in 3Ds. Surgical hooks were then constructed to start up the surgical phase surgical mobilization of the arches and bring occlusion into normal treatment outcome, and **Figure 5** shows the end up with straightening of teeth within orofacial disharmony and unaesthetic smile. Formulating treatment planning in such cases needs mutual collaboration between different health care providers and in particular between orthodontist and maxillofacial surgeon from the very beginning if the treatment objectives and patient's satisfaction are to be realized as in the case presented.

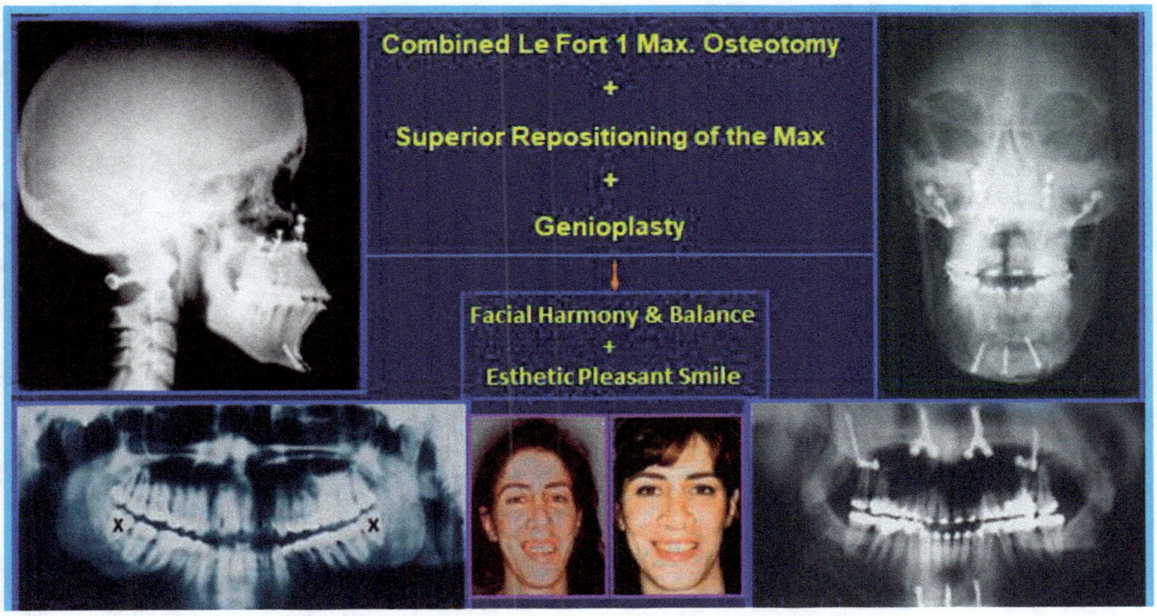

Figure 16. Radiographic representation of LeFort I osteotomy with maxillary superior repositioning and genioplasty for chin augmentation achieved treatment objectives and patient's satisfaction. Phases of treatment (facial esthetics, pleasant smile, and ideal occlusion).

2.3. Case #3

A healthy female patient (23 year old) presented with a chief complaint "I am frustrated with my elongated face, unaesthetic smile, and jam-packed teeth that prevent me from biting objects or chew food efficiently." She was reluctant to wear braces before, but is ready to go through orthodontic treatment to re-establish a pleasant dentofacial appearance.

Diagnosis clinical examination revealed typical long face features with increased lower facial height and almost straight profile. Vertical maxillary excess broke the balance and harmony of the facial parts that caused a clear gummy smile and tipped occlusal plane (**Figure 17**).

Intraorally, the sagittal relationship showed a class III malocclusion with negative overjet and a complex anterior open bite vertically, where second molars are in occlusion (pivoting) and crowded maxillary arch; the transverse relationship exhibited bilateral buccal crossbite, high palatal vault, and narrow maxilla contained in the normal mandibular arch form. There were extraction spaces in the lower arch as appears in the panoramic radiograph **Figure 1**.

2.3.1. Cephalometric assessment of vertical and sagittal features

Jarabak and McNamara lateral cephalometric analyses demonstrated the severe skeletal origin of the dentofacial deformity (**Figure 2**) that cannot be treated by orthodontic approach alone. The vertical maxillary excess caused severe gingival display during full smile and backward rotation of the mandible that surpassed any physiologic eruptive compensation of anterior teeth to develop anterior open bite (**Figure 18**).

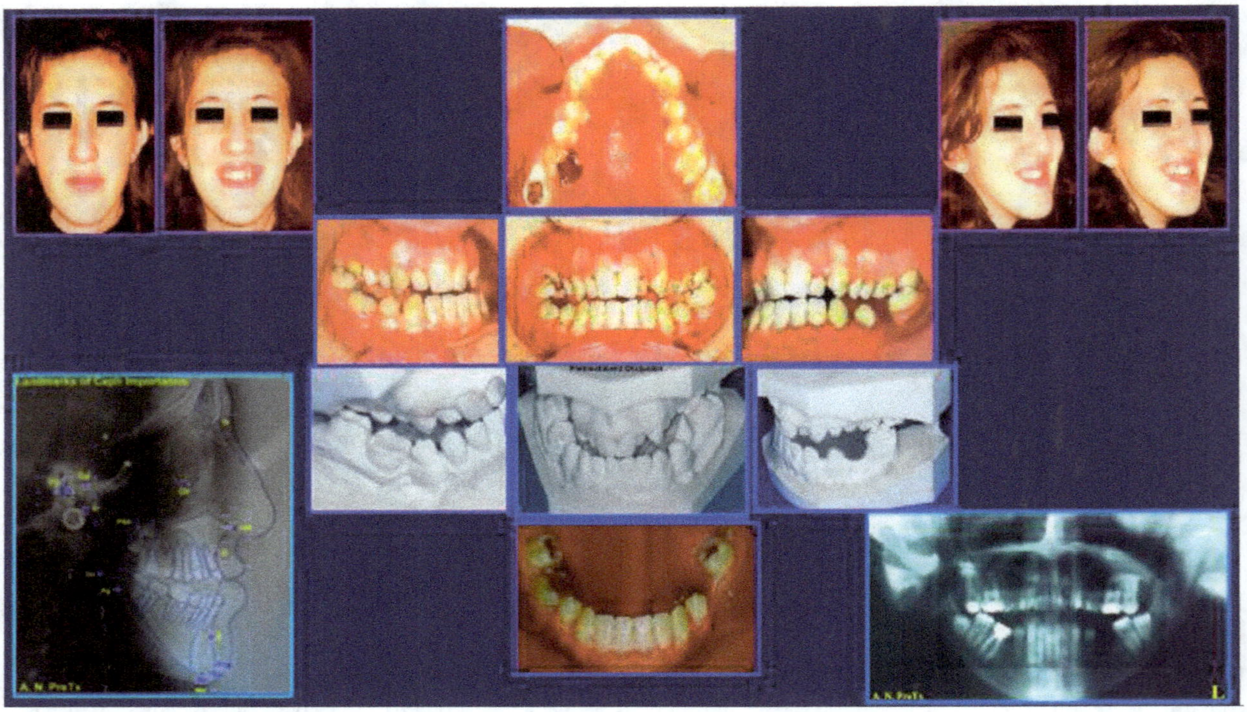

Figure 17. Extra-oral and intra-oral photos showing the dentofacial deformity to be objectively assessed by other diagnostic aids (radiographs).

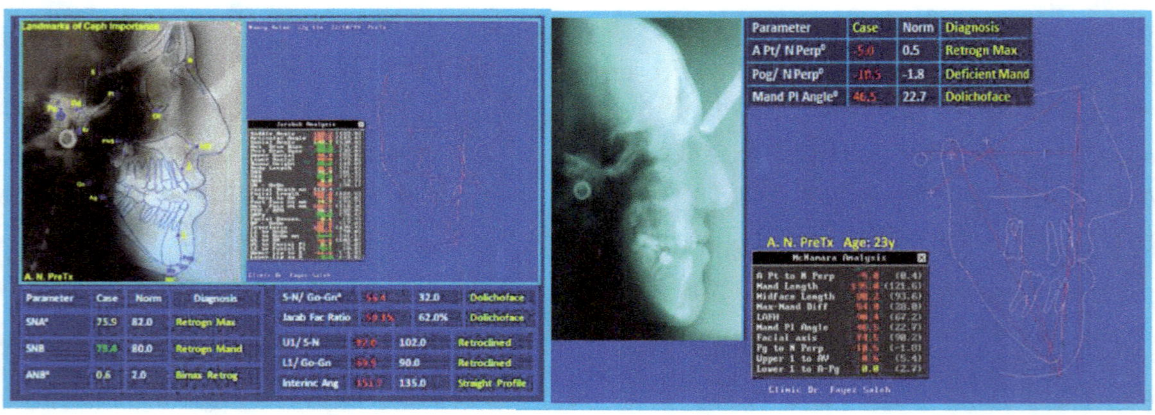

Figure 18. Lateral cephalometric analysis of Jarabak revealing vertical facial height excess, canted occ. plane, straight profile, deficient chin, and high gonial angle.

2.3.2. *Problem listing*

Data collection and analyses (**Figure 3**) endorsed the orthosurgical approach of treatment after joint patient's consultation with the health care team and her enthusiastic approval (**Figure 19**).

2.3.3. *Treatment objectives*

Realistic treatment objectives (**Figure 20**) were strictly reviewed to formulate the appropriate treatment planning, appliance design, and different presurgical orthodontics, surgical, and postsurgical phases of treatment (**Figure 21**).

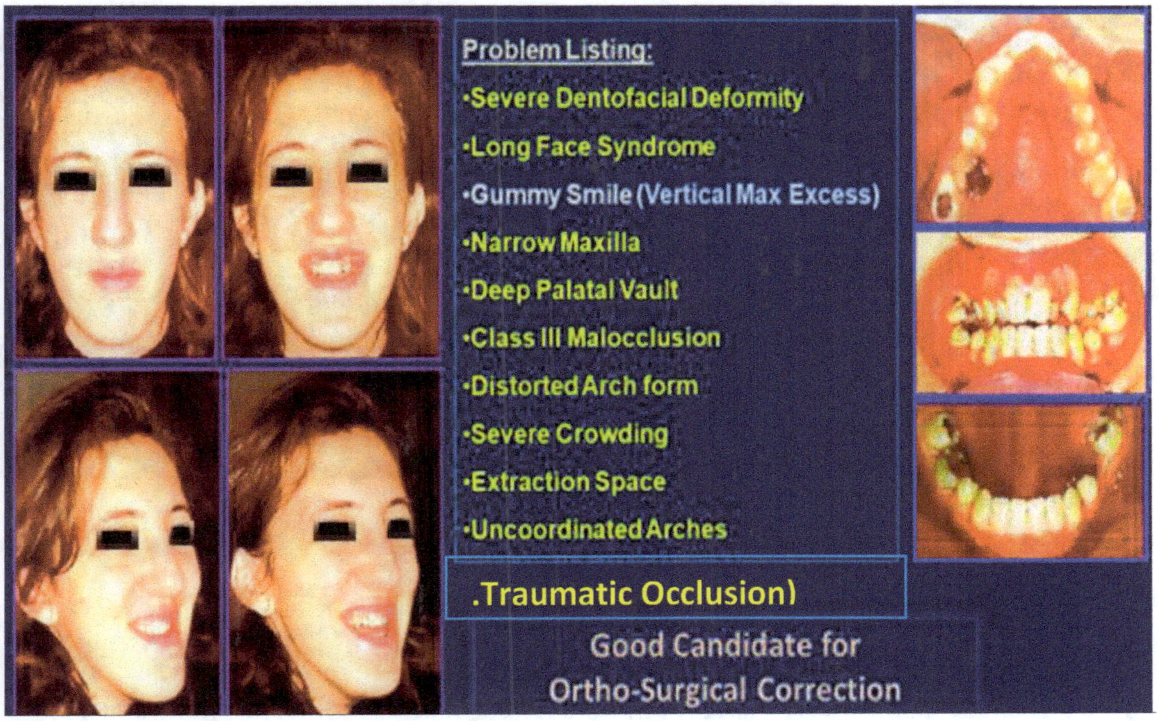

Figure 19. Listing the complex discrepancies of skeletal, dentoalveolar, and soft tissue origin is to justify the orthosurgical approach of interdisciplinary treatment for the benefit of the patient.

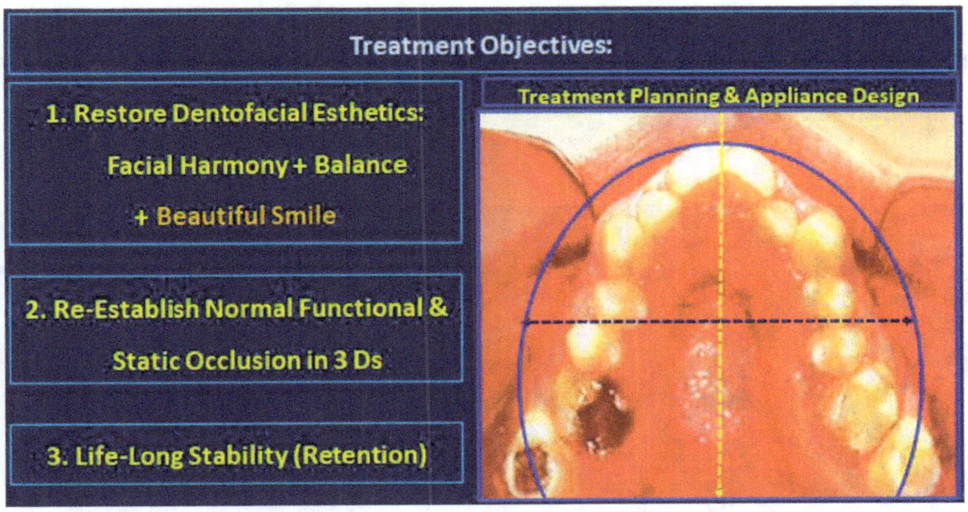

Figure 20. Treatment objectives allowed clinicians to formulate proper treatment planning.

2.3.4. Treatment progress

Maxillary arch expansion with quad helix appliance initiated simultaneously with leveling and alignment of teeth. Almost ideal arch form was attained, and the occlusal planes were flattened. When the presurgical phase was accomplished, surgical hooks were constructed as shown in **Figure 22**. LeFort I maxillary osteotomy with superior maxillary repositioning then took place to be followed by postsurgical detailing of occlusion and prosthetic replacement of the missing teeth.

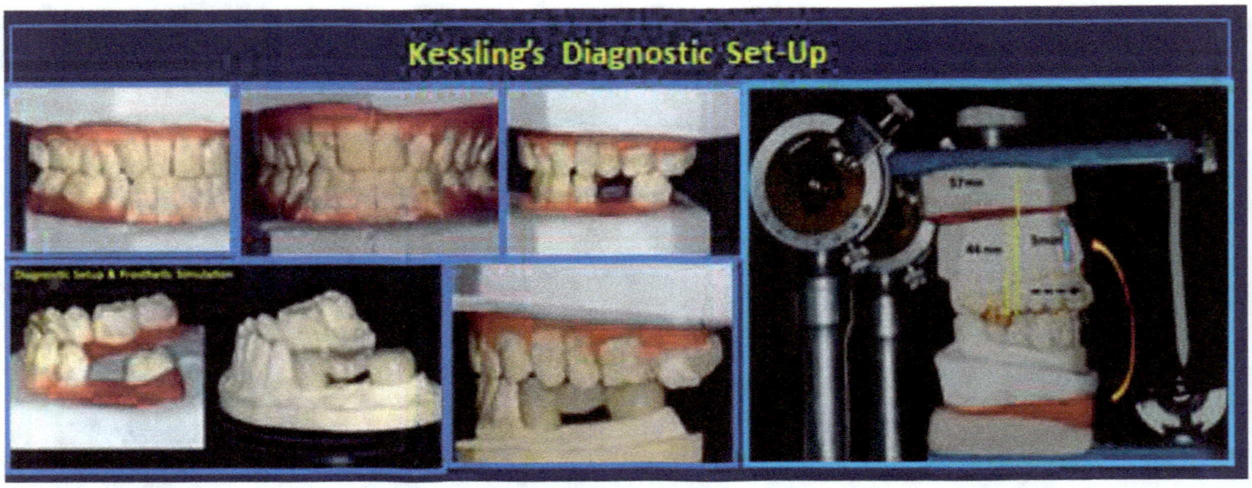

Figure 21. Model surgery and diagnostic set up possible for prosthetic construction.

2.3.5. Results and conclusions

Despite controversy, combined orthosurgical treatment of severe maxillary excess concomitant with facial skeletal disharmony remains the only treatment option. The treatment results as seen in **Figures 22–24** were remarkably promising and satisfactory.

2.4. Case #4

A healthy patient (24 year and 10 month old) presented with a chief complaint "I am unhappy with my unaesthetic smile, lack of biting on my teeth, and prominent chin." The necessary data were collected and analyzed, and the patient was informed that orthodontic treatment

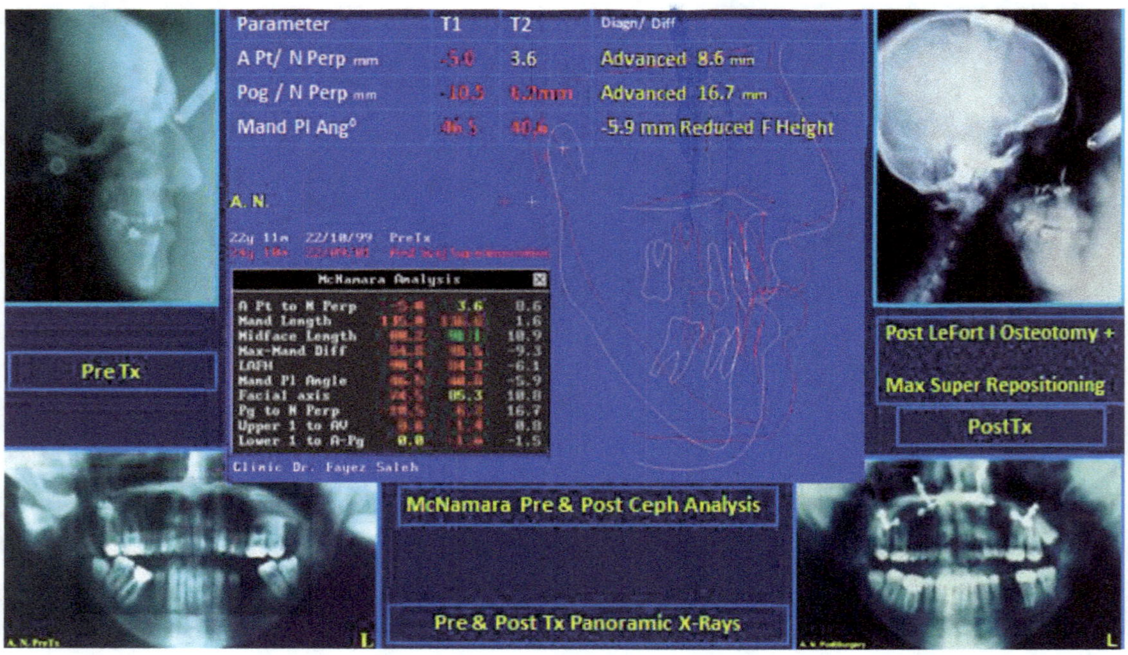

Figure 22. Pre and post treatment cephalometric analysis and panoramic views.

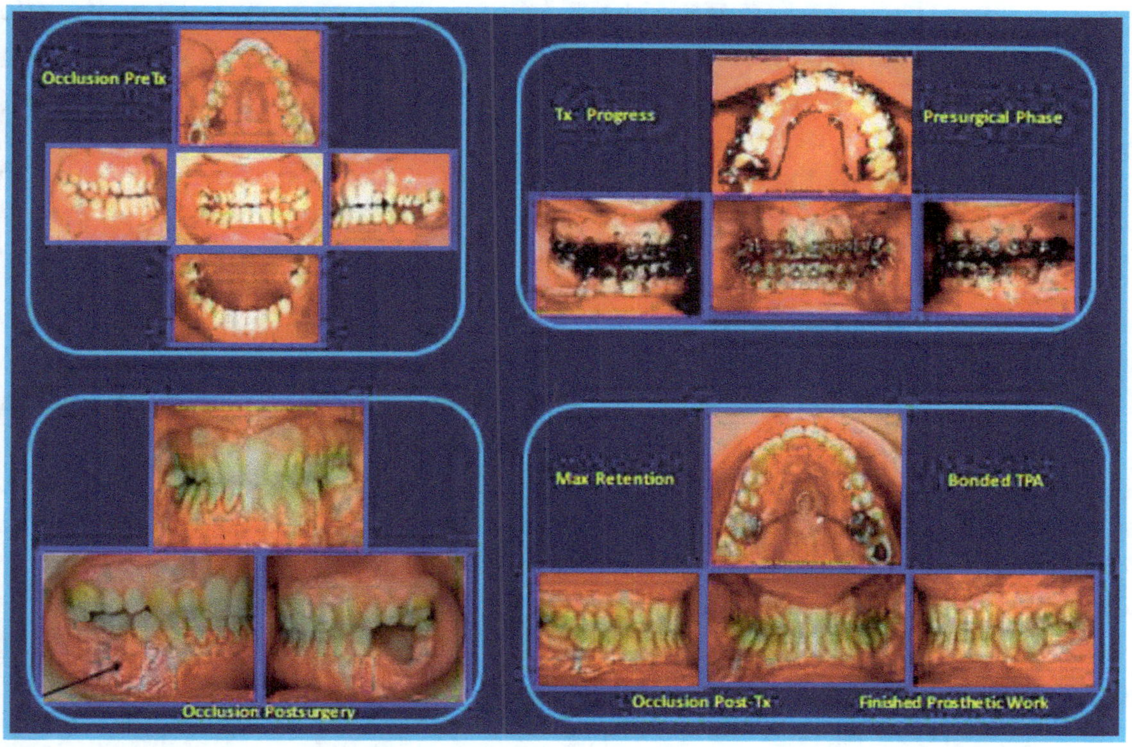

Figure 23. Phases of treatment, pretreatment, presurgical, postsurgical, and post prosthetic replacement of extraction spaces.

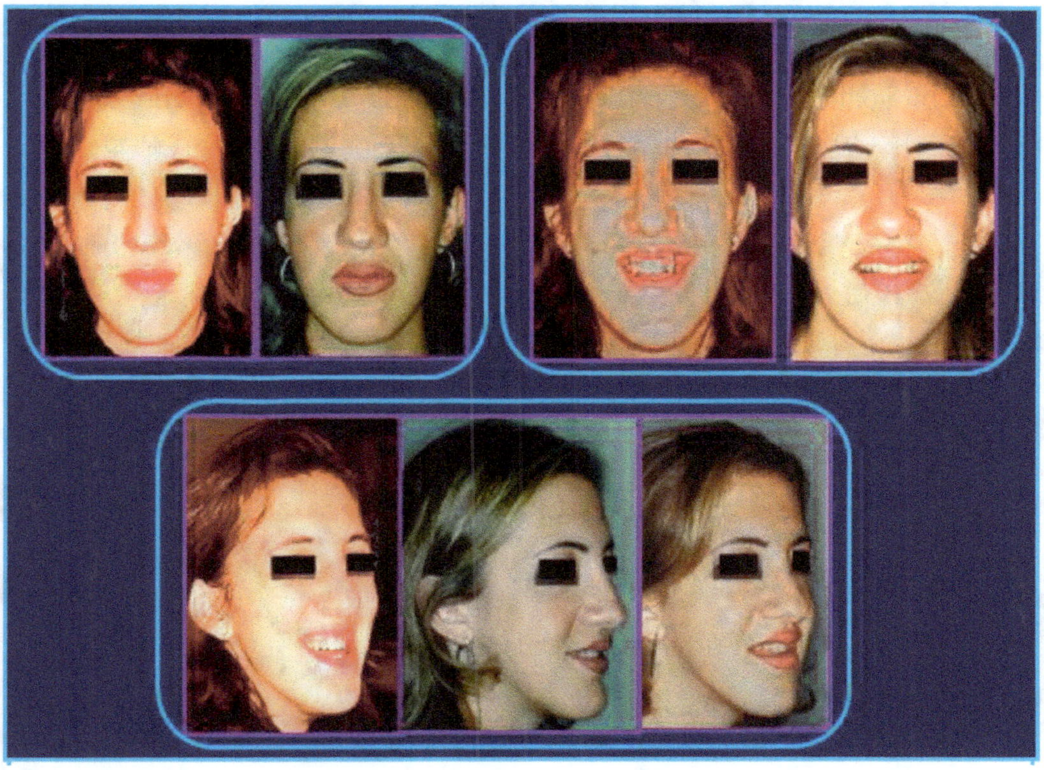

Figure 24. Frontal and lateral photos of the face showing significant esthetic improvement and pleasing smile shaped by combined orthosurgical treatment.

alone cannot be of benefit to you. A combined orthosurgical treatment modality was offered, and a joint meeting with the maxillofacial surgeon was arranged; details of the treatment phases, surgical risk, and cost effectiveness were explained to the patient who showed great interest in undergoing the treatment in a positive manner. The following figures reveal the steps and efforts exerted by the healthcare team and the cooperation of the patient that made the achievement possible.

2.4.1. *Diagnosis*

The diagnostic significance of clinically examining the dentofacial deformities lies in observing the soft and hard tissues functioning, so any abnormality is detected, and further investigations are assigned. Esthetic smile is a function of oral and perioral muscles and their relationship to the teeth and gingiva. Clinical examination of the patient revealed the severity of the skeletal, dentoalveolar, and soft tissues components as listed in **Figure 25**. However, objective judgment of the deformity necessitated other diagnostic aids including radiographs and study models to measure the discrepancy and formulate appropriate.

2.4.2. *Treatment objectives*

To restore normal facial harmony and balance, correct the severe malocclusion, design a pleasant smile, and insure life-long postoperative stability.

2.4.3. *Treatment planning*

Because of the complexity and severity of dentofacial deformity, the healthcare team decided to follow the logic sequence of orthosurgical treatment phases, presurgical orthodontics to be followed by bimaxillary surgical phase. LeFort I osteotomy with superior repositioning of the maxilla intended to reduce the increased facial height and level the tipped back occlusal

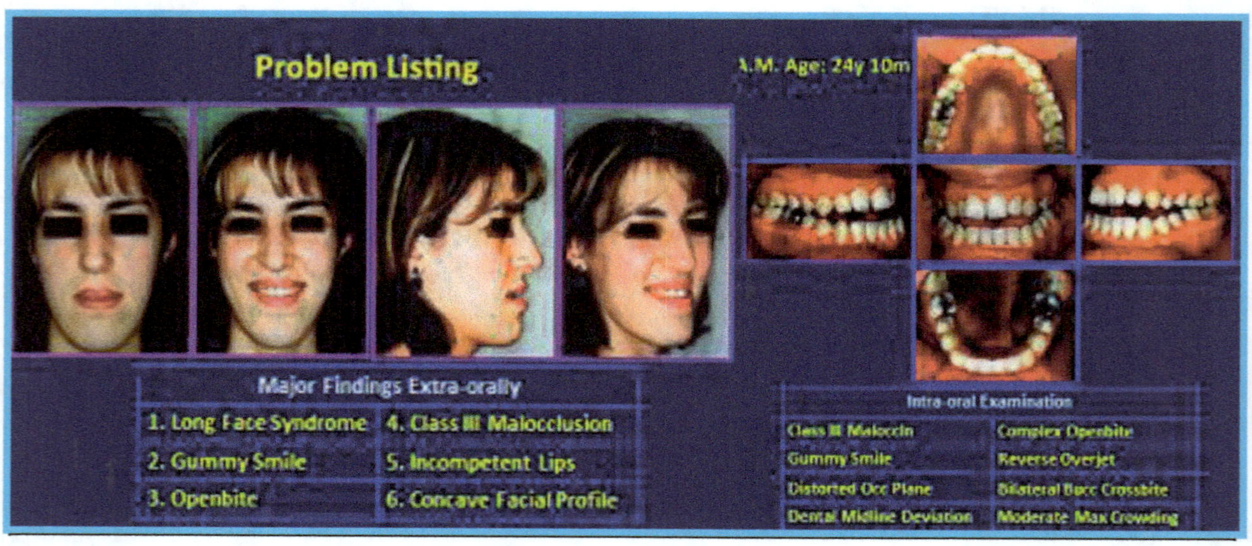

Figure 25. Pretreatment extra and intraoral photos describing the severity of the dentofacial deformity and the problems to be solved.

plane; bilateral sagittal split osteotomy of the mandibular ramus to setback the prognathic mandible bringing narrower mandibular arch in favor of the normal transverse occlusion, anticlockwise rotation aided in correcting the open bite. Retentive means were designed to guarantee stable outcome (**Figures 26–32**).

2.4.4. Conclusions

Mutual collaboration between healthcare providers allows for the proper selection of treatment modality relevant to the dentofacial deformity presented. Bimaxillary surgery helped in

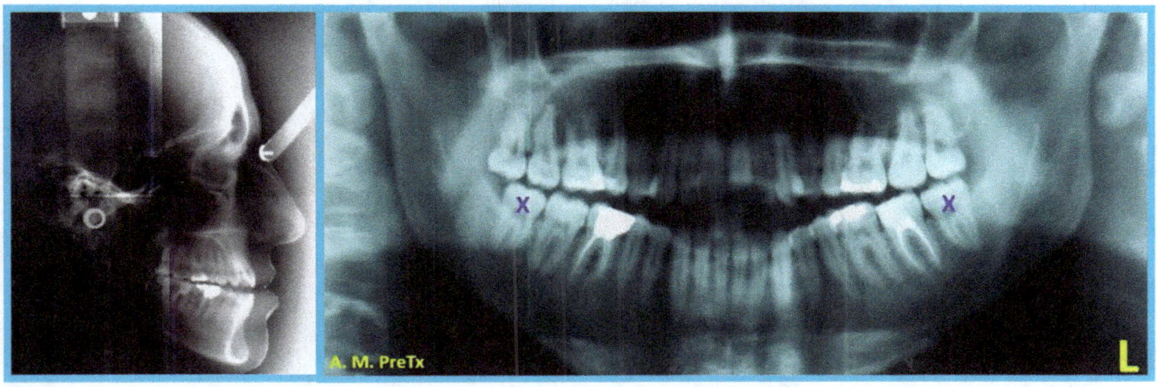

Figure 26. Pretreatment lateral cephalometric and panoramic radiographs (essential diagnostic aids).

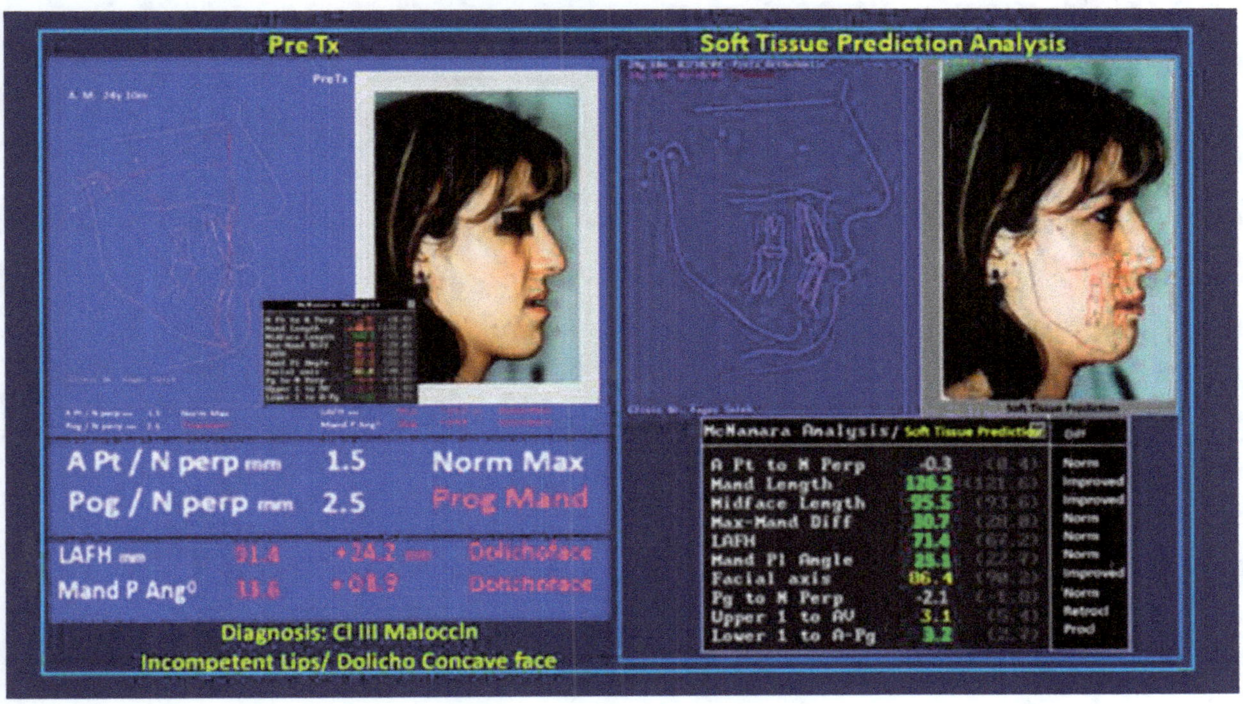

Figure 27. Pretreatment lateral ceph (McNamara) analysis and soft tissue surgical planning (prediction).

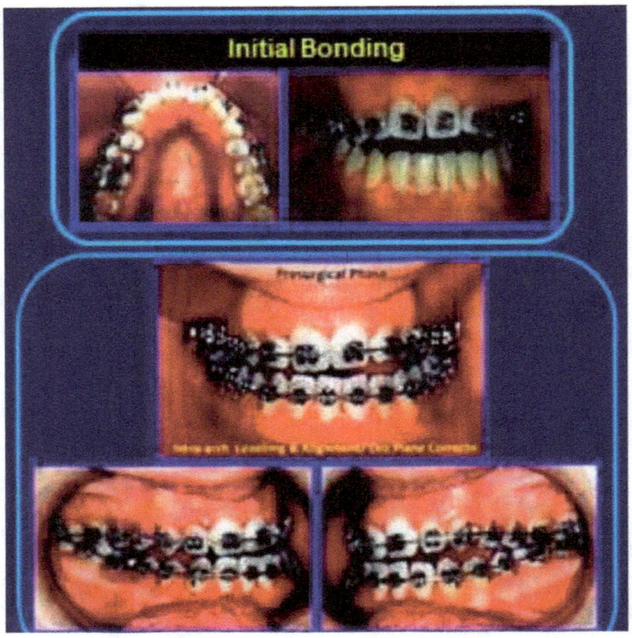

Figure 28. Initial bonding followed by inserting leveling arch wires to prepare the case for surgery.

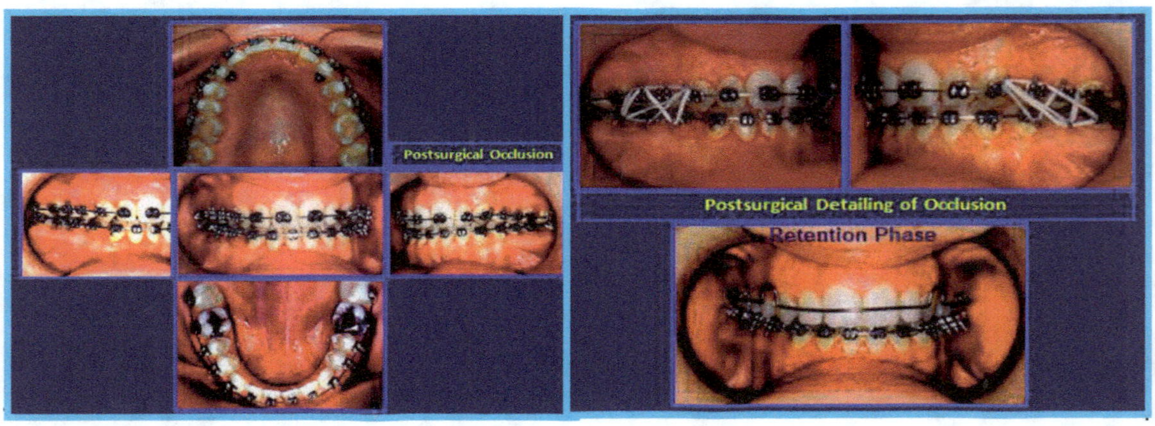

Figure 29. Postsurgical occlusion and the role of inter-maxillary elastics in stabilizing the occlusion and then setup retentive means.

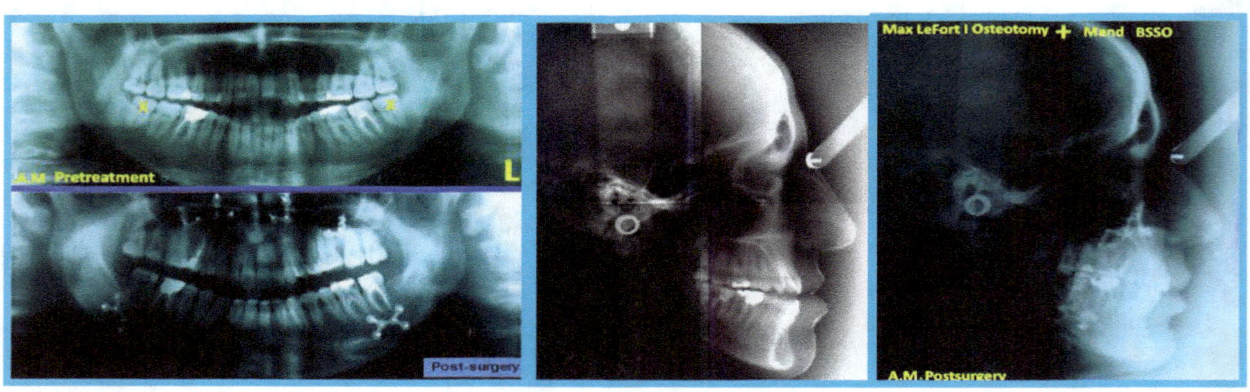

Figure 30. Pre and post cephalometric and panoramic radiographs.

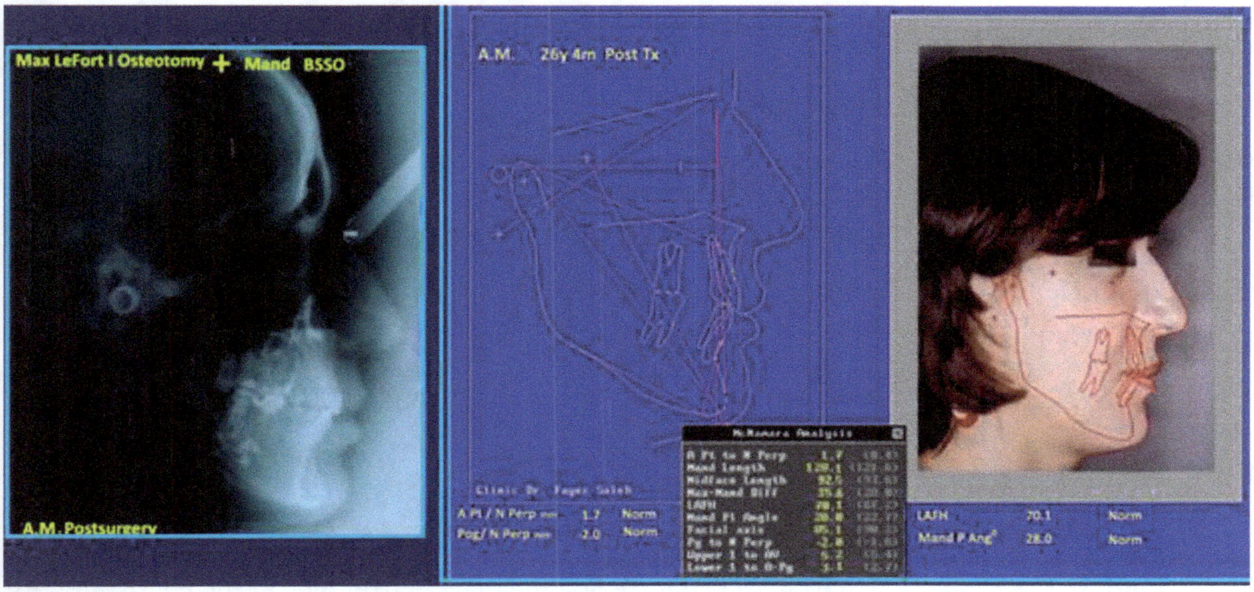

Figure 31. Post treatment cephalometric analysis reflecting the restructural improvement of the profile.

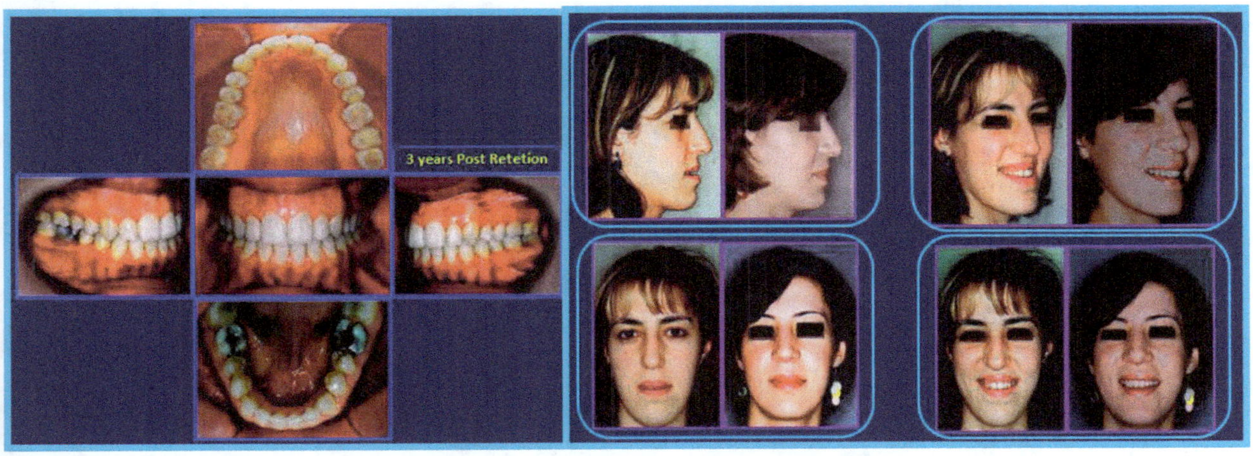

Figure 32. Occlusion 3-year post retention. Pre and post treatment facial features.

restoring harmony and balance of the face and establishing an ideal occlusal relationship. Patient cooperation and her family support were a key factor in achieving the satisfactory treatment outcome. Follow up for 5 year post treatment confirmed the successful procedures performed.

Author details

Fayez Saleh[1]* and Wisam Al Hamadi[2]

*Address all correspondence to: fayez.saleh3@gmail.com

1 Faculty of Dentistry, Beirut Arab University, Beirut, Lebanon

2 Faculty of Dentistry, University of Misan, Iraq

References

[1] Rufenacht CR, Berger RP, Lee RL, Nixon RL, Ricci G, Shavell HM. Fundamentals of Esthetics. Chicago, Illinois: Quintessence Publishing Co, Inc.; 1992

[2] Kallidass P, Srinvias S, Charles A, Davis D, Sushil Charravarthi NC. Smile characteristics in orthodontics: A concept review. International Journal of Orofacial Research. 2017;**2**:1-4

[3] Linder-Aronson S, Woodside DG. Excess Face Height Malocclusion: Etiology, Diagnosis, and Treatment. Chicago, Illinois, USA: Quintessence Publishing Co, Inc.; 2000. pp. 73-90

[4] Moldez MA, Sugawara J, Umemori M, Mtani H, Kawamura H. Long-term dentofacial stability after bimaxillary surgery in skeletal class III open bite patients. The International Journal of Adult Orthodontics & Orthognathic Surgery. 2000;**15**:309-319

[5] Paik C-H, Park H-S, Ahn H-W. Treatment of vertical maxillary excess without open bite in a skeletal class II hyperdivergent patient. The Angle Orthodontist. 2017;**87**(4):625-633

[6] Ishida Y, Ono T. Nonsurgical treatment of an adult with a skeletal class II gummy smile using zygomatic temporary anchorage devices and improved superelastic nickle-titanium alloy wires. American Journal of Orthodontics and Dentofacial Orthopedics. 2017;**152**(5): 693-705

[7] Iraelewicz-Djebali E, Chabre C. Gummy smile: Orthodontic or surgical treatment. Revue d'Orthopédie Dento-Faciale. 2015;**18**:102-120

[8] Conley RS, Legan HL. Correction of severe maxillary excess with anterior open bite and transverse maxillary deficiency. The Angle Orthodontist. 2002;**72**:265-274

[9] Proffit WR, Turvey TA, Phillips C. Orthognathic surgery: Hierarchy of stability. The International Journal of Adult Orthodontics & Orthognathic Surgery. 1996;**11**:191-204

[10] Enacar A, Taner T, Manav O. Effects of single or double jaw surgery on vertical dimension in skeletal class III patients. The International Journal of Adult Orthodontics & Orthognathic Surgery. 2001;**16**:30-35

[11] Proffit WR, Fields HW, Sarver DM, Ackerman JL. Contemporary Orthodontics. 5th ed. Canada: Elsevier-Mosby; 2013

[12] Epker BN, JPM S, Fish LC. Dentofacial Deformities, Integrated Orthodontics and Surgical Correction. 2nd ed. St Louis Missouri, USA: Mosby-Year Book Inc.; 1996

13

Orthodontic Treatment in Children with Cerebral Palsy

María Teresa Abeleira, Mercedes Outumuro, Marcio Diniz, Lucía García-Caballero, Pedro Diz and Jacobo Limeres

Abstract

Cerebral palsy is a permanent neuromuscular motor disorder that gives rise to many functional problems, including impaired swallowing, chewing and speech. Maxillary transverse deficiency and Angle Class II malocclusion are common. Some of these functional problems can be due to maxillary malocclusion. To our knowledge, no case series has yet been published on orthodontic treatment in children with cerebral palsy. In this chapter, we provide an overview of this topic based on the literature and on our own clinical experience. We consider that some patients with cerebral palsy are susceptible to orthodontic treatment. The keys to success are appropriate patient selection, based on anatomical, physiological and behavioural characteristics, and the degree of involvement of parents and caregivers. Among parents of cerebral palsy children undergoing orthodontic therapy, the perceived level of overall satisfaction was very high and expectations were often exceeded; however, these results are conditioned by factors such as the Peer Assessment Rating (PAR) index. Although some authors reported improvements in aesthetics, speech and oral function, an objective assessment of functional improvement is still lacking. In our experience, correction of resting position and management of neuromuscular alterations are essential if successful orthodontic treatment is to be achieved and relapses avoided.

Keywords: cerebral palsy, malocclusion, orthodontic treatment, oral function, special care dentistry

1. Introduction

Cerebral palsy (CP) carries a significant morbidity and has a limited life expectancy [1]. We should therefore ask ourselves the following question: Are these patients susceptible to orthodontic treatment? The main indication for orthodontic treatment is dental malocclusion. In 1956, Lyons [2] had already suggested that CP had effects on dentofacial development and, in particular, on tooth occlusion (to facilitate comprehension, a glossary of orthodontic terms has been included at the end of the chapter [**Box 1**]). The most common malocclusions described in CP patients are overjet and overbite, which have significantly higher prevalences in these patients than in healthy controls matched for sex and race [3]. Overjet ≥ 4 mm has been reported in around 70% of spastic CP children and anterior open bite ≥ 2 mm in up to 90% of cases [4]. Compared with other physical disabilities, there is a particularly high prevalence of open bite in CP; it is estimated that children diagnosed with CP have a threefold greater chance of having open bite than children with other special needs [5]. Paradoxically, when anteroposterior malocclusion is analysed, the prevalence of Angle Class I (normo-occlusion) in patients with CP is higher than in the general population [3]. However, malocclusion in the vertical plane provokes marked functional alterations that, in some cases, could justify performing orthopaedic-orthodontic treatment (**Figure 1**).

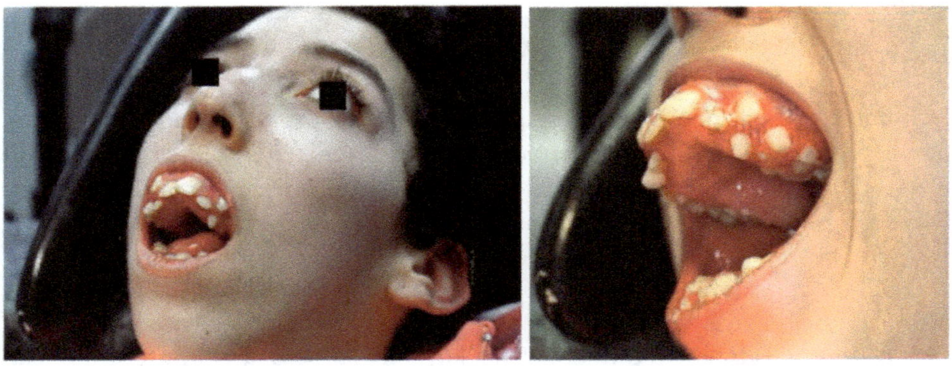

Figure 1. Severe open bite and oral functional impairment in a spastic cerebral palsy patient.

2. Severity of malocclusion

A study carried out in Minas Gerais in Brazil, with the participation of 60 spastic CP children and 60 age-matched controls, showed that some orofacial alterations with functional repercussions were more common in CP children than in the controls: severe lip incompetence was 2.8 times more common, mouth breathing 4.8 times more common and long facies 5.4 times more common [4]. Unfortunately, oral functionality is often left as a secondary issue when discussing the need for orthodontic treatment and many dental practitioners focus treatment on cosmetic objectives. The index most widely used for this purpose is the Dental Aesthetic Index (DAI), published 30 years ago by investigators in the University of Iowa. That index gives us the following classification for malocclusion: mild or absent (DAI score <25), defined (DAI = 26–30), severe (DAI = 31–35) and very severe or debilitating (DAI > 35) [6]. 'Severe' and 'very severe' malocclusions (DAI ≥ 31) are usually considered susceptible to orthodontic correction from a cosmetic point of view [6]. In a study of 44 CP patients of 12–59 years of age performed in Spain, significant differences were observed in the DAI scores for lip incompetence and mouth breathing compared with healthy controls [7]. In that series, resting head position also affected the DAI score; the highest scores were observed in patients with absent resting heading position control, followed by those who held their head permanently in flexion, those who held their head in hyperextension and, finally, those with a resting head position in a vertical axis [7].

A relevant issue is whether CP patients with associated mental disability have a less favourable facial phenotype than those with an intellectual coefficient in the normal range (**Figure 2**). On this subject, a study performed in Leeds, in the United Kingdom, found significantly greater overjet in CP with mental disability (mean of 8.3 versus 5.5 mm) as well as a higher frequency of Angle Class II division 1 (Class II-1) malocclusion (75% versus 36%) [3].

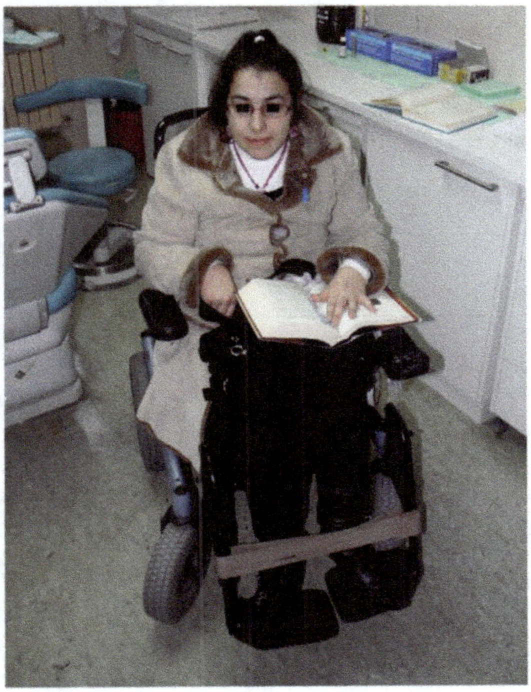

Figure 2. Cerebral palsy is a physical disability and many patients have a normal intelligence.

3. Orthodontic management

No large series of CP patients undergoing orthodontic treatment has been published in the literature, with the exception of a group of 62 adult CP individuals living in Bad Oeynhausen in Bielefeld, Germany; 32% of the patients aged between 18 and 36 years had worn orthodontic appliances, whereas none of the 31 patients aged over 36 years had received treatment. A possible interpretation of such a difference is that it could have been due to the individual initiative of a single dental practitioner or group of practitioners, and the results should therefore be extrapolated with a degree of caution [8]. It has been suggested that the aims of orthodontic treatment in patients with disabilities should focus on optimal aesthetic improvement and enhanced social acceptance, taking into account that an 'ideal' treatment may not be possible [9]. In a review of the literature, we found no studies or case reports that explored the benefits and effects of functional or fixed orthodontic appliance therapy in children with CP [10].

The following basic requirements need to be satisfied when considering orthodontic treatment in children with disabilities: the commitment of the patient and of the parents/carers, adequate oral hygiene, the degree of patient collaboration (behaviour management) and manual dexterity [11]. The criteria for patient selection are detailed in **Table 1**.

• Medical condition
• Malocclusion
• Aesthetic assessment
• Parent/carer commitment
• Child's tolerance to treatment
• Oral hygiene
• Risk/benefit ratio

Table 1. Selection criteria for patients with severe disabilities who are candidates for orthodontic treatment (modified from [9]).

• Impressions using quick-set materials
• Easy bonding of brackets
• Self-etching primer
• Advanced memory wires
• Self-ligating brackets
• Oral functionality
• Advances in orthognathic surgery
• Reversible mini-implant anchorage

Table 2. Technological innovations for dental patients with disabilities (modified with permission from Becker and Shapira [11]).

Certain technological improvements in dentistry in recent years could benefit disabled dental patients in general, including CP patients receiving orthodontic treatment [12] (**Table 2**). These technical innovations and the creation of multidisciplinary teams have made it possible to undertake orthodontic treatment in CP patients with extra-oral appliances (**Figure 3**), fixed multi-bracket appliances (**Figure 4**) and even complex orthodontic treatments and orthognathic surgery (**Figure 5**).

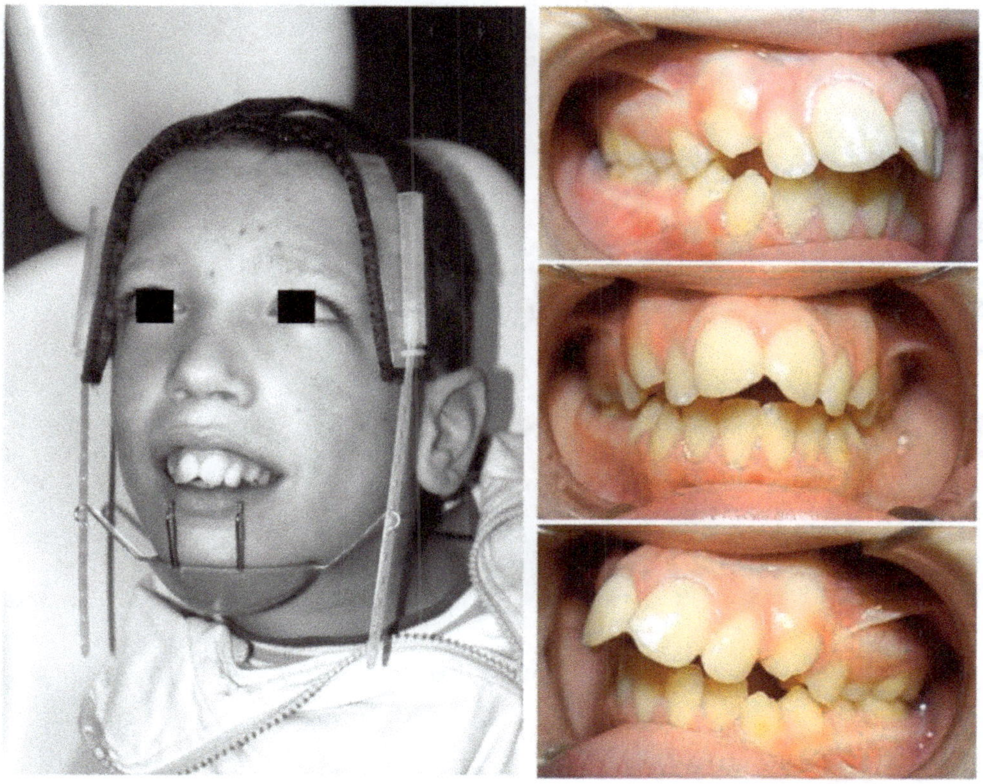

Figure 3. Cerebral palsy patient with severe Class II-1 malocclusion. Initial phase of orthodontic treatment with a face mask.

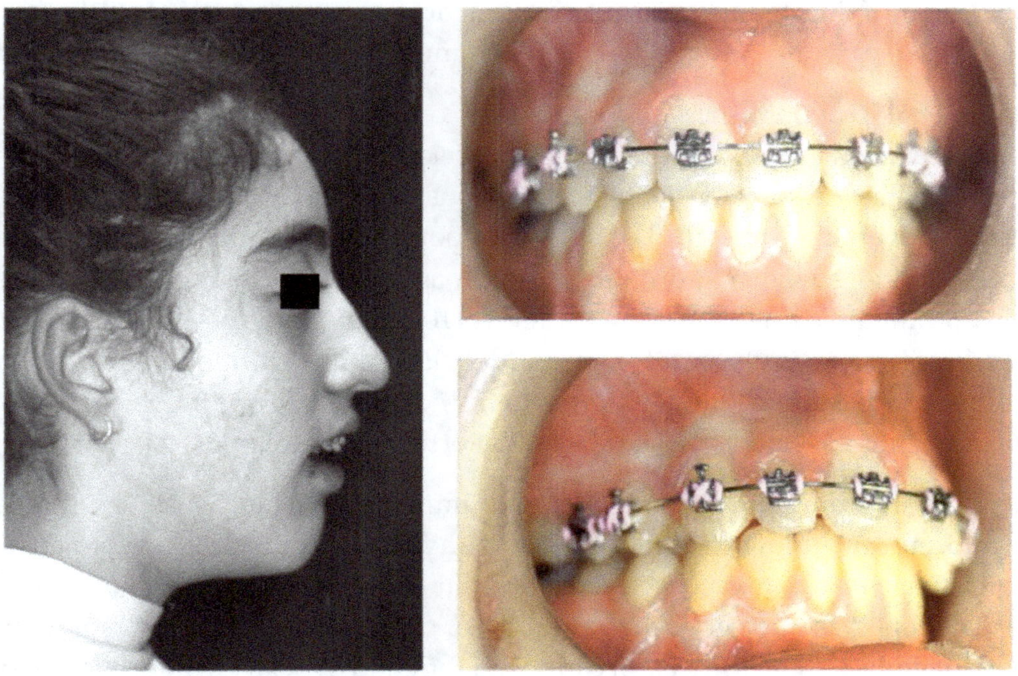

Figure 4. Cerebral palsy patient with Class II-1 malocclusion treated with fixed multi-bracket appliances.

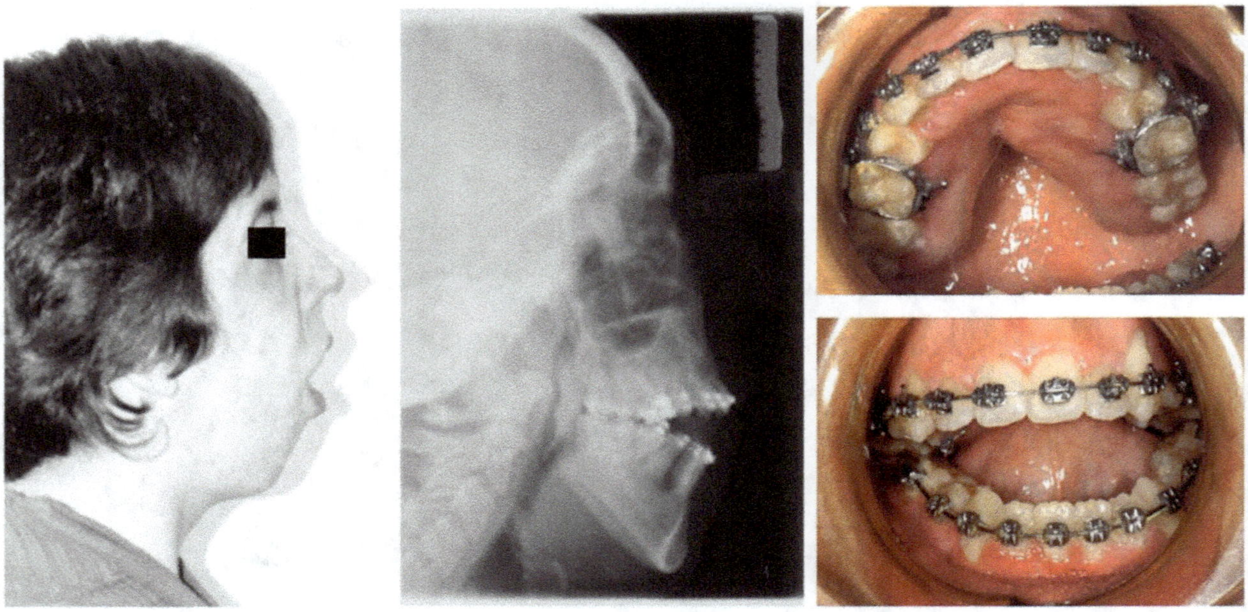

Figure 5. Cerebral palsy patient with open bite treated using fixed multi-bracket appliances before undergoing orthognathic surgery.

4. Identifying success criteria

Evaluation of the results of orthodontic treatment as successful or unsuccessful requires more than simply quantifying the aesthetic improvement. Parameters such as oral functionality, quality of life and, very importantly, relapse rates must also be taken into account.

In 2014, İşcan et al. [10] published a case report of a 12-year-old girl with ataxic CP who had Class II malocclusion, maxillary transverse deficiency and severe crowding. Treatment consisted of maxillary expansion with simultaneous functional therapy, fixed multi-bracket appliances and a vertical chin cup. The authors reported that acceptable occlusion, improvements in swallowing, speech and drooling, better masticatory muscle activity and a reduction in problems of impaired chewing were achieved [10]. That study demonstrated the need to develop tools able to quantify oral functional deficits—similar to the tools used to quantify cosmetic appearance, such as the Dental Aesthetic Index—to provide an objective assessment of the functional improvements accomplished by orthodontic treatment.

A survey of satisfaction and the appreciation of improvements answered by the parents of disabled children—including CP children—who underwent orthodontic treatment made the following findings: results exceeded expectations in 42% of cases, the reaction of friends and relatives was defined as 'they got excited' in 54% of cases, there was a very marked improvement in patient daily activities in 81% of cases, and the child's social life improved significantly according to 45% of respondents [13]. An analysis of the benefits of orthodontic treatment as perceived by the parents of disabled children reported that improvement in quality of life was a response given by 83% of surveyed parents, improvement in social acceptance in 78% of cases and improvement in social integration in 71% of cases. Interestingly, when asked about their desire to enhance dental and facial appearance, only 68% of participants answered 'a lot' and 20% 'a little' [13].

We have found no published studies designed specifically to address the issue of improvement in the quality of life of CP children following orthodontic treatment. In a study performed in Sao Paulo, Brazil, in which the parents of 60 CP children aged 6–14 years were interviewed, it was found that the Child Oral Health-Related Quality of Life Questionnaire (COHRQoL) score was not affected by the presence of malocclusion, dental injuries or dental fluorosis, but, in contrast, there was a significant correlation with a history of dental caries, bruxism and family income [14].

5. Follow-up and relapse prevention

Regular dental check-ups are mandatory in patients with CP because they are more prone to oral health problems related to enamel hypoplasia, pasty food intake, difficulty in maintaining good oral hygiene, drug-induced gingival hyperplasia and periodontal disease [4]. Consequently, parents and caregivers have to receive oral hygiene and diet instructions to avoid carious lesions, and patient will receive professional scaling at regular intervals before, during and after orthodontic treatment, to avoid periodontal disease [15].

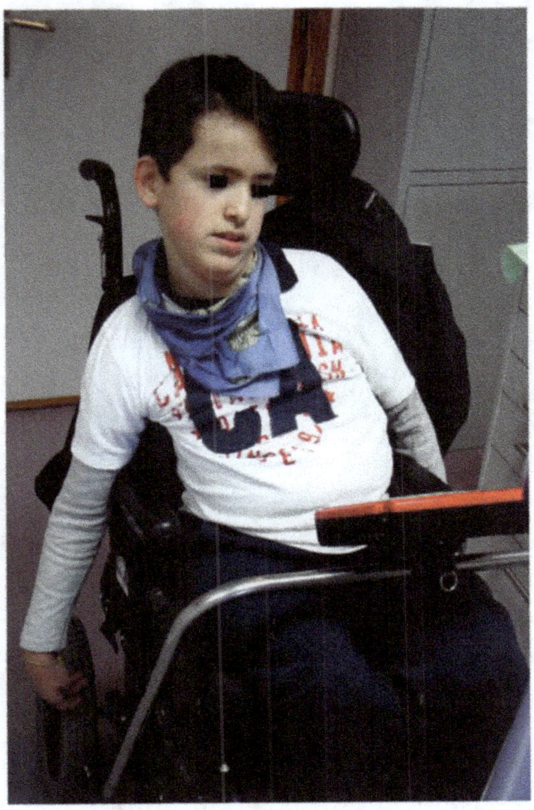

Figure 6. Cerebral palsy patient with severe scoliosis that altered the resting position and affected the occlusal pattern (unilateral open bite).

In an article published in 1927 by Stillwell [16], it was suggested that malocclusion and scoliosis affected posture and that this was a two-way relationship, in that alterations of posture also had repercussions on the teeth and the spine. This factor is probably often underestimated by health professionals, and it needs to be taken into account to be able to assess the risk of relapse. The relationship between malocclusion and vertebral alignment was demonstrated in an experimental model in animals (rats), in which the application of resin to induce unilateral premature tooth contact provoked iatrogenic scoliosis within a few weeks; this alteration was reversible when natural occlusal contact was restored [17]. This relationship is so strong that it has been suggested that the detection of hereditary malocclusions in young children 'allows the identification of a group of children who have a high risk of developing scoliosis in later years' [18]. In a systematic review published in 2011, it was concluded that there is plausible evidence for an increased prevalence of unilateral Angle Class II malocclusions associated with scoliosis and an increased risk of lateral crossbite and midline deviation in children affected by scoliosis [19] (**Figure 6**).

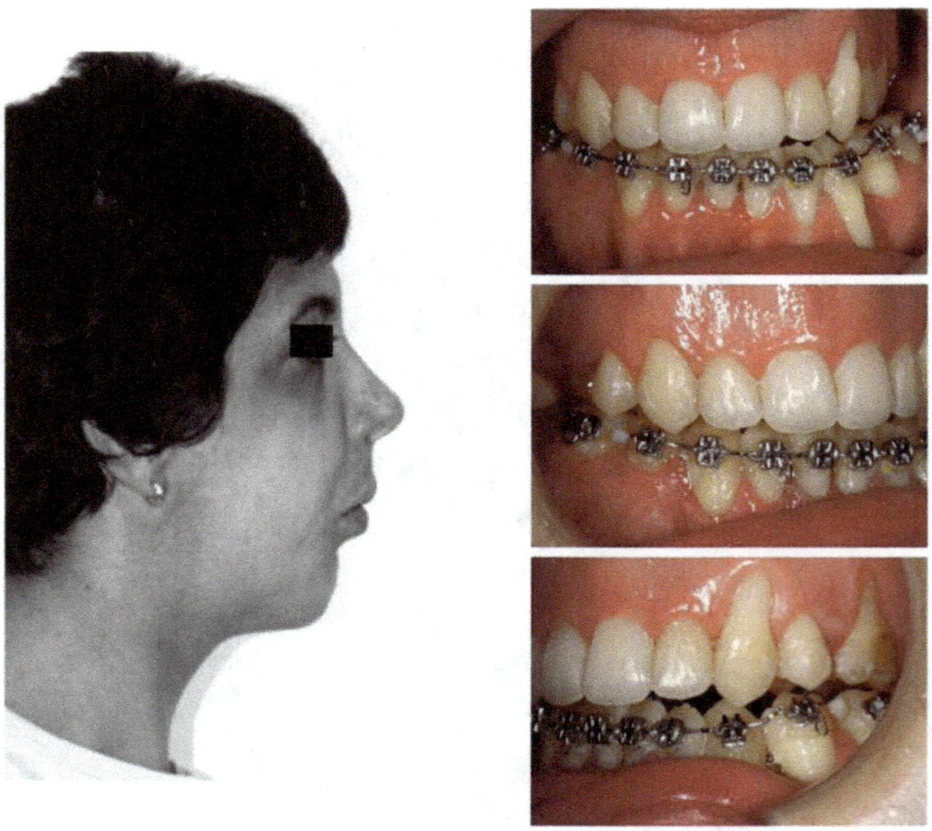

Figure 7. Cerebral palsy patient with open bite relapse after treatment with fixed multi-bracket appliances and orthognathic surgery.

Although the routine use of specific braces to stabilise the spine in CP children was initiated in the second half of the nineteenth century, certain improvements have been made to the modern versions of these braces. Probably the most popular model is the Milwaukee brace, whose effect on dentofacial growth has been described in detail, particularly with regard to abnormal proclination of the upper and lower incisor teeth [20]. Descriptions of cases of orthodontic treatment for malocclusion associated with scoliosis (mainly overjet) have also been published [21].

All these contributions indirectly confirm not only the close two-way relationship between resting position and malocclusion but also introduce a new conditioning factor, neuromuscular alterations, particularly relevant when muscle hypertonicity or spasticity is present. In our experience, these three factors are the principal determinants of relapse, and orthodontic treatment in patients with CP should not be initiated without first evaluating muscle tone and resting position. To illustrate this proposal, we only have to look at the case described by İşcan et al. [10] that we commented above. Their patient presented a certain degree of unilateral posterior open bite in the follow-up photographs. Relapse, even if less severe than the initial occlusal situation, can overshadow the success of a complex treatment, such as in the patient shown in **Figure 5**. After prolonged orthodontic treatment with fixed multi-bracket appliances and bimaxillary orthognathic surgery, that patient developed a relapse with unilateral open bite and marked gingival retraction secondary to muscle hypertonicity (**Figure 7**).

Spasticity of masseter and temporalis muscles causes hypertonia—spastic hypertonia—that aggravates the mandibular malposition (mandible is usually located in a retrograde and posteriorly rotated position) and may promote relapses after orthodontic treatment. It has been shown that intramuscularly injected botulinum toxin type A significantly decreases muscle spasticity [22], which hypothetically may help to prevent relapse in selected cases.

6. Conclusions

Orthodontic treatment is feasible in CP children after careful patient selection, taking into account that success depends not only on obvious factors, such as the type and severity of malocclusion and the degree of patient collaboration, but also on resting position and neuromuscular disturbances. The objective assessment of treatment success requires the application of tools that quantitatively evaluate improvements in the domains of aesthetic appearance, oral functionality and quality of life. Unconventional treatment plans have to be chosen at times, and parents must be thoroughly informed to avoid inappropriate expectations.

Box 1. Glossary of orthodontic terms

Angle's classification system: A method used to classify different types of malocclusion, based on the mesiodistal relationship of the permanent molars on their eruption and locking.

Bracket: A metal, plastic or ceramic element that is glued onto a tooth and that holds a metal wire called an arch wire; this system produces or guides orthodontic tooth movement.

Class I: A malocclusion where the upper teeth line up with your bottom teeth (but the teeth are crooked, crowded or turned).

Class II: A malocclusion where the upper teeth protrude beyond the lower teeth. This is also called 'overbite' or 'buck teeth'.

Class III: A malocclusion in which the lower teeth protrude beyond the upper teeth.

Crossbite: A malocclusion in which some of the upper teeth are inside of the lower teeth when the jaws are closed.

Crowding: An orthodontic problem caused by insufficient space for the teeth.

Fixed appliance: An orthodontic component that is cemented or bonded to the teeth.

Malocclusion: A poor alignment of the upper and lower teeth in the anteroposterior or transverse planes when the jaws are closed.

Overjet: An extension of the incisal or buccal cusp ridges of the upper teeth horizontally (labially or buccally) beyond the ridges of the lower teeth when the jaws are closed normally.

Overbite: An extension of the incisal ridges of the upper anterior teeth below the incisal ridges of the corresponding lower teeth when the jaws are closed normally.

Open bite: A malocclusion that occurs in the vertical plane, characterized by lack of vertical overlap between the maxillary and mandibular dentition.

Self-ligating brackets: Ligatureless bracket systems that have a mechanical device built into the bracket to close off the edgewise slot.

Author details

María Teresa Abeleira, Mercedes Outumuro, Marcio Diniz, Lucía García-Caballero, Pedro Diz* and Jacobo Limeres

*Address all correspondence to: pedro.diz@usc.es

Special Needs Unit and OMEQUI Research Group, School of Medicine and Dentistry, Santiago de Compostela University, Santiago de Compostela, Galicia, Spain

References

[1] Himmelmann, K., Sundh, V. (2015). Survival with cerebral palsy over five decades in western Sweden. *Developmental Medicine & Child Neurology*, 57(8), 762–767.

[2] Lyons, D.C. (1956). An evaluation of the effects of cerebral palsy on dentofacial development, especially occlusion of the teeth. *Journal of Pediatrics*, 49(4), 432–436.

[3] Franklin, D.L., Luther,F., Curzon, M.E. (1996). The prevalence of malocclusion in children with cerebral palsy. *European Journal of Orthodontics*, 18(6), 637–643.

[4] Miamoto, C.B., Ramos-Jorge, M.L., Pereira, L.J., Paiva, S.M., Pordeus, I.A., Marques, L.S. (2010). Severity of malocclusion in patients with cerebral palsy: determinant factors. *The American Journal of Orthodontics and Dentofacial Orthopedics*, 138(394), e1–e5.

[5] Oliveira, A.C., Paiva, S.M., Martins, M.T., Torres, C.S., Pordeus, I.A. (2011). Prevalence and determinant factors of malocclusion in children with special needs. *European Journal of Orthodontics*, 33(4), 413–418.

[6] Cons, N.C., Jenny, J., Kohout, F.J. (1986). DAI: The Dental Aesthetic Index. Iowa City, Iowa: College of Dentistry, University of Iowa.

[7] Martinez-Mihi, V., Silvestre, F.J., Orellana, L.M., Silvestre-Rangil, J. (2014). Resting position of the head and malocclusion in a group of patients with cerebral palsy. *Journal of Clinical and Experimental Dentistry*, 6(1), e1–e6.

[8] Asdaghi Mamaghani, S.M., Bode, H., Ehmer, U. (2008). Orofacial findings in conjunction with infantile cerebral paralysis in adults of two different age groups a cross-sectional study. *Journal of Orofacial Orthopedics*, 69(4), 240–256.

[9] Chadwick, S.M., Asher-Mcdade, C. (1997). The orthodontic management of patients with profound learning disability. *British Journal of Orthodontics*, 24(2), 117–125.

[10] İşcan, H.N., Metin-Gürsoy, G., Kale-Varlik, S. (2014). Functional and fixed orthodontic treatment in a child with cerebral palsy. *The American Journal of Orthodontics and Dentofacial Orthopedics*, 145(4), 523–533.

[11] Becker, A., Shapira, J. (1996). Orthodontics for the handicapped child. *European Journal of Orthodontics*, 18(1), 55–67.

[12] Musich, D.R. (2006). Orthodontic intervention and patients with Down syndrome. *The Angle Orthodontist*, 76(4), 734–735.

[13] Abeleira, M.T., Pazos, E., Ramos, I., Outumuro, M., Limeres, J., Seoane-Romero, J., Diniz, M., Diz, P. (2014). Orthodontic treatment for disabled children: a survey of parents' attitudes and overall satisfaction. *BMC Oral Health*, 14, 98.

[14] Abanto, J., Ortega, A.O.L., Raggio D.P., Bönecker M., Mendes F.M., Ciamponi A.L. (2014). Impact of oral diseases and disorders on oral-health-related quality of life of children with cerebral palsy. *Special Care in Dentistry*, 34(2), 56–63.

[15] Sabuncuoglu, F.A., Özcan, E. (2014). Orthodontic management of a patient with cerebral palsy: six years follow-up. *Journal of Contemporary Dental Practice*, 15(4), 491–495.

[16] Stillwell, F.S. (1927). The correlation of malocclusion and scoliosis to posture and its effect upon the teeth and spine. *Dental Cosmos*, 69, 154–163.

[17] D′Attilio, M., Filippi, M.R., Femminella, B., Festa, F., Tecco, S. (2005). The influence of an experimentally-induced malocclusion on vertebral alignment in rats: a controlled pilot study. *Cranio*, 23(2), 119–129.

[18] Pećina, M., Lulić-Dukić, O., Pećina-Hrncević, A. (1991). Hereditary orthodontic anomalies and idiopathic scoliosis. *International Orthopedics*, 15(1), 57–59.

[19] Saccucci, M., Tettamanti, L., Mummolo, S., Polimeni, A., Festa, F., Tecco, S. (2011). Scoliosis and dental occlusion: a review of the literature. *Scoliosis*, 6, 15.

[20] Rock, W.P., Baker, R. (1972). The effect of the Milwaukee brace upon dentofacial growth. *The Angle Orthodontist*, 42(2), 96–102.

[21] Hitchcock, H.P. (1969). Treatment of a malocclusion associated with scoliosis. *The Angle Orthodontist*, 39(1), 64–68.

[22] Manzano, F.S., Granero, L.M., Masiero, D., dos, Maria, TB. (2004). Treatment of muscle spasticity in patients with cerebral palsy using BTX-A: a pilot study. *Special Care in Dentistry*, 24(4), 235–239.

14

Ceramic Brackets Revisited

Selma Elekdag-Türk and
Hüdanur Yilmaz (née Huda Ebulkbash)

Abstract

Increasing demand for esthetics during fixed appliance therapy has led to a significant increase in the demand for and use of ceramic brackets. This comprehensive review covers the physical properties as well as rebonding and debonding of polycrystalline and monocrystalline ceramic brackets. Furthermore, this review aims to present the advantages and disadvantages as well as the refinements these brackets underwent since their introduction in the late 1980s. Interestingly, the introduction and development of these brackets were a part of a quickly expanding ceramic technology in many industries. The authors strongly believe that the novice will particularly benefit from this review presenting up-to-date knowledge.

Keywords: review, ceramic brackets, monocrystalline alumina brackets, polycrystalline alumina brackets, rebonding, debonding

1. Introduction

It is interesting to note that ceramic braces entered orthodontics via an indirect route. Translucent polycrystalline alumina (TPA) was developed by NASA (National Aeronautics and Space Administration) and Ceradyne, a leader in advanced ceramics for aerospace, defense, electronics, and industrial use. In 1986, a dental equipment and supply company contacted Ceradyne for an esthetic material to be used in orthodontics. Ceradyne recommended TPA. Shortly, after this contact, namely in 1987, ceramic brackets were introduced. In the same year, i.e., 1987, the production of ceramic brackets reached 300,000 pieces a month [1]. To clarify, 300,000 pieces would translate into 15,000 nonextraction patients per month! Ceramic brackets have progressed substantially since their first introduction over 30 years ago. This article aims to present an up-to-date review of the physical and clinical characteristics, i.e., properties, of ceramic brackets.

2. Ceramic bracket production: a short overview

Most ceramic brackets are produced from aluminum oxide (alumina) particles, and these brackets are available in polycrystalline and monocrystalline forms [2].

Nowadays, the majority of polycrystalline (multiple crystals) brackets are produced by ceramic injection molding (CIM). An outline of CIM is as follows: the aluminum oxide (Al_2O_3) particles are mixed with a binder. This mixture is rendered flowable through heat and pressure application and injected into a bracket mold. The binder is removed, i.e., burned out. Subsequently, sintering—the production of a coherent mass by heating without melting—is carried out. The advantage of CIM is that this technology can manufacture complex and precise items with smooth surfaces in large quantities at fast rates [3].

The production process for monocrystalline (single crystal) ceramic brackets, also referred to as sapphire brackets, is completely different. Here, the Al_2O_3 particles are melted. The resultant mass is slowly cooled to permit a controlled crystallization, leading to the production of a large, single crystal. This large, single crystal in rod or bar form is then milled into brackets with ultrasonic cutting techniques and/or diamond cutting tools. After milling, the monocrystalline brackets are heat-treated to eliminate surface imperfections and to relieve the stress caused by the milling procedure. The production of these brackets is more expensive when compared to the production of polycrystalline brackets. This increased expense is mainly due to the difficulty of milling, i.e., the cutting process [2].

3. Properties of ceramic brackets

3.1. Hardness

Ceramic brackets are known for their hardness. They are notably harder than enamel [4–7]. Thus, contact between enamel and ceramic brackets has to be avoided by all means. This type of contact can lead to severe enamel damage [8]. Particular care has to be exercised with deep bite and/or class II canine relationship patients. If required, bite opening applications must be performed to prevent enamel damage.

3.2. Tensile strength

The ultimate tensile strength, often shortened as tensile strength, is defined as the maximum stress that a material can withstand while being stretched or pulled before failing or breaking [9]. When stress is placed on a ceramic material, its unyielding atomic structure makes the redistribution and the relief of stress close to impossible [2]. Ductile materials, such as metals and polymers, experience plastic deformation before failure [10]. In other words, the elongation of ceramics at failure (brittle fracture) is less than 1%, yet the elongation of stainless steel at failure (ductile fracture) is approximately 20% [11]. Hence, ceramic brackets do not flex. This implies that ceramic brackets are much more likely to fracture than metal brackets under identical conditions [11].

3.3. Fracture toughness

Fracture toughness is a property which describes the ability of a material containing a crack to resist fracture [6, 12]. This is an important material property since the presence of imperfections, such as microscopic scratches, cracks, voids, and pores are not completely avoidable during the fabrication of materials. These microscopic imperfections may or may not be harmful to the material, depending on a number of factors such as the fracture toughness of the material examined, the stress on the material, length of the crack, and resistance of the material to crack propagation as well as the environment of the material [6].

The higher the fracture toughness, the more difficult it is to propagate a crack in that material [12]. The fracture toughness of polycrystalline alumina brackets is higher than the fracture toughness of monocrystalline alumina brackets. This implies that crack propagation is relatively easier in single-crystal alumina brackets when compared with polycrystalline alumina brackets [12]. Polycrystalline brackets have a higher resistance to crack propagation due to crack interaction with grain boundaries (GBs). A GB is the interface between two "grains" (crystals) in a polycrystalline (multiple crystals) material (**Figure 1**). Cracks are impeded at these GBs [10]. Clinical applications that may scratch the surfaces of ceramic brackets may greatly reduce the fracture toughness, thereby predisposing ceramic brackets to eventual fracture [12]. Thus, utmost care has to be taken not to scratch ceramic bracket surfaces with instruments and stainless steel ligature wires during treatment. Also, the clinician should not overstress when ligating with steel ligature wires. This might initiate crack growth and propagation, leading to the eventual fracture of the bracket. Careful ligation is mandatory, and elastomeric modules (ligatures) or coated ligatures are advised to prevent ceramic bracket fractures, particularly tie-wing fractures [6, 13, 14]. Arch wire sequencing also has to be performed carefully. The use of resilient full-size arch wires before the placement of full-size stainless steel arch wires is recommended [7]. Furthermore, the patient has to be advised to restrain from chewing and/or biting on any hard substances [6] as well as from intraoral/lip piercings. A prudent choice is to avoid ceramic brackets with orthognathic surgery patients as well as with patients involved in contact sports.

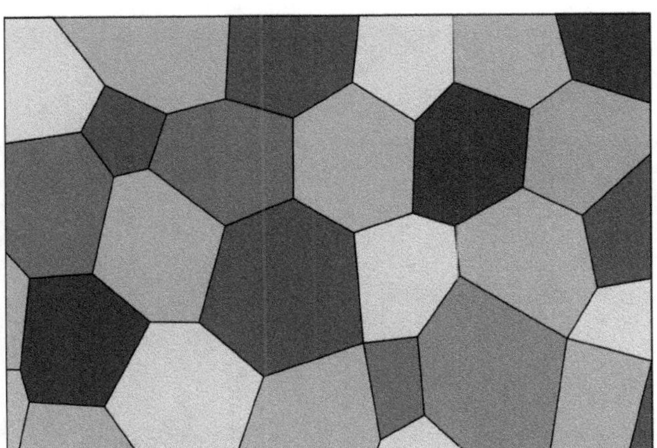

Figure 1. Schematic presentation of "grains" and GBs.

Finally, it should be noted that the exposure of alumina to water or saliva decreases fracture toughness [10]. This characteristic is important to remember when the clinician attempts to extrapolate in vitro results to the clinical setting, i.e., the oral environment.

3.3.1. Tie-wing fracture

Figure 2 pictures a tie-wing fracture of the lower second premolar bracket. Most likely this tie-wing was damaged with pliers during arch wire insertion into the molar tube.

Complete fragmentation of a damaged bracket might occur during arch wire ligation or during the course of treatment. Thus, the removal of an impaired bracket and its replacement with a new bracket is a prudent risk management strategy. The risk of ceramic fragment penetration into the patient's oral soft tissues, inhalation or swallowing by the patient does exist. Ceramics are radiolucent, i.e., ceramic bracket fragments are not visible on radiographs [15].

An interesting in vitro study [16] tested tie-wing fracture strength of polycrystalline and monocrystalline brackets after being exposed to fluoride prophylactic agents (Prevident 5000 and Phos-flur gel; Colgate Pharmaceuticals, Canton, Mass, USA). The researchers stated that the fluoride-alumina surface interaction most likely caused strain in the surface bonds of both types of brackets. Yet, this presumed bond strain only affected the fracture strength of the monocrystalline alumina brackets. The results of this study imply that the use of topical fluoride agents may increase the susceptibility of tie-wing fractures of monocrystalline brackets under clinical conditions and that polycrystalline brackets might be the appropriate choice for poor oral hygiene patients that require fluoride prophylactic agents. The authors [16] pointed out that this outcome was most likely related to the inhibition of cracks at the GBs of the polycrystalline microstructure.

The tie-wing complex of polycrystalline ceramic brackets can be manufactured as either semitwin or true twin. Semitwin differs from true twin by having an isthmus of ceramic joining the mesial and distal tie-wings, i.e., the mesial and distal tie-wings are not four independent projections from the bracket base as with the true twin configuration (**Figure 3**). This semitwin configuration has been stated to possess a better tie-wing fracture strength. It has been proposed that such a ceramic connector produces a cross-stabilizing effect [13, 17].

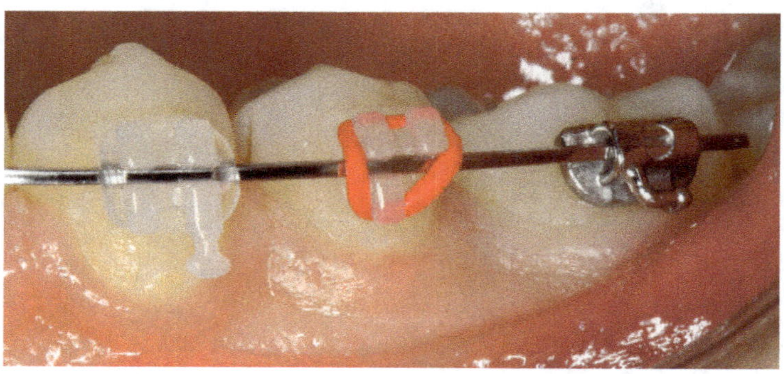

Figure 2. Distogingival tie-wing fracture (the red elastic ligature was used to accentuate this fracture).

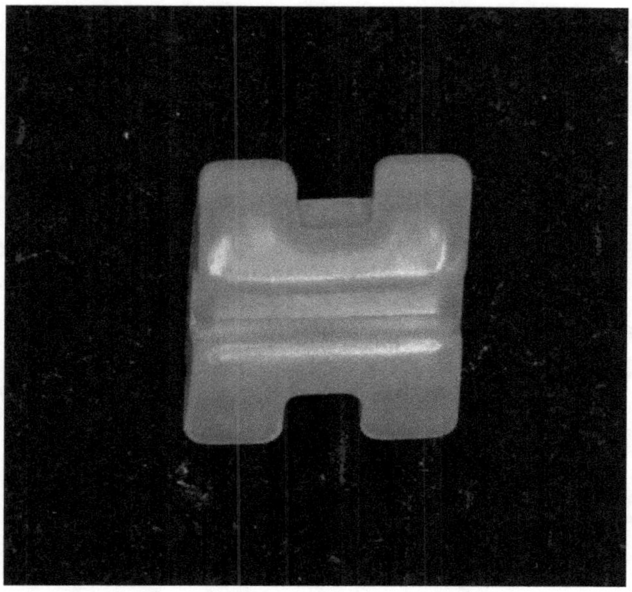

Figure 3. The semitwin tie-wing complex.

3.4. Friction

When polycrystalline ceramics were compared with monocrystalline ceramics, it was concluded that polycrystalline ceramics have a higher coefficient of friction. In fact, more than a decade ago, it was pointed out that monocrystalline brackets have frictional characteristics close to metal brackets [4].

To overcome the problem of frictional resistance of polycrystalline brackets, manufacturers carried out numerous modifications. Polycrystalline ceramic brackets with metal inserts in the arch wire slot (metal slots) were developed [18]. Nevertheless, it was reported that the sharp edges of the metal insert may "dig into" the softer arch wire material, thus increasing resistance to sliding and thereby reducing the efficiency of tooth movement [7, 19]. Another modification was the addition of bumps along the floor of the polycrystalline ceramic bracket slot. Nevertheless, these bumps were not effective in reducing frictional resistance [20].

A recent study, including ceramic and metal brackets that were manufactured by different production methods, including CIM and metal injection molding (MIM), concluded that the manufacturing technologies do not present a critical difference regarding friction [3]. It was reiterated that the complex phenomenon of friction depends on a multitude of factors, such as the bracket/ligature/arch wire combinations, the surface quality of the arch wire/bracket slot, the bracket design, and the force exerted by the ligature on the arch wire [3].

3.5. Optics

The optical properties of ceramic brackets provide an attractive option for a great number of patients. As previously mentioned, polycrystalline ceramic brackets possess a microstructure of crystal GBs. This microstructure reflects light, resulting in some degree of opacity. In contrast, single-crystal brackets lack GBs, thus permitting the passage of light, making these brackets basically clear [2, 10, 21].

As mentioned above, monocrystalline brackets have more optical clarity than polycrystalline brackets (**Figure 4**). Whether this difference is of essential importance from an esthetic point of view is a decision to be made by the orthodontist as well as the patient [2].

Apart from esthetics, the optical properties of ceramic brackets have been shown to affect the amount of light transmitted through these brackets during photocuring. The amount of light transmitted through ceramic brackets affects the curing efficiency of the light-cured adhesive. Polycrystalline brackets and polycrystalline brackets with a polymer mesh base were found to block direct light transmittance to a greater extent than monocrystalline brackets. It was pointed out that the color-coded holders designed for identification and handling of ceramic brackets also hinder light transmittance. The use of clear holders with colored edges has been suggested [22].

3.6. Color stability

The color stability of ceramic brackets throughout orthodontic treatment is an important characteristic. It has been stated that ceramic brackets, both monocrystalline and polycrystalline, undergo a color change when subjected to coffee, black tea, coke, and red wine [21, 23, 24]. It has to be pointed out that these are in vitro findings. In vivo studies concerning the color stability of ceramic brackets are lacking.

3.7. Plaque accumulation

Limited information is available about which bracket material (ceramic versus metal brackets) is less prone to the adhesion of bacteria and plaque accumulation. A clinical study performed by Lindel et al. [25] concluded that ceramic brackets exhibit less long-term biofilm accumulation than metal brackets. It was emphasized that future research should aim to determine whether the difference in biofilm accumulation between ceramic and metal brackets has a clinically significant effect on the development of decalcifications. Lindel et al. [25] pointed out that the results obtained from this type of future research might have a strong effect when choosing bracket material in patients with insufficient oral hygiene habits.

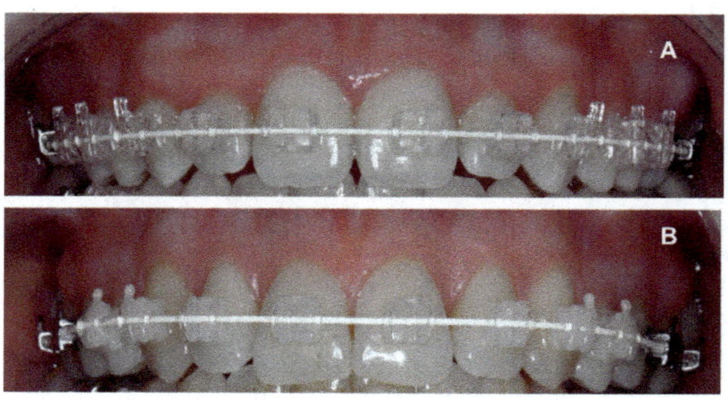

Figure 4. Intraoral image of monocrystalline (A) and polycrystalline (B) ceramic brackets.

3.8. Biocompatibility

Biocompatibility is the ability of a material to provide successful service in a host while causing minimal response [9]. It has been stated that conventional ceramic brackets are chemically stable (inert) in the oral environment and that they exhibit excellent biocompatibility with oral tissues [5].

In 2012, Retamoso et al. [26] carried out an in vitro cytotoxicity study evaluating various orthodontic brackets. These researchers reported that monocrystalline ceramic brackets had good biocompatibility. On the other hand, polycrystalline ceramic brackets with metal slots demonstrated some toxic effects. It was pointed out that the metallic slot was the essential factor responsible for a decrease of cell viability due to nickel ion release. They [26] concluded that it is essential to continue with studies evaluating cytotoxicity. If toxicity of any material is proven, alternative materials have to be used.

3.9. Magnetic resonance imaging (MRI) compatibility

Orthodontists are often asked to remove fixed orthodontic appliances prior to an MRI scan—a diagnostic tool that does not expose the patient to radiation—particularly when looking for pathology in the head and neck region or when information regarding the articular disc is required [10, 27].

Beau et al. [27] provided a detailed flowchart concerning the indications for the removal of fixed orthodontic appliances prior to MRI scans of the head and neck region. According to this flowchart, ceramic brackets do not have to be removed prior to an MRI scan. They are MRI-safe. However, ceramic brackets with any metal components, such as stainless steel slots, have to be removed if the region under examination is adjacent to these brackets. Stainless steel causes extensive artifacts, which may degrade image quality beyond clinical acceptability. The authors [27] pointed out that they did not include arch wires or removable appliances in their research, since these can be easily removed prior to an MRI scan.

4. Characteristics of ceramic bracket bases

Several retention mechanisms were developed for the attachment of ceramic bracket bases to the adhesive. These are chemical retention, mechanical retention, and a combination of both methods [21, 28]. The first developed method was the chemical retention method. This method, now obsolete, used a coating of glass on the flat ceramic bracket base and then a silane coupler to achieve a chemical bond between the glass-coated bracket base and the adhesive. The silane molecule is a bifunctional molecule; that is, one end reacted with the glass coating on the bracket base, while the other end reacted with the adhesive [11, 29]. It was pointed out that the chemical retention mechanism produced very strong bonds that harmed the tooth surface in the form of cracks and enamel tear-outs during debracketing [4, 7, 11, 29–32].

Almost three decades ago, Ghafari and Chen [33] compared the performance of chemical retention ceramic brackets to silane-treated grooved base ceramic brackets (a combination of chemical and mechanical retention). They [33] concluded that mechanical retention might reduce the negative side effects of debracketing by favoring failure within the adhesive, thus protecting the integrity of the enamel surface, i.e., the health of the tooth, as well as the integrity of the ceramic bracket.

The reports about iatrogenic tooth damage during debracketing impelled manufacturers to make changes in the base designs of ceramic brackets, relying more on mechanical retention for bond strength. In fact, the majority of ceramic brackets available today are purely mechanically retained brackets [4, 30, 34]. Mechanical retention is achieved by creating undercuts or grooves in the base of the bracket. These undercuts make a mechanical interlock with the adhesive bonding agent possible [28].

Currently, many different mechanical base designs are available, such as microcrystalline base design with a stress concentrator, button-structured base design, ball-base design with gingival ball reduction, dovetail base design, laser-structured base design, and "portal" bonding base design [4, 15, 35, 36].

An additional, interesting base design is the application of a thin layer of polymer onto the ceramic bracket base [19]. Thus, bonding takes place between the enamel and the flexible polymer mesh base. Encouraging in vitro results concerning the enamel surface after debracketing were obtained [30, 37, 38].

At this point, only two published clinical studies [14, 39] with a purely mechanical retention mechanism were encountered. There is a need for clinical studies, particularly randomized clinical studies, i.e., the gold standard for evaluating clinical procedures.

5. Rebonding of ceramic brackets

Although some major orthodontic supply companies explicitly state in their instruction sheets that their ceramic brackets are for single use only, several laboratory studies suggested various techniques for the reuse, i.e., the rebonding, of ceramic brackets [40–44]. For reuse, the bracket has to be intact in the first place.

It has been pointed out that the appropriate term is "reuse" or "recondition" instead of "recycle," since the term "recycled" implies the manufacturing of new brackets from the raw material of the original, failed brackets [12]. Nevertheless, the literature usually refers to these brackets as "recycled."

An in vitro study [43], carried out in 2016, investigated the "recycling" of polycrystalline ceramic brackets with a microcrystalline base via the following three methods: first is the erbium-doped yttrium aluminum garnet (Er:YAG) laser, and the other two are traditional methods, i.e., flaming and sandblasting. Sandblasting (50 μm Al_2O_3 particles) damaged the delicate bracket base structure and demonstrated significantly less bond strength than new brackets. The flaming procedure yielded a bond strength that was similar to that of new ceramic brackets. However, flaming affected the esthetics of these brackets, i.e., these brackets ended up faded and dark. Er:YAG lasers completely removed the adhesive remnants from the ceramic bracket bases without damaging the base structure. Furthermore, the shear bond strength of Er:YAG laser "recycled" brackets was similar to that of new brackets. It was pointed out that the laser method may be preferred over other "recycling" methods.

Yassaei et al. [44] also concluded that the Er:YAG laser presents an efficient way for "recycling" ceramic brackets. These researchers used polycrystalline ceramic brackets with a dovetailed base in their in vitro study.

6. Debonding of ceramic brackets

Debonding usually refers to the removal of orthodontic brackets and the residual adhesives from the tooth enamel at the end of fixed appliance treatment [45].

Ceramic brackets lack flexibility. In other words, the rigid ceramic and the rigid enamel have little ability to dissipate stress when exposed to debracketing forces at the end of treatment. Thus, bracket fracture and/or enamel damage may occur during debracketing [2, 11].

Several approaches aiming to minimize the side effects associated with the debracketing of ceramic brackets exist. These are the conventional (mechanical), ultrasonic, electrothermal, and laser techniques [11, 21].

6.1. Mechanical debracketing

Three mechanical debracketing techniques have been described. These are lift-off, wrenching, and delamination [46]. The first technique uses a lift-off debracketing instrument (LODI). This pistol-grip plier is placed over the bracket, and a debracketing force is applied to the tie-wings of the bracket. It has been pointed out that the LODI cannot be used with ceramic brackets due to their brittleness [39]. The wrenching technique uses a special tool that produces a wrenching or torsional force at the base of the bracket [46]. This approach, providing a rotational shear force, can be likened to the turning of a door knob.

The delamination technique was the first technique introduced and is still reported to be the most widely accepted ceramic bracket removal technique [11, 15]. This technique involves the application of a slow squeezing force with the sharp blades of the debracketing pliers placed on the enamel surface and within the adhesive, thereby producing a wedging effect (**Figure 5**).

It has been stated that such a force—produced by a slow, gradual compression—would seem to offer the best chance for inducing crack propagation within the adhesive, leading to a cohesive failure, thus minimizing the risk of enamel damage as well as the risk of bracket fracture. A cohesive bond failure is a failure through a single material, where cohesive forces between the same atomic species are present [2, 11, 21, 46].

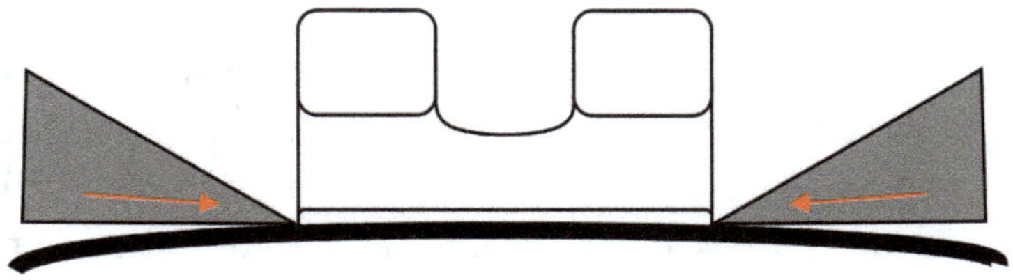

Figure 5. Schematic presentation of the delamination technique.

In 1993, Bishara and Fehr [47] evaluated the force levels produced with wide and narrow blades during ceramic bracket removal from human maxillary molar teeth. The wide blades and narrow blades were 3.2 and 2 mm, respectively. Polycrystalline ceramic brackets relying on a combination of mechanical and chemical retention were used. The findings of this in vitro study indicated that the narrow blades produced a significantly lower mean debracketing force, namely 120 kg/cm^2 than the wider blades (150 kg/cm^2). Bishara and Fehr [47] concluded that such a significant reduction (20%) in the debracketing force places less stress on the enamel surface, thereby reducing the risk of enamel damage. It has been reported and reiterated that debracketing forces larger than 138 kg/cm^2, i.e., 13.53 MPa should be avoided [11, 48, 49].

In 2000, Arici and Minors [50] carried out an in vitro study with four different methods of debracketing. They pointed out that reducing the contact area, i.e., contact area between the plier blades and the adhesive, to a minimum reduces the force necessary to initiate ceramic bracket removal. Macroscopically, no enamel damage and no bracket fractures were reported. Arici and Minors [50] used primary bovine mandibular incisor teeth and polycrystalline ceramic brackets with chemical retention. They concluded that their findings basically corroborate the findings of Bishara and Fehr [47].

Following the introduction of ceramic brackets, more than 30 years ago, serious complications during debracketing were encountered [4, 7, 11, 13, 51, 52]. Many in vitro studies, to assist in the development of more reliable and clinically safe ceramic brackets, followed. The reduction of ceramic debracketing forces, thereby protecting enamel integrity as well as bracket integrity, was the aim of these studies [11, 47, 48, 50].

Nowadays, the majority of ceramic bracket manufacturers present detailed debracketing instructions. In fact, many manufacturers have introduced debracketing instruments specifically designed for their bracket brand. These manufacturers claim that their brackets can be removed as easily and as safely as metal brackets as long as the orthodontist meticulously follows these instructions [4, 11, 13, 15]. As a risk management strategy, ceramic brackets that are not accompanied by detailed instructions for bonding and debracketing should definitely not be used.

Any shortcomings related to ceramic brackets should be reported immediately to the manufacturer [7]. "First, do no harm" should serve as the fundamental guiding principle for anyone engaged in health care [53].

6.2. Precautions for mechanical debracketing

Bonding a ceramic bracket to a compromised tooth, such as a brittle, nonvital tooth (endodontically treated tooth), a tooth with developmental defects, a tooth with demineralized enamel, a tooth with enamel cracks and/or a large restoration, should be avoided as much as possible. This type of tooth is under greater risk for enamel damage when compared with a healthy tooth during mechanical debracketing [21, 39]. Care also has to be exercised with porcelain restorations, such as crowns and veneers [51].

During the bonding procedure, excess adhesive flash (EAF) must be removed with an explorer before the adhesive has set or with burs after setting. Only meticulous EAF removal allows the sharp-edged plier blades of the debracketing instrument to be fully seated on the enamel during ceramic bracket removal. This produces a safe force transmission and crack propagation through the adhesive, resulting in a cohesive failure within the adhesive, thereby protecting enamel as well as bracket integrity [2, 11, 21]. Furthermore, EAF removal improves esthetics by providing a clean and neat appearance.

It should be noted that a flash-free adhesive-coated appliance system was introduced. This innovative technology does not necessitate flash removal [54].

Unfortunately, debracketing may lead to bracket fracture. Bracket fragments may detach (loose fragments) or remain attached on the enamel surface. Low-speed or high-speed grinding of the bracket fragments with no water coolant may bring forth permanent damage and necrosis of the dental pulps. Therefore, water cooling is absolutely necessary during the grinding/removal of ceramic bracket fragments [10, 55]. Furthermore, high-volume suction next to the area of grinding has been emphasized in order to minimize the spreading of ceramic particles [10, 55]. These particles have been reported to cause irritation of the eyes as well as itching of the hands [55]. After the removal of these fragments, the clinician can proceed with adhesive remnant removal.

Loose, fractured ceramic bracket fragments may create serious problems, such as aspiration or ingestion of these radiolucent fragments. Furthermore, during debracketing, the "popping off" of fragments may occur. This may subject the patient as well as the orthodontist to eye injury. The use of protective eyewear and a mask is indispensable for the orthodontist. The patient should be given protective eyewear as well [21, 34, 56].

The force applied during debracketing may cause discomfort. Therefore, the orthodontist should always support the teeth with his or her fingers or make the patient bite firmly into a cotton roll during debracketing. Biting firmly into a cotton roll and/or gauze not only minimizes discomfort but also minimizes the risk of brackets and/or fragments from getting displaced into the oral cavity [21, 34]. Colored cotton rolls may facilitate the detection of fractured ceramic bracket fragments.

If pliers are used for debracketing, Bishara and Fehr [21] advised the renewal of the plier blades after the removal of 50 brackets. Pliers with nonexchangeable blades should be sharpened on a regular basis [21]. Sharp-edged plier blades are required for safe debracketing, i.e., for the induction of crack propagation within the bonding adhesive rather than the enamel or the ceramic bracket. The orthodontist should never delegate ceramic bracket debracketing to auxiliaries [21, 56].

It has been emphasized that every informed consent form signed by the patient/parents (and the orthodontist) should specifically outline the potential risks of ceramic brackets, particularly in an ever-increasing litigious society [56]. Also, the brand of the ceramic bracket should always be recorded on the patient's file. This is of particular importance in the case of transfer to another orthodontist.

6.3. Adjunctive methods proposed for mechanical debracketing

Larmour and Chadwick [57] evaluated the ability of a commercial debonding agent, post-debonding agent (P-de-A) (Oradent Ltd., Eton, Berks, UK). This green gel, containing a derivative of peppermint oil, was claimed to facilitate ceramic bracket debracketing and adhesive residue removal. The manufacturer of P-de-A advised an application time of 1–2 min to soften the resin. Nevertheless, the P-de-A research results did not support these claims [57, 58].

In 1997, Arici et al. [59, 60] proposed the use of a crushable porous ceramic lamella as a means of facilitating debracketing. These porous lamellae were attached to the bracket base with adhesive resin. Subsequently, these bracket/lamella assemblies were bonded to the enamel of the experimental teeth (bovine incisor teeth). The authors [60] of this in vitro study reported the safe removal of these ceramic bracket/lamella assemblies, i.e., no fractures of the ceramic bracket or any evidence of enamel damage was observed. Commercial production of this type of ceramic bracket/lamella assembly was not undertaken.

In 1998, Larmour et al. [61] evaluated the possibility of reducing the complications of ceramic bracket debracketing by introducing a notch in the composite bond layer. A section of Mylar® matrix strip (0.01 mm thick and 0.75 mm wide) was placed within the bonding agent in this ex vivo investigation. After the bonding agent had set, the matrix strip was removed creating a "notched" bond layer. Larmour et al. [61] concluded that notching the bonding agent does facilitate ceramic bracket removal. Nevertheless, they emphasized that this modification is not feasible in a clinical setting due to the time needed and the technical difficulty of creating a "notched" bond layer. Furthermore, they cautioned that such a "notched" adhesive layer may lead to plaque accumulation.

In 2003, Carter [62] suggested that a hot-water bath might facilitate ceramic bracket debracketing. Patients were given a cup of hot water, supplied from a coffeemaker, and were asked to hold this water in their mouths for 1 min without swallowing. Subsequently, debracketing with suitable pliers was performed. Carter [62] emphasized that since 1986 no enamel fracture or any other iatrogenic damage occurred with this application in his clinic. Unfortunately, the exact temperature of this "hot-water bath" was not stated.

6.4. Ultrasonic debracketing

It was reported that the ultrasonic debracketing technique presents a decreased probability of enamel damage as well as a decreased probability of bracket fracture. Also, the residual adhesive remaining after debracketing can be removed with the same ultrasonic tip. Nevertheless, the debracketing time is the longest when compared with the mechanical or electrothermal debracketing techniques. It was reported that the debracketing time of the ultrasonic debonding technique is 38–50 s per bracket, when compared with 1 s per bracket with the mechanical debracketing technique. Furthermore, the contact between the "hard" ceramic bracket and the ultrasonic tip has been reported to cause wear of this expensive tip. During the ultrasonic debracketing procedure, water spray is mandatory to prevent pulp damage. This method requires further testing and is not yet recommended for clinical use [11, 21]. No clinical studies were encountered upon a literature search.

6.5. Electrothermal debracketing

In 1986, Sheridan et al. [63] were the first who described electrothermal debracketing (ETD) for the removal of metallic brackets.

With ceramic brackets, ETD has been reported to cause a reduced incidence of bracket fracture. The reduced incidence of bracket fracture is ascribed to the small amount of force needed to break the bond after the heat-induced tip has promoted bond failure by softening/weakening the adhesive material. A relatively short debracketing time per bracket (2 ± 1 s) was reported. The possibility of pulp damage has been mentioned. Fortunately, no signs of irreversible pulp damage with ETD were described [11, 64–66]. Patient acceptance was generally positive [64].

6.6. Laser debracketing

Different types of lasers have been used for the debracketing of ceramic brackets [67]. The application of laser irradiation causes the softening of the adhesive material. This seems to be quite similar to ETD; however, with laser-assisted debracketing, the amount of thermal energy delivered to the ceramic bracket can be carefully controlled, thereby preventing the possibility of overheating [21, 68]. The time spent for ceramic bracket removal with the laser-based technique is 1–5 s. Debracketing forces are significantly reduced with lasers. As a result, enamel damage and bracket fracture risks are significantly reduced [67, 69]. The high cost of this device may be a disadvantage for the orthodontist [11, 21].

7. Last but not least

The physical properties as well as rebonding and debonding of monocrystalline and polycrystalline alumina ceramic brackets were reviewed. Ceramic brackets fabricated from polycrystalline zirconium oxide (zirconia) were not mentioned. Thus, we would like to add a short paragraph about these brackets for the interested reader.

Zirconia ceramic brackets, manufactured in Japan and Australia, have attracted interest in the past [12]. Nevertheless, problems concerning color (yellowish tint) and opacity (nontranslucency) were reported approximately three decades ago [12, 70]. Furthermore, no significant advantage of zirconia brackets over alumina brackets with regard to their frictional characteristics were reported [71]. Limited published research on zirconia (zirconium oxide) brackets exists [72].

8. Conclusion

In an increasingly demanding and litigious society, it is mandatory for the orthodontist to use carefully designed ceramic brackets. As a simple risk management strategy, ceramic brackets that are not accompanied by detailed instructions for bonding and bracket removal should definitely not be used. These products might not have been exposed to appropriate, detailed testing procedures prior to their sale. Thus, be alert and keep updated!

Author details

Selma Elekdag-Türk[1†*] and Hüdanur Yilmaz (née Huda Ebulkbash)[2]

*Address all correspondence to: elekdagturk@yahoo.com

1 Faculty of Dentistry, Department of Orthodontics, University of Ondokuz Mayis, Samsun, Republic of Turkey

2 Anadolu Mahallesi, Samsun, Republic of Turkey

† I, Selma, dedicate this chapter to the memory of my grandmother, Anna Kirschner (1915–2004). My heart will always miss you....

References

[1] Available from: https://spacetechdevelopment.weebly.com/invisible-braces.html

[2] Swartz ML. Ceramic brackets. Journal of Clinical Orthodontics. 1988;**22**:82-88

[3] Reimann S, Bourauel C, Weber A, Dirk C, Lietz T. Friction behavior of ceramic injection-molded (CIM) brackets. Journal of Orofacial Orthopedics. 2016;**77**:262-271

[4] Russell JS. Aesthetic orthodontic brackets. Journal of Orthodontics. 2005;**32**:146-163

[5] Gautam P, Valiathan A. Ceramic brackets: In search of an ideal! Biomaterials and Artificial Organs. 2007;**20**:122-126

[6] Scott GE Jr. Fracture toughness and surface cracks—The key to understanding ceramic brackets. The Angle Orthodontist. 1988;**58**:5-8

[7] Birnie D. Ceramic brackets. British Journal of Orthodontics. 1990;**17**:71-74

[8] Viazis AD, DeLong R, Bevis RR, Douglas WH, Speidel TM. Enamel surface abrasion from ceramic orthodontic brackets: A special case report. American Journal of Orthodontics and Dentofacial Orthopedics. 1989;**96**:514-518

[9] O'Brien WJ. Dental Materials and Their Selection. 2nd ed. Chicago: Quintessence; 1997. p. 16, 199

[10] Graber LW, Vanarsdall RL Jr, Vig KWL. Orthodontics Current Principles and Techniques. 5th ed. Philadelphia: Mosby/Elsevier; 2012. p. 114, 749-755, 1028-1030

[11] Graber TM, Eliades T, Athanasiou AE, editors. Risk Management in Orthodontics: Experts' Guide to Malpractice. Chicago: Quintessence; 2004. pp. 36-40

[12] Brantley WA, Eliades T, editors. Orthodontic Materials: Scientific and Clinical Aspects. Stuttgart: Thieme; 2001. p. 22, 23, 146, 151, 159, 160

[13] Karamouzos A, Athanasiou AE, Papadopoulos MA. Clinical characteristics and properties of ceramic brackets: A comprehensive review. American Journal of Orthodontics and Dentofacial Orthopedics. 1997;**112**:34-40

[14] Verstrynge A, Ghesquiere A, Willems G. Clinical comparison of an adhesive precoated vs. an uncoated ceramic bracket system. Orthodontics & Craniofacial Research. 2004;**7**:15-20

[15] Jena AK, Duggal R, Mehrotra AK. Physical properties and clinical characteristics of ceramic brackets; a comprehensive review. Biomaterials and Artificial Organs. 2007;**20**:101-115

[16] Sanchez DJ, Walker MP, Kula K, Williams KB, Eick JD. Fluoride prophylactic agents effect on ceramic bracket tie-wing fracture strength. The Angle Orthodontist. 2008;**78**:524-530

[17] Johnson G, Walker MP, Kula K. Fracture strength of ceramic bracket tie wings subjected to tension. The Angle Orthodontist. 2005;**75**:95-100

[18] Proffit WR, Fields HW, Sarver DM, Ackerman JL. Contemporary Orthodontics. 5th ed. Vol. 2013. St. Louis: Mosby/Elsevier. pp. 370-372

[19] Devanathan D. Design and Development of Ultimate Ceramic Brackets. La Porte: TP Orthodontic, Inc; 2003; 996-372E Apr

[20] Thorstenson GA, Kusy RP. Resistance to sliding of orthodontic brackets with bumps in the slot floors and walls: Effects of second-order angulation. Dental Materials. 2004;**20**:881-892

[21] Bishara SE, Fehr DE. Ceramic brackets: Something old, something new, a review. Seminars in Orthodontics. 1997;**3**:178-188

[22] Eliades T, Johnston WM, Eliades G. Direct light transmission through ceramic brackets. American Journal of Orthodontics and Dentofacial Orthopedics. 1995;**107**:11-19

[23] de Oliveira CB, Maia LG, Santos-Pinto A, Gandini Junior LG. In vitro study of color stability of polycrystalline and monocrystalline ceramic brackets. Dental Press Journal of Orthodontics. 2014;**19**:114-121

[24] Guignone BC, Silva LK, Soares RV, Akaki E, Goiato MC, Pithon MM, Oliveira DD. Color stability of ceramic brackets immersed in potentially staining solutions. Dental Press Journal of Orthodontics. 2015;**20**:32-38

[25] Lindel ID, Elter C, Heuer W, Heidenblut T, Stiesch M, Schwestka-Polly R, Demling AP. Comparative analysis of long-term biofilm formation on metal and ceramic brackets. The Angle Orthodontist. 2011;**81**:907-914

[26] Retamoso LB, Luz TB, Marinowic DR, Machado DC, De Menezes LM, Freitas MP, Oshima HM. Cytotoxicity of esthetic, metallic, and nickel-free orthodontic brackets: Cellular behavior and viability. American Journal of Orthodontics and Dentofacial Orthopedics. 2012;**142**:70-74

[27] Beau A, Bossard D, Gebeile-Chauty S. Magnetic resonance imaging artefacts and fixed orthodontic attachments. European Journal of Orthodontics. 2015;**37**:105-110

[28] Bishara SE, Fehr DE, Jakobsen JR. A comparative study of the debonding strengths of different ceramic brackets, enamel conditioners, and adhesives. American Journal of Orthodontics and Dentofacial Orthopedics. 1993;**104**:170-179

[29] Bishara SE, Trulove TS. Comparisons of different debonding techniques for ceramic brackets: An in vitro study. Part I. Background and methods. American Journal of Orthodontics and Dentofacial Orthopedics. 1990;**98**:145-153

[30] Kitahara-Céia FM, Mucha JN, Marques dos Santos PA. Assessment of enamel damage after removal of ceramic brackets. American Journal of Orthodontics and Dentofacial Orthopedics. 2008;**134**:548-555

[31] Ødegaard J, Segner D. Shear bond strength of metal brackets compared with a new ceramic bracket. American Journal of Orthodontics and Dentofacial Orthopedics. 1988; **94**:201-206

[32] Winchester LJ. Bond strengths of five different ceramic brackets: An in vitro study. European Journal of Orthodontics. 1991;**13**:293-305

[33] Ghafari J, Chen SS. Mechanical and SEM study of debonding two types of ceramic brackets (abstract). Journal of Dental Research. 1990;**69**:338

[34] Ghafari J. Problems associated with ceramic brackets suggest limiting use to selected teeth. The Angle Orthodontist. 1992;**62**:145-152

[35] Dentaurum. Available from: http://www.discovery pearl ceramic bracket line [Accessed: January 03, 2018]

[36] G&H Orthodontics. Available from: http://www.vapor ceramic bracket system [Accessed: January 03, 2018]

[37] Elekdag-Turk S, Isci D, Ozkalayci N, Turk T. Debonding characteristics of a polymer mesh base ceramic bracket bonded with two different conditioning methods. European Journal of Orthodontics. 2009;**31**:84-89

[38] Lemke K, Xu X, Hagan JL, Armbruster PC, Ballard RW. Bond strengths and debonding characteristics of two types of polycrystalline ceramic brackets. Australian Orthodontic Journal. 2010;**26**:134-140

[39] Cochrane NJ, Lo TWG, Adams GG, Schneider PM. Quantitative analysis of enamel on debonded orthodontic brackets. American Journal of Orthodontics and Dentofacial Orthopedics. 2017;**152**:312-319

[40] Lew KK, Djeng SK. Recycling ceramic brackets. Journal of Clinical Orthodontics. 1990; **24**:44-47

[41] Lew KK, Chew CL, Lee KW. A comparison of shear bond strengths between new and recycled ceramic brackets. European Journal of Orthodontics. 1991;**13**:306-310

[42] Chung CH, Friedman SD, Mante FK. Shear bond strength of rebonded mechanically retentive ceramic brackets. American Journal of Orthodontics and Dentofacial Orthopedics. 2002;**122**:282-287

[43] Han RQ, Yang K, Ji LF, Ling C. Analysis of shear bond strength and morphology of Er:YAG laser-recycled ceramic orthodontic brackets. BioMed Research International. 2016: 6 pp. Article ID 7276287

[44] Yassaei S, Aghili H, Hosseinzadeh Firouzabadi A, Meshkani H. Effect of Er:YAG laser and sandblasting in recycling of ceramic brackets. Journal of Lasers in Medical Sciences. 2017;**8**:17-21

[45] Oliver RG. The effect of different methods of bracket removal on the amount of residual adhesive. American Journal of Orthodontics and Dentofacial Orthopedics. 1988;**93**:196-200

[46] Sinha PK, Nanda RS. The effect of different bonding and debonding techniques on debonding ceramic orthodontic brackets. American Journal of Orthodontics and Dentofacial Orthopedics. 1997;**112**:132-137

[47] Bishara SE, Fehr DE. Comparisons of the effectiveness of pliers with narrow and wide blades in debonding ceramic brackets. American Journal of Orthodontics and Dentofacial Orthopedics. 1993;**103**:253-257

[48] Bishara SE, Fonseca JM, Fehr DE, Boyer DB. Debonding forces applied to ceramic brackets simulating clinical conditions. The Angle Orthodontist. 1994;**64**:277-282

[49] Retief DH. Failure at the dental adhesive-etched enamel interface. Journal of Oral Rehabilitation. 1974;**1**:265-284

[50] Arici S, Minors C. The force levels required to mechanically debond ceramic brackets: An *in vitro* comparative study. European Journal of Orthodontics. 2000;**22**:327-334

[51] Machen DE. Legal aspects of orthodontic practice: Risk management concepts. Ceramic bracket update. American Journal of Orthodontics and Dentofacial Orthopedics. 1990;**98**:185-186

[52] Bishara SE. Ceramic brackets and the need to develop national standards. American Journal of Orthodontics and Dentofacial Orthopedics. 2000;**117**:595-597

[53] Keim RG. Primum non nocere. Journal of Clinical Orthodontics. 2008;**42**:193-194

[54] Cinader DK, Aung M, Ugai R, Conley A. APC™ flash-free adhesive: A technical overview. Orthodontic Perspectives Innova. 2013;**XX**(1):7-9

[55] Vukovich ME, Wood DP, Daley TD. Heat generated by grinding during removal of ceramic brackets. American Journal of Orthodontics and Dentofacial Orthopedics. 1991; **99**:505-512

[56] Abdelkarim A, Jerrold L. Risk management strategies in orthodontics. Part 1: Clinical considerations. American Journal of Orthodontics and Dentofacial Orthopedics. 2015;**148**:345-349

[57] Larmour CJ, Chadwick RG. Effects of a commercial orthodontic debonding agent upon the surface microhardness of two orthodontic bonding resins. Journal of Dentistry. 1995;**23**:37-40

[58] Larmour CJ, McCabe JF, Gordon PH. An ex vivo investigation into the effects of chemical solvents on the debond behaviour of ceramic orthodontic brackets. British Journal of Orthodontics. 1998;**25**:35-39

[59] Arici S, Minors CJ, Messer PF. Porous ceramic lamellae for orthodontic ceramic brackets: Part I: Fabrication and characterization. Journal of Materials Science. Materials in Medicine. 1997;**8**:441-446

[60] Arici S, Minors CJ, Messer PF. Porous ceramic lamellae for orthodontic ceramic brackets: Part II: *In vitro* performance testing. Journal of Materials Science. Materials in Medicine. 1997;**8**:447-453

[61] Larmour CJ, McCabe JF, Gordon PH. Notching of orthodontic bonding resin to facilitate ceramic bracket debond--an *ex vivo* investigation. British Journal of Orthodontics. 1998;**25**:289-291

[62] Carter RN. Hot-water bath facilitates ceramic debracketing. Journal of Clinical Orthodontics. 2003;**37**:620

[63] Sheridan JJ, Brawley G, Hastings J. Electrothermal debracketing. Part I. An in vitro study. American Journal of Orthodontics. 1986;**89**:21-27

[64] Dovgan JS, Walton RE, Bishara SE. Electrothermal debracketing: Patient acceptance and effects on the dental pulp. American Journal of Orthodontics and Dentofacial Orthopedics. 1995;**108**:249-255

[65] Jost-Brinkmann PG, Radlanski RJ, Artun J, Loidl H. Risk of pulp damage due to temperature increase during thermodebonding of ceramic brackets. European Journal of Orthodontics. 1997;**19**:623-628

[66] Kailasam V, Valiathan A, Rao N. Histological evaluation after electrothermal debonding of ceramic brackets. Indian Journal of Dental Research. 2014;**25**:143-146

[67] Ghazanfari R, Nokhbatolfoghahaei H, Alikhasi M. Laser-aided ceramic bracket debonding: A comprehensive review. Journal of Lasers in Medical Sciences. 2016;**7**:2-11

[68] Ma T, Marangoni RD, Flint W. In vitro comparison of debonding force and intrapulpal temperature changes during ceramic orthodontic bracket removal using a carbon dioxide laser. American Journal of Orthodontics and Dentofacial Orthopedics. 1997;**111**:203-210

[69] Azzeh E, Feldon PJ. Laser debonding of ceramic brackets: A comprehensive review. American Journal of Orthodontics and Dentofacial Orthopedics. 2003;**123**:79-83

[70] Springate SD, Winchester LJ. An evaluation of zirconium oxide brackets: A preliminary laboratory and clinical report. British Journal of Orthodontics. 1991;**18**:203-208

[71] Keith O, Kusy RP, Whitley JQ. Zirconia brackets: An evaluation of morphology and coefficients of friction. American Journal of Orthodontics and Dentofacial Orthopedics. 1994;**106**:605-614

[72] Alrejaye N, Pober R, Giordano R II. Torsional strength of computer-aided design/computer-aided manufacturing-fabricated esthetic orthodontic brackets. The Angle Orthodontist. 2017;**87**:125-130

Permissions

All chapters in this book were first published in CAO, by InTech Open; hereby published with permission under the Creative Commons Attribution License or equivalent. Every chapter published in this book has been scrutinized by our experts. Their significance has been extensively debated. The topics covered herein carry significant findings which will fuel the growth of the discipline. They may even be implemented as practical applications or may be referred to as a beginning point for another development.

The contributors of this book come from diverse backgrounds, making this book a truly international effort. This book will bring forth new frontiers with its revolutionizing research information and detailed analysis of the nascent developments around the world.

We would like to thank all the contributing authors for lending their expertise to make the book truly unique. They have played a crucial role in the development of this book. Without their invaluable contributions this book wouldn't have been possible. They have made vital efforts to compile up to date information on the varied aspects of this subject to make this book a valuable addition to the collection of many professionals and students.

This book was conceptualized with the vision of imparting up-to-date information and advanced data in this field. To ensure the same, a matchless editorial board was set up. Every individual on the board went through rigorous rounds of assessment to prove their worth. After which they invested a large part of their time researching and compiling the most relevant data for our readers.

The editorial board has been involved in producing this book since its inception. They have spent rigorous hours researching and exploring the diverse topics which have resulted in the successful publishing of this book. They have passed on their knowledge of decades through this book. To expedite this challenging task, the publisher supported the team at every step. A small team of assistant editors was also appointed to further simplify the editing procedure and attain best results for the readers.

Apart from the editorial board, the designing team has also invested a significant amount of their time in understanding the subject and creating the most relevant covers. They scrutinized every image to scout for the most suitable representation of the subject and create an appropriate cover for the book.

The publishing team has been an ardent support to the editorial, designing and production team. Their endless efforts to recruit the best for this project, has resulted in the accomplishment of this book. They are a veteran in the field of academics and their pool of knowledge is as vast as their experience in printing. Their expertise and guidance has proved useful at every step. Their uncompromising quality standards have made this book an exceptional effort. Their encouragement from time to time has been an inspiration for everyone.

The publisher and the editorial board hope that this book will prove to be a valuable piece of knowledge for researchers, students, practitioners and scholars across the globe.

List of Contributors

Anand K. Patil
Department of Orthodontics and Dentofacial Orthodontics, SDM College of Dental Sciences and Hospital, Karnataka, India

Amrit Singh Maan
SDM College of Dental Sciences and Hospital, Dharwad, Karnataka, India

Ayşe Gülşen
Department of Plastic Reconstructive and Esthetic Surgery, University of Gazi, Ankara,Turkey

Bakr M.Rabie
Faculty of Dentistry, The University of Hong Kong, Hong Kong

Jeremy Ho and Qianfeng Li
The University of Hong Kong, Hong Kong

Marcos Jimmy Carruitero Honores
Department of Orthodontics, Bauru Dental School, University of São Paulo, Brazil

Amila Vujacic
The Faculty of Medicine, The University of Pristina, Kosovska Mitrovica, Serbia

Jasna Pavlovic
School of Medicine, University of Pristina, Kosovska Mitrovica, Serbia

Aleksandra Konic-Ristic
School of Agriculture and Food Science, Dublin, Ireland

Phimon Atsawasuwan
Department of Orthodontics, University of Illinois at Chicago, Chicago, Illinois, United States

Sajjad Shirazi
Department of Oral Biology, University of Illinois at Chicago, Chicago, Illinois, United States

Dental and Periodontal Research Center, Tabriz University of Medical Sciences, Iran

Handan Tuğçe Oğuz
Private Orthodontics Clinic, Ankara, Turkey

Esra Bolat
Department of Orthodontics, Faculty of Dentistry, Akdeniz University, Antalya, Turkey

Mustafa Sancar Atac
Faculty of Dentistry, Gazi University, Department of Oral and Maxillofacial Surgery, Ankara, Turkey

Emine Kaygısız and Tuba Tortop
Faculty of Dentistry, Department of Orthodontics, Gazi University, Ankara, Turkey

Aslıhan Uzel
Department of Orthodontics, Faculty of Dentistry, Cukurova University, Adana, Turkey

Fayez Saleh
Faculty of Dentistry, Beirut Arab University, Beirut, Lebanon

Wisam Al Hamadi
Faculty of Dentistry, University of Misan, Iraq

María Teresa Abeleira, Mercedes Outumuro, Marcio Diniz, Lucía García-Caballero, Pedro Diz and Jacobo Limeres
Special Needs Unit and OMEQUI Research Group, School of Medicine and Dentistry, Santiagode Compostela University, Santiago de Compostela, Galicia, Spain

Selma Elekdag-Türk
Faculty of Dentistry, Department of Orthodontics, University of Ondokuz Mayis, Samsun, Republic of Turkey

Hüdanur Yilmaz (née Huda Ebulkbash)
Anadolu Mahallesi, Samsun, Republic of Turkey

Index